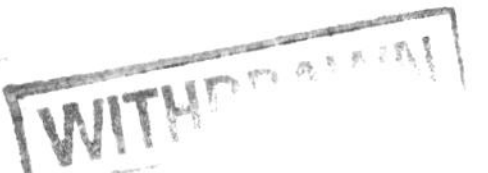

Fine Afferent Nerve Fibers and Pain

edited by
R. F. Schmidt, H.-G. Schaible, C. Vahle-Hinz

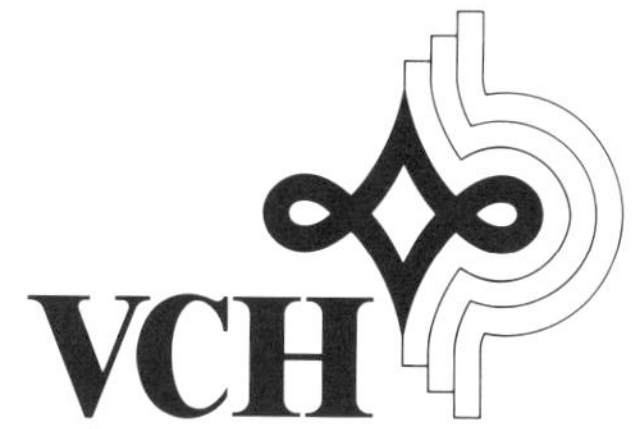

Distribution:

VCH Verlagsgesellschaft, Postfach 1260/1280, D-6940 Weinheim (Federal Republic of Germany)

USA und Canada: VCH Publishers, Suite 909, 220 East 23rd Street, New York, NY 10010-4606 (USA)

ISBN 3-527-15349-7 (VCH Verlagsgesellschaft) ISBN 0-89573-668-3 (VCH Publishers)

Fine Afferent Nerve Fibers and Pain

edited by

R. F. Schmidt, H.-G. Schaible, C. Vahle-Hinz

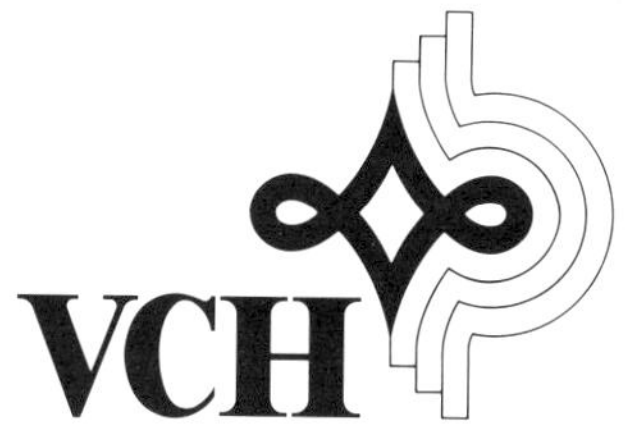

Prof. Dr. med. Robert F. Schmidt
Physiologisches Institut
der Universität Würzburg
Röntgenring 9
D-8700 Würzburg
Federal Republic of Germany

Dr. rer. nat. Christiane Vahle-Hinz
Physiologisches Institut
der Universität Würzburg
Röntgenring 9
D-8700 Würzburg
Federal Republic of Germany

Priv.-Doz. Dr. med. Hans-Georg Schaible
Physiologisches Institut
der Universität Würzburg
Röntgenring 9
D-8700 Würzburg
Federal Republic of Germany

The authors and publisher have made every effort to ensure that drug selection and dosage described in this book are in accord with current recommendations and practice at the time of publication. However, in view of changes in regulations and ongoing research with regard to drug actions and therapeutic schemes – but also in view of potential typographical errors – neither the authors nor the publisher are to be held responsible for the accuracy of the statements made. Rather, the reader is urged to study the package insert for indications, dosage, warnings and precautions before administering a drug. This is particularly important when the drug under considerations is new or infrequently used.

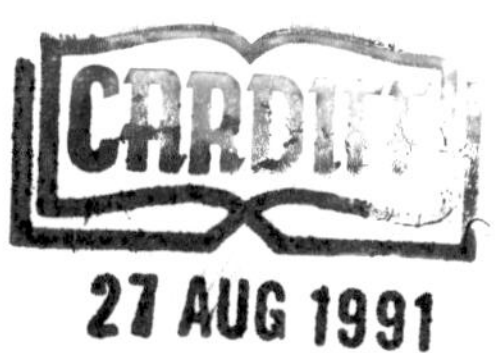

Editorial Director: Silvia Osteen
Production Manager: Peter J. Biel

Library of Congress Card No. 87-15625

Deutsche Bibliothek Cataloguing-in-Publication Data

Fine afferent nerve fibers and pain / ed. by R. F. Schmidt ... –
Weinheim ; New York : VCH, 1987.
ISBN 3-527-15349-7 (Weinheim)
ISBN 0-89573-668-3 (New York)

NE: Schmidt, Robert F. [Hrsg.]

Composition: Hagedornsatz, D-6806 Viernheim
Printing: Zechnersche Buchdruckerei, D-6720 Speyer
Bockbinding: J. Schäffer GmbH & Co. KG, D-6178 Grünstadt
Printed in the Federal Republic of Germany

Preface

Fine myelinated and unmyelinated afferent fibers form the vast majority of all afferents in mammalian nerves. For instance, articular nerves contain four times as many fine than thick afferent nerve fibers, and similar proportions hold for cutaneous and visceral nerves. Judging from these numbers alone, it may be predicted that fine afferents play a much more important role in somatovisceral sensation than is presently appreciated in the neuroscience community where in recent times fine afferent fibers attracted less attention than they deserved. Fortunately for those with a longstanding engagement in this field the tides are changing. This book is a most remarkable sign for this change, indicating an increasing interest in the properties, function and mode of operation of fine afferent nerve fibers.

Traditionally, fine afferent nerve fibers have been thought to be preferentially or exclusively involved in the transmission of information about the noxious or potentially noxious quality of stimuli to the organism, i.e. that they are "pain fibers". Thus, studies on fine afferents have mainly been carried out by scientists with an interest in the neurobiological mechanisms of nociception and pain. In consequence, our knowledge is advanced most in this field of fine fiber physiology. Therefore, it comes as no surprise that the overwhelming majority of the contributions in this book is devoted to studies of the significance of fine afferent activity for nociception and pain. In this respect it is a state of the art survey of impressing actuality on the intricate relations between fine afferent nerve fibers, their spinal and supraspinal relais stations, and the processing and handling of pain-inducing stimuli. At present there is no better and certainly no faster way to gain firsthand knowledge of this field than to study this book.

A wide variety of methods, such as histological, morphological, physiological, and neurochemical procedures, were used to investigate the receptive and other peripheral properties of fine afferent nerve fibers, the impact of their activity on spinal and supraspinal structures, and the clinical and therapeutic implications of these findings. Particularly remarkable are the efforts of several laboratories to explore the functional properties of fine afferents in hitherto "forgotten" areas such as the dura mater, the uterus and other visceral organs, and the great number of reports dealing with pathophysiological aspects of fine fiber activity. As a result, we have reached a new level of understanding for several aspects of cutaneous, deep and visceral pain, and of the pain during inflammatory states.

The book has a short but remarkable history. Less than a year ago its cradle was a symposium on "Role of fine afferent nerve fibers in somatovisceral sensation". As a satellite to the XXXth International Congress of Physiological Sciences (IUPS) in Vancouver this symposium took place – thanks to the outstanding efforts of our Canadian colleagues Jim Nagy and Lyn Polson – in the beautiful mountain resort of Lake Louise in the summer of 1986 (a photograph of the participants is shown on page XXII). Instead of assembling the manuscripts to publish them as proceedings of this meeting the participants decided to engage in a rigorous anonymous cross-refereeing of the manuscripts with the goal in mind, to create a carefully reviewed and edited monograph on the neurobiology of fine afferent nerve fibers and pain. This task and the consequent rewriting of the reviewed manuscripts was done with such enthusiasm and efficiency that it took only one year from the end of the Lake Louise meeting for the book to be published.

The publisher, VCH Verlagsgesellschaft, particularly its editorial director, Silvia Osteen, and the production manager, Peter Biel, took no small part in this speedy performance. We thank them for their efforts, as well as everybody else who participated in the many stages this book went through – from its conception to its completion.

Würzburg, July 1987

R. F. Schmidt H.-G. Schaible C. Vahle-Hinz

Contents

I Morphology of Fine Afferents and Their Peripheral and Central Terminals

II Receptive Properties of Fine Afferents in Normal and Injured Tissue

IV Synaptic Transmission and Modulation in the Dorsal Horn

V Spinal and Supraspinal Processing of Fine Afferent Activity

List of Contributors

Altschuler R. A.
NINCDS
Bethesda, MD 20205
USA

Andres K. H.
Institut für Anatomie der
Ruhr-Universität Bochum
D-4630 Bochum
FRG

Baranowski R.
Dept. of Physiology
University College London
Gower St.
London WC1E 6BT
U. K.

Battaglia G.
Departments of Anatomy
and Physiology
University of North Carolina
at Chapel Hill
Chapel Hill, NC 27514
USA

Baxendale R. H.
Institute of Physiology
The University
Glasgow G12 8QQ
Scotland U. K.

Benoist J. M.
I. N. S. E. R. M. U 161,
2 rue d'Alésia
F-75014 Paris
France

Berberich P.
Anatomisches Institut III
Universität Heidelberg
Im Neuenheimer Feld 307
D-6900 Heidelberg
FRG

Berkley K. J.
Department of Psychology
Florida State University
Tallahassee
Florida 32306-1051
USA

Bowsher D.
Pain Relief Foundation and
Department of Neurological Sciences
University of Liverpool
Liverpool L69 3BX
U. K.

Brock L.
Pain Relief Foundation and
Department of Neurological Sciences
University of Liverpool
Liverpool L69 3BX
U. K.

Broton J. G.
Dept. of Physiology
Faculty of Medicine
University of Toronto
Toronto, Ontario M5S 1A8
Canada

Cant R.
Institute of Physiology
University of Glasgow
G12 8QQ
Scotland

Casale E.
Dept. of Physiology, University of North Carolina at Chapel Hill
Chapel Hill, NC 27514
USA

Cervero F.
Dept. of Physiology
University of Bristol
Medical School
University Walk
Bristol BS8 1TD
U.K.

Chung J. M.
Marine Biomedical Institute and Department of Anatomy & Neurosciences
University of Texas Medical Branch
200 University Blvd.
Galveston, Texas 77550
USA

Chung K.
Marine Biomedical Institute and Depts. of Anatomy & Neurosciences and Physiology & Biophysics
University of Texas Medical Branch
Galveston, Texas 77550-2772
USA

Coggeshall R. E.
Marine Biomedical Institute and Depts. of Anatomy & Neuroscience and Physiology & Biophysics
University of Texas Medical Branch
Galveston, Texas 77550-2772
USA

Coimbra A.
Institute of Histology and Embryology
Faculty of Medicine
and the Center of
Experimental Morphology
of the University (INIC)
P-4200 Porto
Portugal

Comstock, W. J.
Dept. of Neurology
Good Samaritan Hospital
Neurological Sciences Center
Portland, Oregon 97210
USA

Dalsgaard C.-J.
Department of Anatomy
Karolinska Institutet
Box 60400
S-104 01 Stockholm
Sweden

Davis K. D.
Dept. Physiology
Univ. of Toronto
Toronto, Ontario
Canada M5S 1A8

Dostrovsky J. O.
Dept. Physiology
Univ. of Toronto
Toronto, Ontario
Canada M5S 1A8

Downie J.W.
Marine Biomedical Institute and
Department of Anatomy & Neurosciences
University of Texas Medical Branch
200 University Blvd.
Galveston, Texas 77550
USA

Düring M. von
Institut für Anatomie der
Ruhr-Universität Bochum
D-4630 Bochum
FRG

El-Yassir N.
University Department of Preclinical
Veterinary Sciences
Royal (Dick) School of Veterinary Studies
Summerhall
Edinburgh EH9 1QH
U.K.

Ferrell W. R.
Institute of Physiology
University of Glasgow
Glasgow G12 8QQ
Scotland

Ferrington D. G.
Marine Biomedical Institute and
Department of Anatomy & Neurosciences
University of Texas Medical Branch
200 University Blvd.
Galveston, Texas 77550
USA

Fitzgerald M.
Dept. of Anatomy & Embryology
University College London
Gower Street
London WC1E 6 BT
U.K.

Fleetwood-Walker S. M.
University Department of Preclinical
Veterinary Sciences
Royal (Dick) School of Veterinary Studies
Summerhall
Edinburgh EH9 1QH
U.K.

Foote J.
Faculty of Medicine
Memorial University of Newfoundland,
St. John's
Newfoundland
Canada A1B 3V6

Freund I.
Physiologisches Institut
der Universität Würzburg
Röntgenring 9
D-8700 Würzburg
FRG

Gamse R.
Institut für experimentelle und
klinische Pharmakologie
Universität Graz
A-8010 Graz
Austria

Gebhart G. F.
Department of Pharmacology
College of Medicine
University of Iowa
Iowa City, Iowa 52242
USA

Guilbaud, G.
I. N. S. E. R. M. U161
2 rue d'Alésia
F-75014 Paris
France

Handwerker H. O.
Institut für Physiologie und
Biokybernetik
Universitätsstr. 17
D-8520 Erlangen
FRG

Harti G.
Max-Planck-Institut für
physiologische und klinische Forschung
W. G. Kerckhoff-Institut
Parkstr. 1
D-6350 Bad Nauheim
FRG

Headley P. M.
Department of Physiology
Medical School
University of Bristol
University Walk
Bristol BS8 1TD
U.K.

Hildebrand C.
Department of Anatomy
Karolinska Institutet
Box 60400
S-104 01 Stockholm
Sweden

Hoheisel U.
Anatomisches Institut III
Universität Heidelberg
Im Neuenheimer Feld 307
D-6900 Heidelberg
FRG

Honda C. N.
Marine Biomedical Institute and
Department of Anatomy & Neurosciences
University of Texas Medical Branch
200 University Blvd.
Galveston, Texas 77550
USA

and
Dept. of Anatomy and Neurobiology
University of California College of Medicine
Irvine, CA 927 14
USA

Hope P. J.
University Department of Preclinical
Veterinary Sciences
Royal (Dick) School of Veterinary Studies
Summerhall
Edinburgh EH9 1QH
U. K.

Jeftinija S.
Department of Veterinary Anatomy
Iowa State University
Ames, IA 50011
USA

Jyväsjärvi E.
Department of Physiology
University of Helsinki
Siltavuorenpenger 20 J
SF-00170 Helsinki
Finland

Kangrga I.
Department of Veterinary Physiology
and Pharmacology
Iowa State University
Ames, IA 50011
USA

Kayser V.
I. N. S. E. R. M. U. 161
2 rue d'Alésia
F-75014 Paris
France

Klemm F.
II. Physiologisches Institut
der Universität Heidelberg
Im Neuenheimer Feld
D-6900 Heidelberg
FRG

Kniffki K.-D.
Physiologisches Institut
der Universität Würzburg
Röntgenring 9
D-8700 Würzburg
FRG

Koschorke G.-M.
II. Physiologisches Institut
Universität Heidelberg
Im Neuenheimer Feld 326
D-6900 Heidelberg
FRG

Koyama N.
Department of Physiology
Medical College of Shiga
Seta
Otsu 520-21
Japan

Kruger L.
Departments of Anatomy and
Anesthesiology and the
Ahmanson Laboratory of the
Brain Research Institute,
UCLA Center for Health Sciences
Los Angeles, CA 90024
USA

Kumazawa T.
Dept. of Nervous and Sensory Functions
Research Institute of Environmental
Medicine
Nagoya University
Nagoya 464
Japan

Lahuerta J.
Pain Reflief Foundation and
Department of Neurological Sciences
University of Liverpool
Liverpool L69 3BX
U.K.

Lang E.
II. Physiologisches Institut
der Universität Heidelberg
Im Neuenheimer Feld
D-6900 Heidelberg
FRG

Lawson S.N.
Department of Physiology
Medical School
University of Bristol
University Walk
Bristol BS8 1 TD
U.K.

Light A.R.
Dept. of Physiology, University of
North Carolina at Chapel Hill
Chapel Hill, NC 27514
USA

Lundberg L.
Department of Clinical Neurophysiology
University Hospital
S-751 85 Uppsala
Sweden

Lynn B.
Dept. of Physiology
University College London
Gower St.
London WC1E 6BT
U.K.

Magerl W.
II. Physiologisches Institut
der Universität Heidelberg
Im Neuenheimer Feld
D-6900 Heidelberg
FRG

Marchettini P.
Dept. of Neurology
University of Milano
I-Milano
Italy

Masuda T.
Department of Physiology
Medical College of Shiga
Seta
Otsu 520-21
Japan

Mayer Ch.
Department of Clinical Neuropharmacology
Max-Planck-Institute for Psychiatry
Kraepelinstr. 2
D-8000 München 40
FRG

McCarthy P. W.
Department of Physiology
Medical School
University of Bristol
University Walk
Bristol BS8 1TD
U. K.

McMahon S. B.
Sherrington School of Physiology
U. M. D. S. - St. Thoma's Campus
London SE1 7EH
U. K.

Mense S.
Anatomisches Institut III
Universität Heidelberg
Im Neuenheimer Feld 307
D-6900 Heidelberg
FRG

Mitchell R.
MRC Brain Metabolism Unit
University Department of Pharmacology
1 George Square
Edinburgh
EH8 9JZ
U. K.

Mizumura K.
Dept. of Nervous and Sensory Functions
Research Institute of Environmental
Medicine
Nagoya University
Nagoya 464
Japan

Molony V.
University Department of Preclinical
Veterinary Sciences
Royal (Dick) School of Veterinary Studies
Summerhall
Edinburgh EH9 1QH
U. K.

Murase K.
Information and Computer Sciences
Toyohashi University of Technology
Tempaku
Toyohashi 440
Japan

Muszynski K.
Institut für Anatomie der
Ruhr-Universität Bochum
D-4630 Bochum
FRG

Neil A.
I. N. S. E. R. M. U.161, 2 rue d'Alésia
F-75014 Paris
France

Ness T. J.
Department of Pharmacology
College of Medicine
University of Iowa
Iowa City, Iowa 52242
USA

Nizamuddin G.
Dept. of Neurology
University of Wisconsin
Madison
Wisconsin
USA

Ochoa J. L.
Dept. of Neurology
Good Samaritan Hospital
Neurological Sciences Center
Portland
Oregon 97210
USA

Parsons Ch. G.
Department of Physiology
Medical School
University Walk
Bristol BS8 1TD
U. K.

Petrusz P.
Department of Anatomy
University of North Carolina
at Chapel Hill
Chapel Hill, NC 27514
USA

Pierau Fr.-K.
Max-Planck-Institut
für physiologische und klinische Forschung
W. G. Kerckhoff-Institut
Parkstr. 1
D-6350 Bad Nauheim
FRG

Pignatelli D.
Institute of Histology and Embryology
Faculty of Medicine
and the Center of
Experimental Morphology
of the University (INIC)
P-4200 Porto
Portugal

Randić M.
Veterinary Physiology and Pharmacology
Iowa State University
Ames, IA 50011
USA

Risling M.
Department of Anatomy
Karolinska Institutet
Box 60400
S-104 01 Stockholm
Sweden

Robbins A.
Department of Psychology
Florida State University
Tallahassee
Florida 32306-1051
USA

and
Department of Physiology
Tokyo Metropolitan Institute
of Gerontology
35-2 Sakaecho
Itabashiku
Tokyo 173
JAPAN

Robinson J.
Faculty of Medicine
Memorial University of Newfoundland
St. John's
Newfoundland
Canada AlB 3V6

Russell N. J. W.
Bioscience Dept. II
ICI Pharmaceuticals Division
Alderley Park
Macclesfield
Cheshire, SK10 4TG
U. K.

Rustioni A.
Departments of Anatomy and Physiology
University of North Carolina
at Chapel Hill
Chapel Hill, NC 27514
USA

Ryu P. D.
Dept. of Veterinary Physiology
and Pharmacology
Iowa State University
Ames, IA 50011
USA

Sann H.
Max-Planck-Institut für
physiologische und klinische Forschung
W. G. Kerckhoff-Institut
Parkstr. 1
D-6350 Bad Nauheim
FRG

Sato J.
Dept. of Nervous and Sensory Functions
Research Institute of Environmental Medicine
Nagoya University
Nagoya 464
Japan

Sato Y.
Department of Psychology
Florida State University
Tallahassee
Florida 32306-1051
USA

Schaible H.-G.
Physiologisches Institut
der Universität Würzburg
Röntgenring 9
D-8700 Würzburg
FRG

Schmidt R. F.
Physiologisches Institut
der Universität Würzburg
Röntgenring 9
D-8700 Würzburg
FRG

Scott T. M.
Faculty of Medicine
Memorial University of Newfoundland
St. John's
Newfoundland
Canada A1B 3V6

Sedivec M.
Dept. of Biology
Appalacian State University
Boone, NC. 28608
USA

Sharkey K. A.
Department of Physiology
University of Bristol
The Medical School
University Walk
Bristol BS8 1TD
U. K.

Skeppar P.
Anatomisches Institut III
Universität Heidelberg
Im Neuenheimer Feld 307
D-6900 Heidelberg
FRG

Sorkin L. S.
Marine Biomedical Institute and
Department of Anatomy & Neuroscience
University of Texas Medical Branch
200 University Blvd.
Galveston, Texas 77550
USA

Steedman W. M.
Department of Preclinical Veterinary Sciences
Royal (Dick) School of Veterinary Studies
University of Edinburgh
Summerhall
Edinburgh EH9 1QH
U. K.

Surmeier D. J.
Marine Biomedical Institute and
Dept. of Anatomy & Neurosciences
University of Texas Medical Branch
200 University Blvd.
Galveston, Texas 77550
USA
and
Dept. of Anatomy and Neurobiology
University of Tennessee
Memphis, TN 38163
USA

Taguchi H.
Department of Physiology
Medical College of Shiga
Seta
Otsu 520–21
Japan

Tattersall J. E. H.
Department of Physiology
University of Bristol
The Medical School
University Walk
Bristol BS8 1TD
U.K.

Torebjörk E.
Department of Clinical Neurophysiology
University Hospital
S-751 85 Uppsala
Sweden

Urban L.
Department of Anatomy
University Medical School
H-4012 Debrecen
Hungary

Usui S.
Information and Computer Sciences
Toyohashi University of Technology
Tempaku
Toyohashi 440
Japan

Vahle-Hinz C.
Physiologisches Institut
der Universität Würzburg
Röntgenring 9
D-8700 Würzburg
FRG

Waddell P. J.
Department of Physiology
Medical School
University of Bristol
University Walk
Bristol BS8 1TD
U.K.

Wall P. D.
Cerebral Functions Group
University College London
London WC1E 6BT
U.K.

Warma N. K.
Dept. of Physiology
Faculty of Medicine
University of Toronto
Toronto, Ontario, M5S 1A8
Canada

West D. C.
University College
Cardiff CF1 1XL
U.K.

Westerman R. A.
II. Physiologisches Institut
der Universität Heidelberg
Im Neuenheimer Feld
D-6900 Heidelberg
FRG

Willis W. D.
Marine Biomedical Institute and
Department of Anatomy
& Neurosciences
University of Texas Medical Branch
200 University Blvd.
Galveston, Texas 77550
USA

Woolf C. J.
Department of Anatomy
University College London
London WC1E 6BT
U.K.

Yokota T.
Department of Physiology
Medical College of Shiga
Seta
Otsu 520-21
Japan

Zieglgänsberger W.
Department of Clinical
Neuropharmacology
Max-Planck-Institut für Psychiatrie
Kraepelinstr. 2
D-8000 München 40
FRG

Zimmermann M.
II. Physiologisches Institut
Universität Heidelberg
Im Neuenheimer Feld 326
D-6900 Heidelberg
FRG

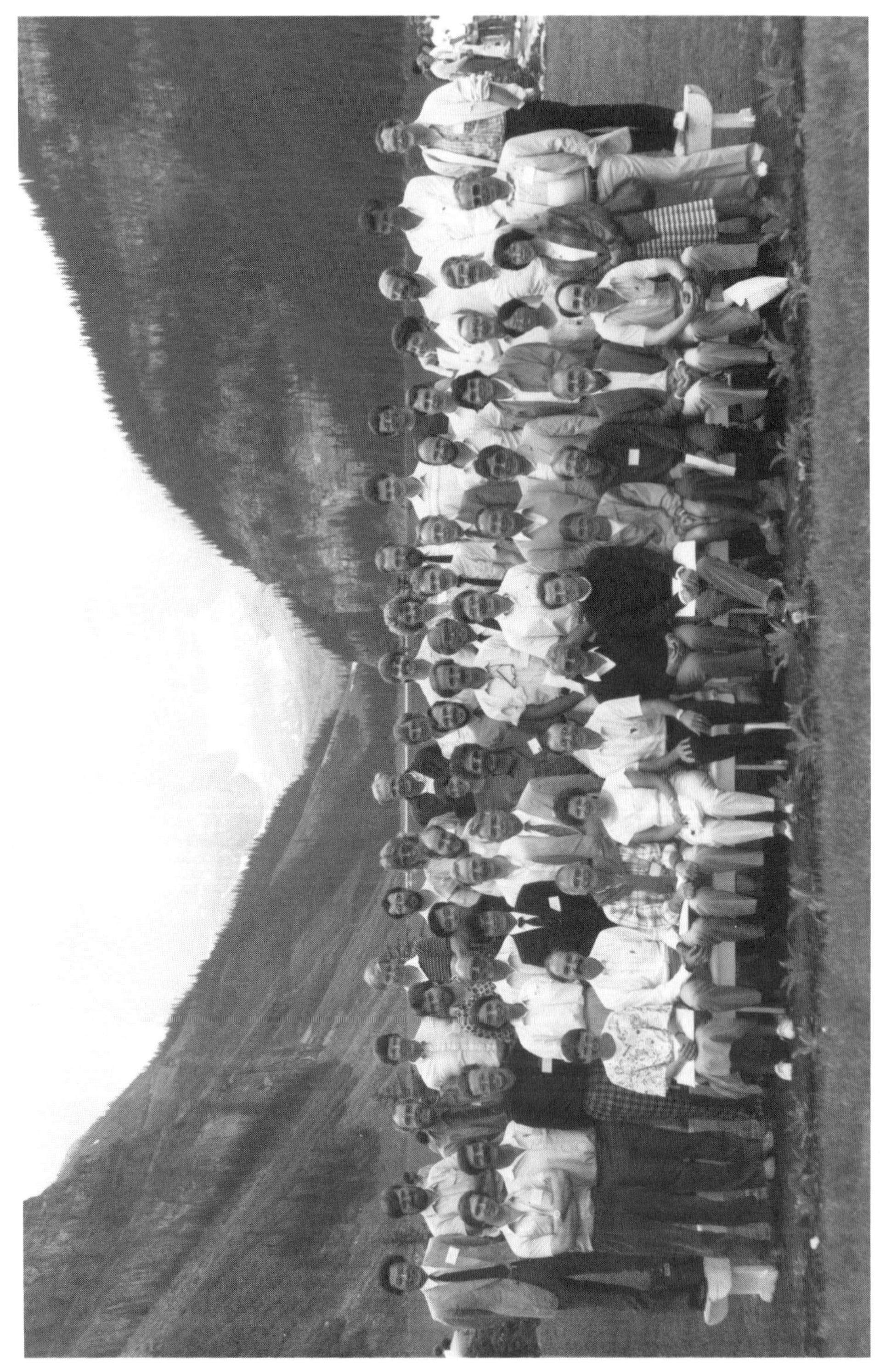

1	Sato	11	Vahle-Hinz	21	Schaible	31	Zieglgänsberger	41	Molander	51	Davis
2	Scott	12	Lynn	22	Berkley	32	Cervero	42	Seltzer	52	Dostrovski
3	Molony	13	Baranowski	23	McMahon	33	Ochoa	43	Bowsher	53	Schmidt
4	Briggs	14	Headley	24	Torebjörk	34	Kumazawa	44	Mizumura	54	Lele
5	Grigg	15	Guilbaud	25	Taguchi	35	Gebhart	45	Mense	55	Polson
6	Sharkey	16	Pierau	26	Asato	36	Jyväsjärvi	46	Tadaki	56	Nagy
7	Lawson	17	Giesler	27	Baxendale	37	Grant	47	Handwerker	57	Zimmermann
8	Coggeshall	18	Risling	28	McCarthy	38	Willis	48	Fitzgerald	58	Baumann
9	Steedman	19	Ferrell	29	Yokota	39	Honda	49	Schwen		
10	Ness	20	Russell	30	Hope	40	Woolf	50	Kruger		

1 Morphological Correlates of "Free" Nerve Endings – A Reappraisal of Thin Sensory Axon Classification

L. Kruger

If science can be described properly as an organized body of knowledge, the functional properties, associations, and morphological features of axons encumbered with the designation "free nerve ending" provide a remarkable example of failure to achieve rigorous scientific definition. It is not merely a matter of semantic niceties and exactitude, but rather a longstanding obfuscation of what probably constitutes the most numerous type of sense organs in mammals. The variety and complexity of functional roles subserved by unmyelinated sensory (C) axons provide sufficient incentive for a re-examination of several basic questions that have become ingrained into our scientific literature. The tacit assumption that sensory endings associated with "pain," currently called "nociceptors," can be equated with a class of sense organs that merit the descriptor "free," is subject to serious challenge. This presentation aims at presaging an emerging new taxonomy based on modern principles of classification. A brief examination of the history of the concept of "free" endings and a more comprehensive account of recent information should establish the basis for development of a new terminology, for there is ample evidence that the peripheral terminals of unmyelinated sensory axons do not comprise a single homogeneous class on either morphological or functional grounds.

Justification for the term "free nerve ending" derives from three key observations made by the nineteenth century: (1) Unmyelinated fibers do not acquire a corpuscular or specialized encapsulated structure at their distal ends, nor do they have an association with cells suspected of participation in sensory processes, such as Merkel cells. (2) Axonal metallic impregnation or "staining" with silver, gold, or osmium rarely revealed a specific and exclusive association with other cells and thus these endings might logically be considered "free." (3) The unmyelinated "free" terminal pattern appeared to be the sole or predominant morphological variant in those structures from which a sensory report of "pain" was elicited on excitation in human subjects, e.g., cornea, dental pulp, periosteum, viscera, and tympanic membrane.

One might quibble with some details, but these early observations are essentially sound and account for general acceptance that "pain endings" and "free nerve endings" constitute the same entity and that these terms could be used interchangeably. Contemporary use of the term "free" can be defended on the grounds that a specialized membrane contact and thickening has yet to be discovered in electron microscopy of C fiber endings, though clearly demonstrable for specialized **myelinated** axon terminals such as those contacting Merkel cells or Pacinian corpuscles (Gottschaldt 1985).

The alternative view that neither C fibers nor "free" nerve endings constitute a distinct class on functional grounds has gradually become more persuasive as a result of numerous modern findings, including the expanding application of biochemical "markers." However, it is unlikely that each new label uncovered by immunohistochemistry will provide a new taxon. If we are to devise a rational new nomenclature, it becomes crucial to define the generalized, the exclusive, and the specialized properties of all peripheral somatosensory neurons.

Dorsal root ganglion cells can be conveniently divided into two main classes on the basis of soma size. The large neurons emit larger diameter axons ensheathed by layers of Schwann cell plasmalemma constituting "myelin," and their distal terminals are often, but not always, associated with corpuscular or epithelial cells forming highly specialized sense organs, most of which respond exquisitely to some feature of mechanical perturbation. Although the division is inexact and the spectrum of cell body and axon diameter shifts with animal species, rostrocaudal level of the neuraxis, etc., the smaller-diameter ganglion cells emit the generally larger population of small-diameter axons that cluster to share a single Schwann cell. The incomplete Schwann sheath over axons in connective tissues is reserved for thin fibers with terminals that are "free" except for an intact basal lamina surround (Munger and Halata 1983), but even the distinction between clusters of "free" endings and a corpuscular structure is sometimes difficult, as shown for genital corpuscles by Halata and Munger (1986). Aside from some reservations about sharply separating the thinnest myelinated axons from their unmyelinated cohorts, this dichotomy works fairly well on functional grounds.

The thin axon population originating from small (or B) ganglion cells also displays a variety of biochemical features that sharply distinguish them from large myelinated components. The richest basis for establishing new functional classes can be found in the expression of multiple neurotransmitters and/or neuromodulators. The number of cytochemical "markers" specific to B cells and unmyelinated axons is growing rapidly and includes at least the following groups: (1) neuropeptides, (2) amino acids, (3) 5'-nucleotides, (4) cytoplasmic enzymes, e.g., specific acid phosphatase isoenzymes, (5) cell surface complex oligosaccharides, (6) monoclonal antibodies directed toward a variety of antigens, (7) catecholamines, and (8) viral genomes, often without producing viral particles, a phenomenon known as "viral latency." This minimal list reflects the range of phenotypic diversity of B neurons, and it should be evident that these categories must exhibit varying degrees of overlap and that within the exceptionally rich category of neuropeptides exclusively found in thin-fiber neurons, colocalization of two or more peptides in the **same** cell is also a common feature.

A systematic classification based on a given class of metabolic enzymes or transmitters might be constructed, and if an immunologic subclassification were to be superimposed, an enormous variety of neuron classes would emerge. This could be multiplied further by combining purely morphological variants with cytochemical labels (e.g., Dodd and Jessell, 1985; Kruger et al. 1985; Lawson et al. 1985; Sommer et al. 1985). The significance of some functional classes is reflected in different laminar terminal patterns in the dorsal horn of the spinal cord and although the distal correlates in peripheral tissues have barely been explored, a new cytochemical basis for sense organ classification is likely to emerge in the near future. Ignoring details for a moment, a striking principle derives from contrasting the vastness of C fiber diversity with the highly conservative, strict specialization of myelinated sensitive mechanoreceptors.

In an evolutionary sense, specialization represents the more advanced condition, whereas the more primitive "prototypic" neural system is required to archieve the full range of essential tasks with a minimal number of elements. The lack of specialization does not equate with lack of differentiation; rather, it denotes preservation of an exuberant versatility of the kind best exemplified by the small sensory ganglion (B) cell; the quintessential multifunctional prototypic neuron.

Peripheral axon terminals should presumably mirror the fine structural, immunohistochemical, and metabolic variety of B cell somata and further parallel the several types of C fiber sense organs and their differential laminar projection into the spinal cord (Hunt and Rossi 1985). The **lack of specialization** in terminals is inferred from the absence of corpuscular structures and lack of "synaptic-like" membrane thickening or contacts (Gottschaldt 1985); once again, in marked contrast to the highly specialized terminals of myelinated axons. The **diversity** of the prototypic sensory neuron is realized through the impressive promiscuity of peripheral terminals in the variety of tissues and cells encountered.

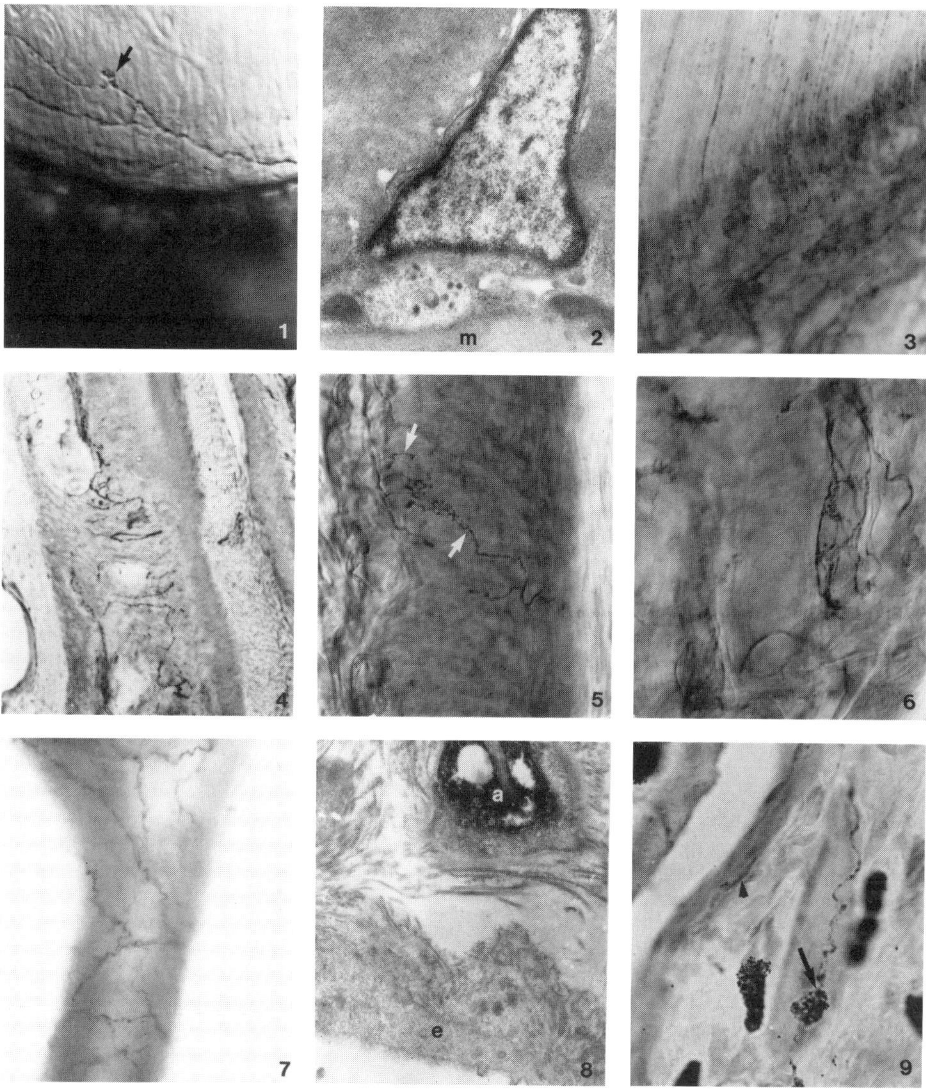

Fig. 1. Peptidergic thin fibers in rat tissues. **1** A whole-mount preparation of the mucosal surface of the tympanic membrane revealing calcitonin gene-related peptide immunoreactive (CGRP-IR) C fibers and a terminal (arrow). **2** Electron micrograph of a tympanic membrane ending containing dense-core vesicles on the mucosal basal lamina (m). **3** CGRP-IR axons from the dental pulp, entering the dental tubules (above). **4** CGRP-IR axons of the periosteum of forelimb. **5** CGRP-IR axons (arrows) penetrating from the dermis (left) into the epidermis (arrows) extending almost to the stratum corneum (right). **6** CGRP-IR innervation surrounding a small artery in the dermis. **7** A whole-mount preparation of CGRP-IR axons in the adventitia of a large mesenteric blood vessel. **8** Electron micrograph of a CGRP-IR axonal profile (a) approaching the endothelium (e) of a small dermal blood vessel. **9** Dermal axons in the region of a mast cell (arrow) and arterial wall (arrowhead) in this case showing neuropeptide Y immunoreactivity with patterns similar to those observed for substance P and CGRP immunoreactivity

The richness and nature of epithelial innervation by unmyelinated fibers, especially in structures from which painful sensations can be generated in the absence of other sensory modalities, accounts for the most common use of the term "free ending" and its presumptive association with pain in contemporary textbooks. The derivation of such axons from "sensory" ganglion cells has been established in some tissues by axonal transport labeling methods and the application of specific neurotoxins (e.g., Byers and Yeh 1984; Kruger et al. 1985; Yeh and Kruger 1984). Visualization of many of these fibers can be achieved by standard immunohistochemical labeling for several of the peptides found in small sensory neurons. The most ubiquitous of these, calcitonin gene-related peptide (CGRP), is conveniently absent from sympathetic axons and the antibody labeling sufficiently robust to enable identification of true "endings" in whole-mount preparations of cornea and the mucosal surface of the tympanic membrane (Fig. 1.1–2) (Colin and Kruger 1986). CGRP labeling is also evident in decalcified tissue sections of tooth and bone (Kruger et al. 1986b), with remarkable richness in dentinal tubules and periosteum (Fig. 1.3–4) and numerous sensory fibers penetrating the epidermis (Fig. 1.5) paralleling those with substance P (SP) immunoreactivity (Kruger et al. 1985), which colocalizes with CGRP-immunoreactive (CGRP-IR) axons (Gibbins et al. 1985; Lee et al. 1985). Parenthetically, it might be worth noting that the presence of intraepidermal SP and CGRP immunoreactivity is not paralleled by evidence of specific, high-affinity receptor binding sites for these peptides within the epidermis (Kruger et al. 1986). It should also be emphasized that the peptidergic intraepidermal innervation (Fig. 1.5) constitutes only a portion (of undetermined magnitude) of the total C fiber innervation and that some peptides (e.g., SP and somatostatin) are found in distinct populations (Hökfelt et al. 1976) and may be released separately by different types of noxious stimuli (Kuraishi et al. 1985).

The rich unmyelinated axonal array found in the adventitia of a wide range of blood vessels (Fig. 1.6) includes sympathetic noradrenergic postganglionic fibers. There is also a non-noradrenergic sympathetic innervation (Morris et al. 1985) and a dense innervation by neuropeptide Y (NPY) -IR fibers (Fig. 1.9). Most surprising, however, is the demonstration of an exceptionally vast supply of **sensory** C fibers revealed by CGRP immunoreactivity, an example of which is shown in a whole-mount preparation developed by my colleague Catia Sternini (Fig. 1.7). It is feasible to demonstrate more directly that perivasular fibers are indeed derived from sensory ganglion cells, and we have successfully labeled this innervation by injecting an enzyme-lectin conjutate (HRP-WGA) into dorsal root ganglia and tracing it to a perivascular contact.

The functional significance of these observations is a subject of intensive inquiry. The first and most obvious crucial question is whether vascular endings are actually sensory. Sensory fibers labeled by axonal transport have been traced to presumptive terminals. The presence of vesicles, especially of the dense-core variety often associated with peptides, and mitochondria (Fig. 1.8) are the only criteria available supporting the notion that these are indeed terminals. Despite extensive search, my colleague Yung Yeh has not yet found a single putative terminal displaying a contact or membrane specialization of synaptic nature. This should not be surprising, as this is the rule for sympathetic endings, and if peptidergic vasomotor actions require dispersed rather than focal chemical membrane effects, the same "nonsynaptic" principle would apply to all vascular innervation. This appeal to parsimony is reinforced by extensive and persuasive evidence that these **sensory** peptidergic axons also exert an **efferent** action. The "axon reflex" of Bayliss can account for the long-known peripheral vasodilatation and plasma extravasation shown to depend on C fibers by Hinsey and Gasser (1930) and more recently demonstrated to involve only nociceptor afferent fibers by Kenins (1981) through combining electrical recording and stimulation of single fibers. The participation of (SP) in "antidromic vasodilatation" and plasma extravasation has been affirmed by use of antagonists and by capsaicin depletion. The more recently discovered novel peptide, CGRP, is found in the same axons as SP, but is far more powerful than SP as a vasodilator (Brain et al. 1985) and is found in a larger number of thin afferent axons. While these two vasoactive neuropeptides may prove only representative of the many effector substances in afferent axons, their presence in a select population of thin axons implicated in nociceptor function is an important clue to the vicarious activities of "sensory" fibers.

The next question is whether each C **afferent** perivascular axon terminal is functionally **efferent**. Mantyh et al. (1985) have been studying specific, high-affinity peptide receptor binding sites in autoradiographic sections of the entire body , and together we have given detailed attention to the integumentary localization of peptide receptor binding sites. The most striking finding has been the richness of **perivascular** peptide receptor binding sites, in contrast to their apparent absence in epidermis and other epithelia rich in peptidergic C fibers. Thus, the evidence for a perivascular **efferent** or cytokine function becomes increasingly persuasive, whereas the generally inferred sense organ role of these endings is relatively tenuous. Within the epidermis, where effector cells are absent, functional peptide receptors would seem superfluous, but conversely, a sensory role C fibers seems essential.

Before considering the implications of such dichotomies, there remains the problem of classifying the vast array of afferent C fibers distributed among the connective tissues of the body. Some of these may exert specific effects in relation to cellular elements. For example, we have evidence of SP-IR and CGRP-IR as well as NPY-IR axons in apparently nonrandom relation to mast cells (Fig. 1.9), although specialized contacts have not been observed, consistent with our preceding account of vascular relations. Vasodilatation mediated by peptidergic C fibers via mast cell histamine release (Foreman et al. 1982; Lembeck and Gamse 1982) suggests that this arrangement is not fortuitous. Neuropeptides are also known to exert regulatory effects on sweat glands, leukocytes, and lymphocytes. The modulation of function in immunocompetent cells by peptides present in small DRG cells (Payan et al. 1984), and the presence of receptors for these peptides on lymphocytes and leukocytic macrophages (Payan and Goetzl 1985), indicate a diverse range of effector functions mediated by the numerous axons distributed "freely" in tissue fluid and surrounded largely by collagen fibers. These "free" nerve endings found throughout the connective tissues of the body are difficult to categorize on strictly morphological grounds, because even the presence of vesicles and mitochondria in small-diameter axonal profiles seen in the electron microscope may not denote a functional "terminal." Similar profiles can be found in nerve bundles surrounded by perineurium. For the present, we should recognize the uncertain validity of relegating any of these endings to an afferent or efferent role or perhaps even both simultaneously.

These findings may be summarized by the hypothesis that small sensory ganglion cells represent the ultimate exemplars of the "prototype." In the evolution of a nervous system, one of the first requirements is a means of detecting stimuli that threaten or produce tissue damage. Such elements are retained as the dominant sense organs of the body in large numbers in all mammals and constitute the "nociceptors" of modern parlance. In the "prototypic" (i.e., primitive and/or neotenic) condition, these neurons assumed an increasing variety of functional roles, in contrast to the fast-conducting, myelinated axons subserving the highly specialized sense organs arising during vertebrate evolution. The remarkable feature of "prototypic" neurons is that a single cell can subserve a multiplicity of functions, an expression of what Bertrand Russell called the "laws of cosmic laziness." Versatility in a single neuron is relatively rare, but it requires fewer cells and, perhaps more importantly, provides for functionally inextricable linkages. For the nociceptive system, the practical requirements must include tissue protection and repair. Phenotypic expression of multiple transmitters and modulators in single neurons enables this unique class of sensory fiber to exercise control of circulation, immune response to the challenge of those new antigens associated with damage and/or infection, and mobilization of the metabolic events underlying the inflammatory reaction. Such a "prototypic" neuron is the antithesis of assigning a single transmitter and a single functional role for each cell. No sense organs other than nociceptors are known to invoke complex efferent mechanisms without recruiting additional and highly specialized neurons for effector tasks. Another extraordinary consequence of the cytochemical versatility of individual nociceptive neurons is the possibility for different axonal branches of the same cell to perform different functions, i.e., one branch might exert efferent vascular control while another could form a terminal sense organ. It is also possible that a single axonal terminal may serve both as a sense organ and as a complex effector initiating a multiplicity of events, but there is no direct evidence for this conjecture. Modification of local events at separate terminals by receptor regulation provides for an epigenetic mechanism of long-term functional perturbation of a single neuron that can be selective in relation to different surrounding tissues.

This survey of the morphological properties and relations of the sensory thin-fiber system makes no pretense of being exhaustive – though perhaps exhausting at this point. But it would be remiss to summarize the unique anatomy of the "prototypic" nociceptive neuron without noting a few other exceptional features that distinguish these neurons.

The recent report that neurogenesis of sensory ganglion cells continues throughout adult life in rats (Devor and Govrin-Lippman 1985), largely in the small neurons, is most unexpected. The increase in neuron number is slow enough to evade detection by observing mitoses or ^{3}H-thymidine incorporation, a property that is exceptionally rare in mammals, although exhibited by the relatively primitive olfactory system (Altman 1969; Graziadei and Monti Graziadei 1979) and common in lower vertebrates in which recovery of function results from generation of new neurons. Thus the injury that often accompanies nociception may be compensated for by adding to the unmyelinated axon population.

Other exotic traits that also deserve brief "honorable mention" include the observation that numerous unmyelinated axons enter the ventral root and generally loop back to finally enter the cord via the dorsal root (Risling et al. 1984), thereby providing a longer and slower route to the spinal cord for many C fibers. Some individual neurons display dichotomous distal axons innervating viscera and skin (Bahr et al. 1981; Taylor and Pierau 1982). Although this may be rare, it might provide a peripheral basis for the phenomenon of referred pain. Finally, it should be noted that unmyelinated sensory axons appear to transport botanical markers in a selective fashion related to specific cell-surface glycoconjugates (Dodd and Jessell 1985) that enables them to be labeled independently of myelinated axons (Mori 1986; Swett 1985).

The numerous remarkable morphological features cited above do not require an entirely new classification, in that one could argue that all sensory ganglion cells with thin axons share several features lacking in other neurons, thus constituting a distinct idiosyncratic set. The distal endings differ from other axon terminals by the absence of a specialized membrane contact, and in this sense the term "free" ending is not totally inappropriate. A subclassification might be devised based on the differential cytochemical characterization of each neuron, or perhaps more logically, for the separate "free endings" of the same cell, depending on the cellular territory and molecular receptor population associated with each terminal.

In a lighter vein, one can offer a somewhat facetious argument for retaining the term "free" pertaining to C fiber function in the same sense that neurons emitting unmyelinated sensory axons are probably the most promiscuous of all cells in the mammalian nervous system; this implies the general use of "promiscuous" denoting multiplicity and variety of associations. On functional grounds, the multiplicity of separate physiological classes of C fibers and of a variety of quite different activities for individual neurons can be defended with alacrity by enumerating several remarkable features of sensory C fibers, including the following:

1. Several classes of transducers: these include sense organs responsive to cooling or to warming, sensitive mechanoreceptors, and a variety of nociceptors, including a predominant "polymodal" type.

2. "Sensitization" of nociceptors: a process wherein successive identical stimuli elicit more impulses or the threshold for successuve stimuli is lowered, in contrast to the "adaptation" recovery process displayed by all other sense organs.

3. A variety of "efferent" functions, alluded to in the preceding account of morphological specialization in terms of multiple neurotransmitters and/or neuromodulators, especially peptides. A sensory C fiber role can be demonstrated in the control of circulation, the immune response, and the neurogenic component of inflammatory reactions.

4. Regulation of mitogenesis: a recently discovered effect of specific tachykinins (e.g., substances P and K) on tissue repair by a "growth" effect on non-neural cell multiplication in peripheral tissues (Nilsson et al. 1985).

5. "Abnormal" patterns of electrical activity, including the pathological excitation associated with "neuroma" formation, evidence that only C fibers display "ephaptic" interaction in nerve trunks (Meyer et al. 1985) and of impulse generation in both neuron soma and sense organ (Wall and Devor 1983), the latter a general property of DRG cells.

6. Selective neurotoxin susceptibility, e.g., the large-scale elimination of small ganglion cells and C fibers by capsaicin in neonatal rodents.

7. Endocytosis and exocytosis: the evidence for selectivity is indirect and based on the demonstration of an Fc receptor (a generalized macrophage marker), only on small sensory ganglion cells (Dodd et al. 1983), and selective viral uptake (e.g., herpes simplex) and "latent" viral expression associated with sensory reports of pain and burning.

8. Collateral sprouting: this remains a controversial issue, but the best evidence for peripheral invasion of a denervated territory relies on C fiber sprouting, in contrast to minimal evidence of myelinated axon divergence.

Conclusion

Any attempt to summarize the features, functions, and associations of thin sensory axons enumerated in the preceding account must emphasize the heterologous nature of this most remarkably diversified class of neurons. Generalizations about nociceptor axons and "free nerve endings" emerge readily if one accepts the principle of multiplicity of function in single neurons. There is certainly an economy achieved in combining a number of efferent mechanisms of importance in functional recovery following the injurious stimulus that excites nociceptor endings and elicits pain. The biochemical specificities and overlap in a single cell probably reflect the need for mobilizing several related factors. Thus CGRP appears to be the most potent vasodilator, but is clearly less involved in plasma extravasation than SP, which is also a vasodilator and shares with substance K its role in tissue repair. Add to these effects specific peptide regulation of mast cells and release of histamine or the activation of the several elements involved in prostaglandin and leukotriene formation, and it becomes apparent that the neurons specialized for sensory information concerning injury also coordinate and mobilize a host of related events required for recovery and repair. The various species of axonal terminals will be defined in terms of multiple criteria for each ending. These may include both afferent and efferent properties, a rich variety of cytokine agents, and a diversity in the specific receptor molecules generated in each host tissue. Clearly, we are ready for a new descriptive terminology to replace the outmoded concept of an undifferentiated "free" nerve ending.

Summary

Observations based upon electron microscopy and specific chemical markers of unmyelinated sensory axons indicate that the unencapsulated terminal patterns are more varied than the "encapsulated" endings of myelinated axons. Sensory fibers have been traced in relation to a variety of structures without forming intimate or specialized membrane contacts; for instance, intraepithelial axons display specific biochemical and morphological relations of exceptional diversity. Some "free endings" probably subserve nonsensory, i.e., efferent roles independent of afferent information transmission, thus rendering individual small sensory neurons capable of multiple functions.

Acknowledgements. I am indebted to my colleagues Nicholas Brecha, Patrick Mantyh, James Silverman, Catia Sternini, and Yung Yeh, for their contributions to the research and ideas expressed in this paper. The technical and secretarial aid of Sharon Sampogna and Anita Roff is also deeply appreciated. This work was supported by NIH grant NS-5685.

References

ALTMAN J (1968) Autoradiographic and histological studies of postnatal neurogenesis. IV. Cell proliferation and migration in the anterior forebrain, with special reference to persisting neurogenesis in the olfactory bulb. J Comp Neurol 137 : 433–458

BAHR R, BLUMBERG H, JANIG W (1981) Do dichotomizing afferent fibers exist which supply visceral organs as well as somatic structures? A contribution to the problem of refferred pain. Neurosci Lett 24 : 25–28

BRAIN SD, WILLIAMS TJ, TIPPINS JR, MORRIS HR, MACINTYRE I (1985) Calcitonin gene-related peptide is a potent vasodilator. Nature 313 : 54–56

BYERS MR, YEH Y (1984) Fine structure of subepithelial "free" and corpuscular trigeminal nerve endings in anterior hard palate of the rat. Somatosens Res 1 : 265–280

BORGES LF, SIDMAN RL (1982) Axonal transport of lectins in the peripheral nervous system. J Neurosci 2 : 647–653

COLIN S, KRUGER L (1986) Peptidergic nociceptive axon visualization in whole-mount preparations of cornea and tympanic membrane in rat. Brain Res 398 : 199–203

DEVOR M, GOVRIN-LIPPMANN, R (1985) Neurogenesis in adult rat dorsal root ganglia. Neurosci Lett 61 : 189–194

DODD J, JESSELL TM (1985) Lactoseries carbohydrates specify subsets of dorsal root ganglion neurons projecting to the superficial dorsal horn of rat spinal cord. J Neurosci 5 : 3278–3294

DODD J, JAHR CE, HAMILTON PN, HEATH MJS, MATTHEW WD, JESSELL TM (1983) Cytochemical and physiological properties of sensory and dorsal horn neurons that transmit cutaneous sensation. Cold Spring Harbor Symp Quant Biol 48 : 685–695

FOREMAN JC, JORDAN CC, PIOTROWSKI W (1982) Interaction of neurotensin with the substance P receptor mediating histamine release from rat mast cells and the flare in human skin. Br J Pharmacol 77 : 531–539

GIBBINS IL, FURNESS JB, COSTA M, MACINTYRE I, HILLYARD CJ, GIRGIS S (1985) Co-localization of calcitonin gene-related peptide-like immunoreactivity with substance P in cutaneous, vascular and visceral sensory neurons of guinea pigs. Neurosci Lett 57 : 125–130

GOETZL EJ, CHERNOV T, RENOLD F, PAYAN DG (1985) Neuropeptide regulation of the expression of immediate hypersensitivity. J Immunol 135 : 802s–805s

GOTTSCHALDT K-M (1985) Structure and function of avian somatosensory receptors. In: KING AS, MCLELLAND J (eds) Form and function in birds, vol 3. Academic, London, pp 375–461

GRAZIADEI PPC, MONTI GRAZIADEI GA (1979) Neurogenesis and neuron regeneration in the olfactory system of mammals. 1. Morphological aspects of differentiation and structural organization of the olfactory sensory neurons. J Neurocytol 8 : 1–18

HALATA Z, MUNGER BL (1986) The neuroanatomical basis for the protopathic sensibility of the human glans penis. Brain Res 371 : 205–230

HINSEY JC, GASSER HS (1930) The component of the dorsal root mediating vasodilatation and the Sherrington contraction. Am J Physiol 92 : 679–689

Hökfelt T, Elde R, Johansson O, Luft R, Nilsson G, Arimura A (1976) Immunohistochemical evidence for separate populations of somatostatin-containing and substance P-containing primary afferent neurons in the rat. Neuroscience 1:131–136

Hunt SP, Rossi J (1985) Peptide- and non-peptide-containing unmyelinated primary afferents: the parallel processing of nociceptive information. Philos Trans R Soc Lond (Biol) 30:283–290

Kenins P (1981) Identification of the unmyelinated sensory nerves which evoke extravasation in response to antidromic stimulation. Neurosci Lett 25:137–141

Krishtal OA, Marchenko SM, Pidoplichko VI (1983) Receptors for ATP in the membrane of mammalian sensory neurons. Neurosci Lett 35:41–45

Kruger L, Sampogna SL, Rodin BE, Clague J, Brecha N, Yeh Y (1985) Thin-fiber cutaneous innervation and its intraepidermal contribution studied by labeling methods and neurotoxin treatment in rats. Somatosens Res 2:335–356

Kruger L, Sternini C, Brecha N, Mantyh C, Mantyh P (1986a) CGRP immunoreactivity and receptor distribution in the rat central nervous system. Anat Rec 214:69A

Kruger L, Sternini C, Mantyh CR, Mantyh PW, Brecha NC, Silverman JD, Colin S, Yeh Y (1986b) Calcitonin gene-related peptide (CGRP) immunoreactivity and receptor binding sites in relation to specific sensory pathways in the rat. Proc Int Union Physiol Sci 16:328

Kuraishi Y, Hirota N, Sato Y, Hino Y, Satoh M, Takagi H (1985) Evidence that substance P and somatostatin transmit separate information related to pain in the spinal dorsal horn. Brain Res 325:294–298

Lawson SN, Harper LI, Harper AA, Garson JA, Coakham HB, Randle BJ (1985) Monoclonal antibody 2C5: a marker for a subpopulation of small neurones in rat dorsal root ganglia. Neuroscience 16:365–374

Lee Y, Kawai Y, Shiosaka S, Takami K, Kiyama H, Hillyard CJ, Girgis S, MacIntyre I, Emson PC, Tohyama M (1985) Coexistence of calcitonin gene-related peptide and substance P-like peptide in single cells of the trigeminal ganglion of the rat: immunohistochemical analysis. Brain Res 330:194–196

Lembeck F, Gamse R (1982) Substance P in peripheral sensory processes. Ciba Found Symp 91:35–49

Mantyh PW, Mantyh CR, Brecha NC, Kruger L, Sternini C (1985) Autoradiographic localization of calcitonin gene-related peptide binding sites in the rat brain, guinea pig periphery and human spinal cord. Soc Neurosci Abstr 11:415

Meyer RA, Raja SN, Campbell JN (1985) Coupling of action potential activity between unmyelinated fibers in the peripheral nerve of monkey. Science 227:184–187

Mori K (1986) Lectin **Ulex europaeus** agglutinin I specificially labels a subset of primary afferent fibers which project selectively to the superficial dorsal horn of the spinal cord. Brain Res 365:404–408

Morris JL, Gibbins IL, Furness JB, Costa M, Murphy R (1985) Co-localization of neuropeptide Y, vasoactive intestinal polypeptide and dynorphin in non-noradrenergic axons of the guinea pig uterine artery. Neurosco Lett 62:31–38

Munger BL, Halata Z (1983) The sensory innervation of primate facial skin. 1. Hairy skin. Brain Res Rev 5:45–80

Nilsson J, von Euler AM, Dalsgaard CJ (1985) Stimulation of connective tissue cell growth by substance P and substance K. Nature 315:61–63

PAYAN DG, GOETZL EJ (1985) Modulation of lymphocyte function by sensory neuropeptides. J Immunol 135 : 783s-786s

PAYAN DG, LEVINE JD, GOETZL EJ (1984) Modulation of immunity and hypersensitivity by sensory neuropeptides. J Immunol 132 : 1601–1604

PERNOW B (1985) Role of tachykinins in neurogenic inflammation. J Immunol 135 : 812s-815s

RISLING M, DALSGAARD CJ, CUKIERMAN A, CUELLO AC (1984) Electron microscopic and immunohistochemical evidence that unmyelinated ventral root axons make U-turns or enter the spinal pia mater. J Comp Neurol 225 : 53–63

SOMMER EW, KAZIMIERCZAK J, DROZ B (1985) Neuronal subpopulations in the dorsal root ganglion of the mouse as characterized by combination of ultrastrutural and cytochemical features. Brain Res 346 : 310–326

SWETT JE (1985) Differential patterns of labeling in the rat dorsal in the rat dorsal horn and dorsal column nuclei with transganglionic transport of WGA-HRP and HRP. Neurosci Abstr 11 : 120

TAYLOR DCM, PIERAU F-K (1982) Double fluorescence labelling supports electrophysiological evidence for dichotomizing peripheral sensory nerve fibers in rats. Neurosci Lett 33 : 1–6

WALL PD, DEVOR M (1983) Sensory afferent impulses originate from dorsal root ganglia as well as from the periphery in normal and nerve injured rats. Pain 17 : 321–339

YEH Y, KRUGER L (1984) Fine-structural characterization of the somatic innervation of the tympanic membrane in normal, sympathectomized, and neurotoxin-denervated rats. Somatosens Res 1 : 359–378

2 The Innervation of the Dura Mater Encephali of the Rat

K. H. Andres, M. von Düring, K. Muszynski, and R. F. Schmidt

Previous Investigation on the Innervation of the Dural Tissue

In 1826 Arnold was the first to describe "nervi tentorii" coming from the ophthalmic branch of the trigeminal nerve. Later authors, such as von Luschka (1850), Alexander (1875) and many others in this century confirmed and extended these observations (for review see Crosby et al. 1962). Thus, it is now common knowledge that all three branches of the trigeminal nerve contribute to the afferent innervation of the dura mater.

Recent studies have concentrated on the topographical relations between the peripheral termination sites of fine afferents and the location of their perikarya within the Gasserian ganglion (Steiger et al. 1982; Mayberg et al. 1984). The latter authors also demonstrated that the dura mater carries a sympathetic innervation coming from the superior cervical ganglion.

We now report data on the quantitative aspects of the innervation of the dura mater as well as the localization and ultrastructure of the afferent terminals. For further details see Andres et al. (1987).

Our Own Approach: Serial Studies of Decalcified Heads

Sprague-Dawley rats were prepared for EM studies using the techniques of this laboratory (Andres and von Düring 1981). Eight of the rats were used to study the number and distribution of the nerve fibres. After removing the calvarium the convex part of the dura mater, together with the brain tissue, was cut horizontally. Cranial nerves were transsected within the subarachnoid space just before their dural portals. The rest of the brain tissue was removed. The basal and convex part of the dura mater were postfixed with OsO_4. This procedure exhibits the nerve fibre bundles supplying the dura mater, coming from the Gasserian ganglia or the branches of the trigeminal nerve, as thin black outlines. The photo documentation of the specimens with the black nerve fibre bundles allowed a systemic cutting of the nerve fibre after embedding of the whole specimen. In addition, to obtain a complete quantitative analysis of the innervation of the dura mater two heads were decalcified for 2 months in 25% EDTA, pH 7.4, at room temperature under continuous shaking followed by washing in 0.1 M phosphate buffer, pH 7.4. The heads were adjusted in plexiglass frames, surrounded with 4% agarose, cut into 2.5-mm frontal slices using the technique of Andres and von Düring (1981) and postfixed in 2% OsO_4 (Friedrich and Mugnaini 1981). The subsequent dehydration was interrupted at the stage of 70% ethanol for photographic documentation of each slice by the interference reflecting light (IRL) method (Andres and von Düring, 1974, 1977). After embedding in Araldite, series of alternate semithin and ultrathin sections were cut with a Reichert OM U II and LKB Ultrotom III and examined with a Zeiss Photomicroscope II and with a Philips 300 electron microscope. The location of fibre counts and measuring was near the division of the dural nerves from the main trigeminal branches and, peripherally, at the sagittal sinus and the parietal dura mater.

Nerve Supply to Supratentorial Part is from Three Sources

The major dural nerve fascicles stem from all three major branches of the trigeminal nerve (Fig. 1A). The first branch, i.e. the ophthalmic nerve, contributes several fascicles to the dural innervation: The most rostral ones stem from the ethmoidal nerve in its course along the olfactory bulb. The other fascicles branch directly from the ophthalmic nerve, the tentorial nerve being the most prominent. The maxillary and the mandibular nerve contribute several branches (see arrows in Fig. 1A) which leave the nerves just above the Gasserian ganglion.

All the fascicles mentioned above contain myelinated as well as unmyelinated nerve fibres (Fig. 2A). For instance, the branches coming from the ethmoidal nerve contain together about 50 myelinated and 300 unmyelinated axons; the nervus spinosus (consisting of one or two bundles) contains about 160 myelinated and 320 unmyelinated axons; and the nervus tentorius carries about 40 myelinated and 280 unmyelinated axons. Taken together, about 250 myelinated and 800 unmyelinated nerve fibres supply one side of the supratentorial part of the dura mater encephali. The proportion of myelinated to unmyelinated nerve fibres is about 1:3.2.

Fig. 1 A. Topography of innervation and blood supply of the dura mater encephali. Venous sinuses and venous vessels stippled. The dural nerves (large arrows) originate with one or two bundles with the main trigeminal branches. Small arrows indicate bundles of the dural nerve fibres running to the sagittal sinus to form the terminal plexus. Ophthalmic nerve (V_1), maxillary nerve (V_2), mandibular nerve (V_3), ethmoidal nerve (ETH), optic nerve (II), oculomotor nerve (III), trochlear nerve (IV), anterior meningeal artery (AMA), middle meningeal artery (MMA), sagittal sinus (SS), rectus sinus (RS), confluence of sinuses (CS), superior cerebral veins (SCV), inner maxillary vein (MV). (From Andres et al., 1987) **B** Diagram of nerve terminals at the postcapillary venule (PV) with segments of endothelial fenestration (arrows within the vessel). The Schwann cell (SC) contains unmyelinated branches of a myelinated axon and "true" unmyelinated axons (CA). Terminals facing to the connective tissue of the venule (thick arrows), myelinated axon (AA), fibrocyte (F), pericyte (P), basement lamina of the vessel (BL), erythrocyte (E). (Modified from Andres et al., 1987) **C** Diagram of an unencapsulated Ruffini-

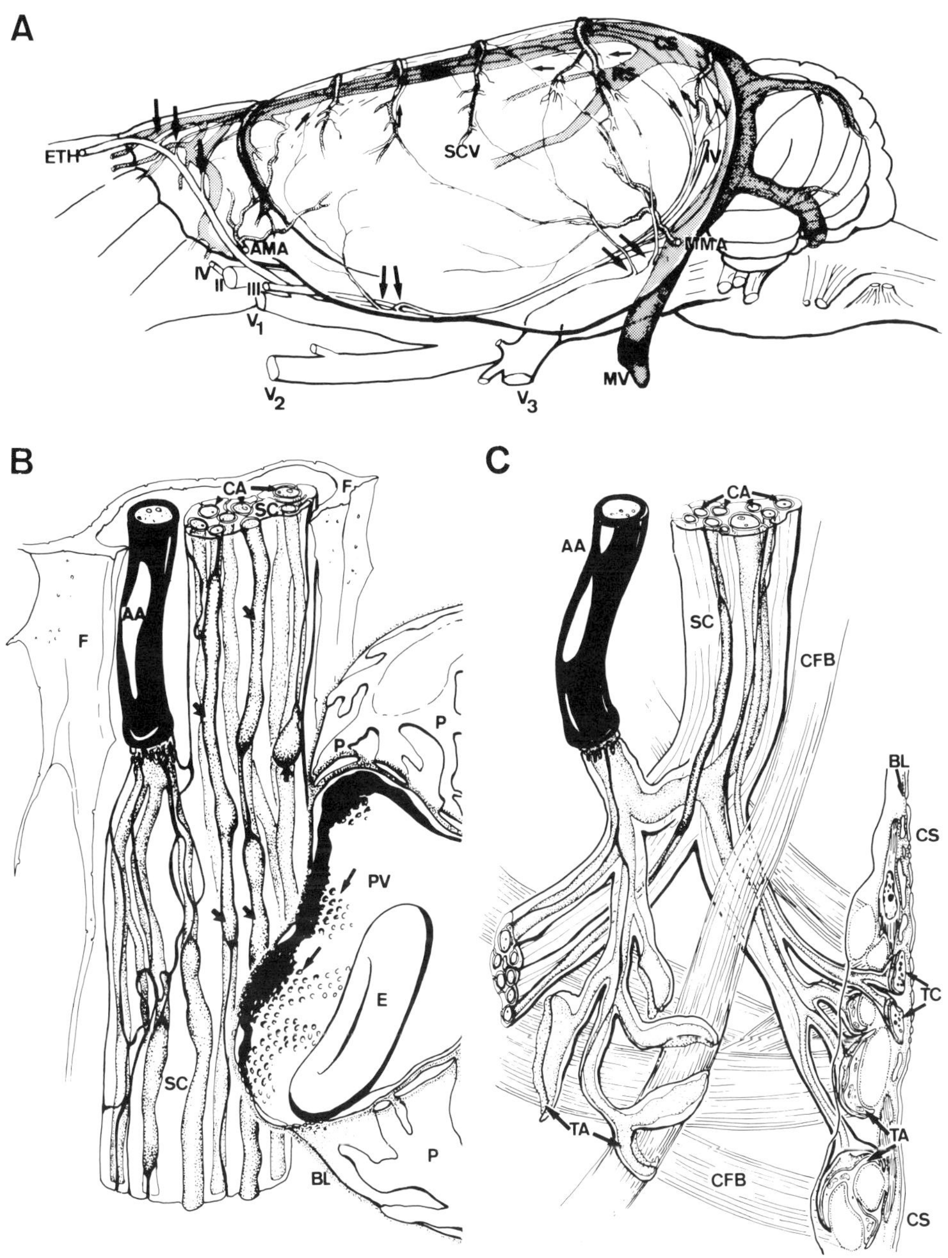

like terminal from a myelinated axon (AA) located in the dense collagenous fibre bundles (CFB) of a cerebral vein entering the confluence of sinuses (CS). Unmyelinated axons (CA) carry along the myelinated axon. Terminals of the myelinated axon (TA) exhibit close contact to the collagenous fibre bundles. The unmyelinated branches of the A axon mix with the C axons in one Schwann cell (SC). Terminals of unmyelinated axons (TC) contact the vessel wall; basement lamella of the vessel wall (BL). Basement lamella of the nerve fibre bundles is not drawn. (Modified from Andres et al., 1987)

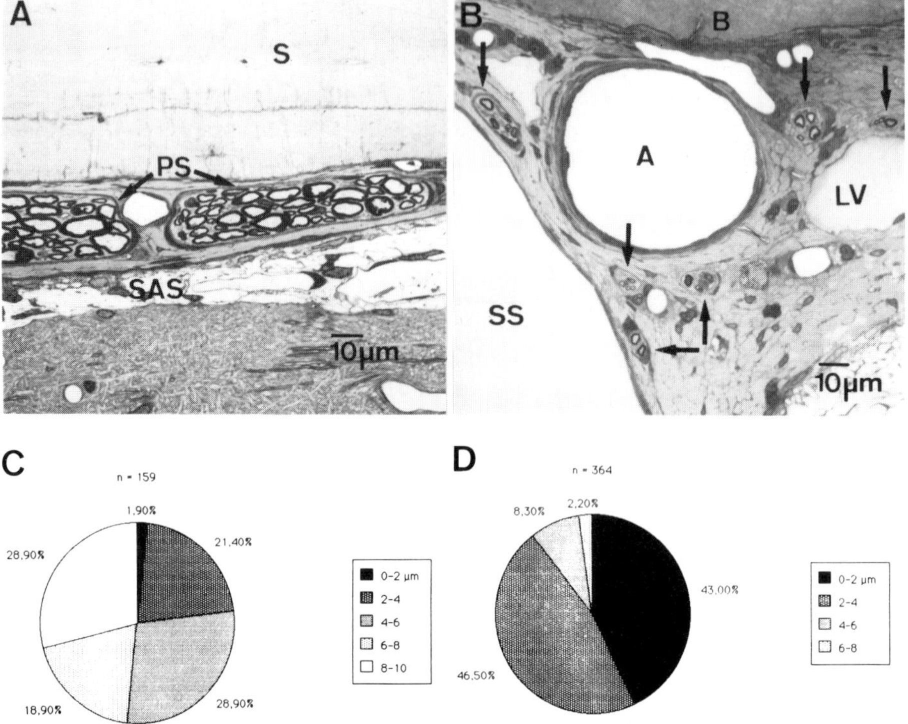

Fig. 2 A. Part of the ramus of the nervus spinosus lying in the dura mater of the squamosa segment with myelinated and unmyelinated nerve fibres. Perineural sheath (PS), squamosa (S), subarachnoid space (SAS). Semithin section, x 600. **B** Nerve fibre bundles (arrows) within the perineural net continuum and different segments of the vascular bed in the dura mater between the lateral and dorsal side of the sagittal sinus (SS) and the cranial bone (B). Lymphatic vessel (LV), branch of meningeal artery (A). Semithin section, x 600. **C** Pie diagram of myelinated nerve fibres in the proximal part of the nervus spinosus of the rat. **D** Pie diagram of myelinated nerve fibres at the peripheral branching of the fibres in the parietal dura mater and at the sagittal sinus.

Myelinated Afferents are Much Finer Distally than Proximally

A comparison of a proximal segment of the spinosus nerve (Fig. 2A) with an area lateral to the sinus sagittalis showing the distal nerve fibre network (Fig. 2B) immediately reveals that on average the myelinated afferents are much finer distally than proximally. A quantitative evaluation is given in Fig. 2C,D. The diameter distribution shown in C was taken from sections of the nervus spinosus just at its origin from the maxillary nerve. There is an equal distribution of nerve fibre diameters in the range from 2 to 10 μm. In contrast, nerve fibre diameters measured in the peripheral perineural net (Fig. 2D) have shifted to a much smaller range, the majority of fibres now having diameters not exceeding 4 μm. The numbers of unmyelinated axons at different segments of the sagittal sinus and the parietal dura mater have increased; the proportion of myelinated to unmyelinated axons has shifted to about 1 : 10.

It was a regular finding that the final unmyelinated segments of the myelinated fibres (which have a length of 200 μm and more) share their Schwann cell with true unmyelinated axons (Fig. 3A–C). Thus, even when using serial sections it was difficult to identify the parent fibre of a given terminal (for an exception see below). The branching of unmyelinated afferents seems to be much more pronounced than that of the myelinated ones, because in the periphery a single myelinated fibre is always accompanied by about 8–15 unmyelinated ones.

Only Unencapsulated Terminals are Observed in the Dura Mater

The terminals in the dura mater are mainly distributed in two locations: (1) in different segments of the vascular bed: arterioles, capillaries, postcapillary venules, venules, venous sinuses and lymphatic vessels; (2) at various sites within the connective tissue compartments of the dura mater: inner periosteal layer, collagenous fibre bundles of meningeal layer, at mesothelial cell layer of subdural space.

The terminals found in different sections of the vascular bed have a rather uniform appearance. Local swellings, accumulations of vesicles and some areas of receptor matrix are the typical characteristics of these terminals (Figs. 1B, 3A, B). The distance between the terminals and the basement lamella of the venules or the endothelial cell of the lymphatic vessels is reduced to 1 μm. Of all the various segments of the vascular bed (nomenclature according to Rhodin 1968) the venules are those showing the most prominent afferent innervation.

The terminals within the different compartments of the dura mater are also quite similar in structure regardless of their fibres of origin. In their ultrastructure they resemble those seen near vessels. Nevertheless, the topography of the terminals and the connective tissue texture build up a different microenvironment. At the more lateral parts of the parietal dura mater the Schwann cells with their terminal axons spread to a width of 30 μm, forming flat 4- to 6-μm-thick processes.

An exception to the rather uniform picture described so far is formed by the unencapsulated Ruffini-like terminals which were found in the connective tissue of the sutures of the cranial bone, at the locations where the superior cerebral veins empty into the sinuses and at the confluences of sinuses (Figs. 1C, 3C). The parent fibres of these endings are all myelinated (Andres et al., 1987). Their final unmyelinated sections are much larger in diameter (about 2 μm) than those of the other types of terminals.

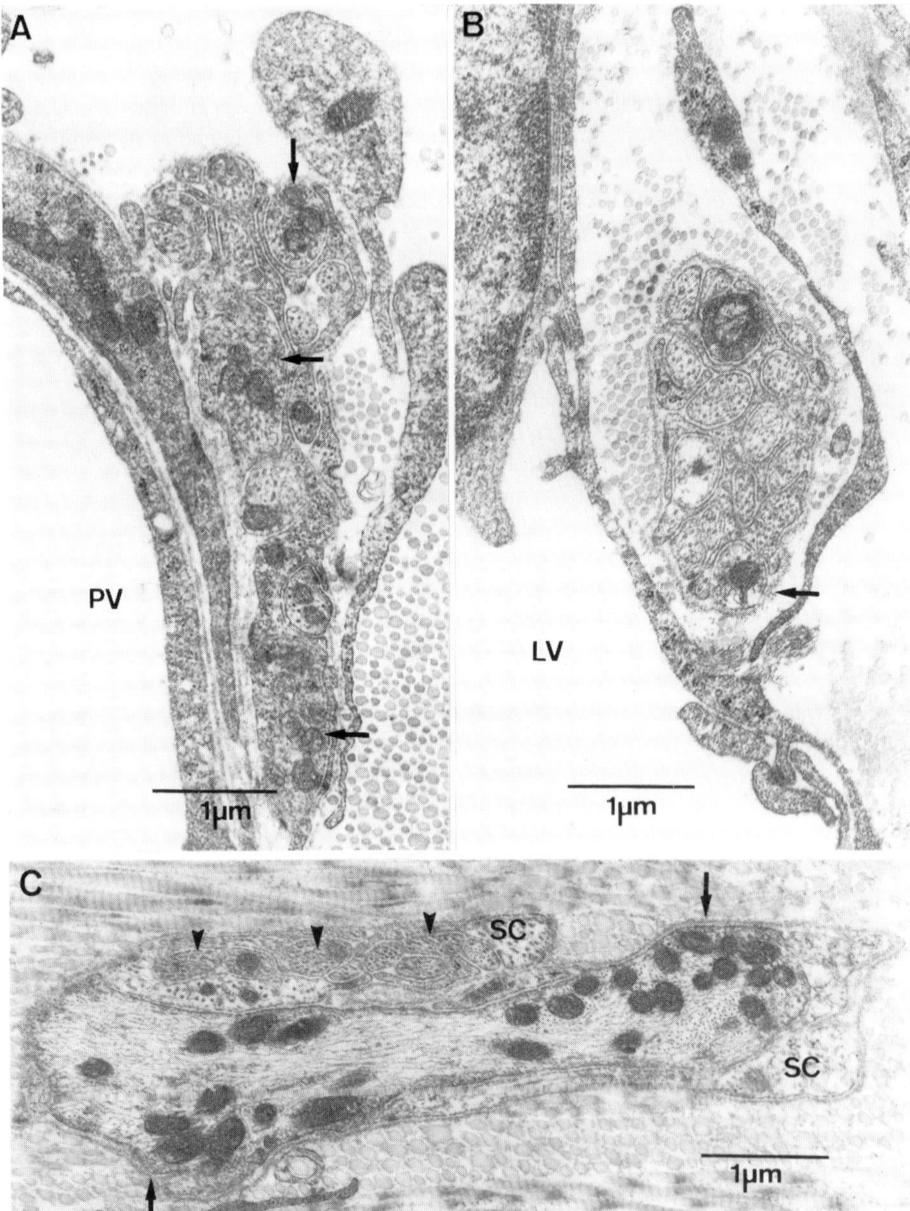

Fig. 3 A. Nerve terminations from myelinated and unmyelinated axons at a postcapillary venule (PV) in the dura mater. Axon profiles with vesicles and receptor matrix (arrows); the other axonal profiles exhibit cytoskeletal elements. EM, x 25 300. **B** Nerve terminations from myelinated and unmyelinated axons at a lymphatic vessel (LV) in the dura mater. One of the axons contacts the connective tissue compartment and exhibits clear vesicles (arrow). EM, x 25 300. **C** Unmyelinated segment of an unencapsulated Ruffini-like terminal (arrows) of a myelinated axon facing the tough collagen fibre bundles of the dura mater at the entrance of a cerebral venous vessel. Several unmyelinated axons accompany the unencapsulated Ruffini-like terminal (arrowheads). EM, x 25 300

Terminals in the Dura Mater may be Mechano- and Chemosensitive

Based on comparative studies the unencapsulated Ruffini-like terminals exhibit all the criteria established for mechanoreceptors. Their position, described above, makes them excellent candidates to measure the stretching of the vascular walls of the sinus region, i.e. the venous pressure and/or flow volume in this area.

The other terminals, both close to the vessels and in the connective tissue proper, lack specific perineural or Schwann cell differentiations which in other tissue have been recognized as characteristic for mechanoreceptors (for review see Iggo and Andres 1982; Iggo 1985). Therefore, it is tempting to speculate that these terminals are mainly or exclusively sensitive to chemical stimulation. Particularly those terminals less than 1 μm from the endothelial cells of the venous vessel wall are in a prominent position to monitor the chemical composition of the blood.

The terminals described in this study may include nociceptors. In man, high-intensity stimulation of the dura mater along the margins of the dural sinuses elicited pain (Penfield and McNaughton 1940; Ray and Wolff 1940; Wirth and van Buren 1971). Thus afferent terminals at these sites may participate in the generation of vascular headaches which could be elicited by either mechanical or chemical events.

Summary

The dura mater encephali of the rat is richly supplied by myelinated and unmyelinated nerve fibres. For the supratentorial part the main nerve supply stems from all three branches of the trigeminal nerve. Finally, 250 myelinated and 800 unmyelinated nerve fibres innervate one side of the supratentorial part. The vascular bed of the dura mater exhibits long postcapillary venules up to 200 μm in length with segments of endothelial fenestration. Lymphatic vessels occur within the dura mater. The perineural sheath builds up a tube-like net containing the myelinated and unmyelinated axons. It is spacious in the parietal dura mater and dense at the sagittal sinus along its extension from rostral to caudal and at the confluence of sinuses. Terminals of both the myelinated and unmyelinated axons are of the unencapsulated type. Unencapsulated Ruffini-like receptors stemming from myelinated A axons are found in the dural connective tissue at sites where superficial cerebral veins enter the sagittal sinus, at the confluence of sinuses and at the sutures of the cranial bones. The terminations of single myelinated axons together with unmyelinated axons mingle in their final course in one Schwann cell to build up multiaxonal units or terminations (up to 15 axonal profiles). Morphological differentiation is made on the basis of the topography of these terminations; firstly, in different segments of the vascular bed:

postcapillary venule, venule, sinus wall, lymphatic vessel wall; and secondly, within the dura mater: inner periosteal layer, collagenous fibre bundles of meningeal layer, at mesothelial cell layer of subdural space.

Acknowledgements. The authors wish to thank Mrs. Luzie Augustinowski for her skilled technical assistance and Mrs. Hannelore Finkensiep for photographical work.

References

Alexander WT (1875) Bemerkungen über die Nerven der Dura mater. Arch Mikrosk Anat 11 : 231–234

Andres KH, von Düring M (1974) Interferenzphänomene am osmierten Präparat für die systematische elektronenmikroskopische Untersuchung. Mikroskopie 3 : 139–149

Andres KH, von Düring M (1977) Interference phenomen on osmium tetroxide-fixed specimens for systematic electron microscopy. In: Hayat A (ed) Principles and techniques of electron microscopy. Van Nostrand Reinhold, New York, pp 246–261

Andres KH, von Düring M (1981) General methods for characterization of brain regions. In: Heym C, Forssmann WG (eds) Techniques in neuroanatomical research. Springer, Berlin Heidelberg New York, pp 100–108

Andres KH, von Düring M, Schmidt RF (1985) Sensory innervation of the Achilles tendon by group III and IV afferent fibers. Anat Embryol (Berl) 172 : 145–156

Andres KH, von Düring M, Muszynski K, Schmidt RF (1987) Nerve fibres and their terminals of the dura mater encephali of the rat. Anat Embryol 175 : 289–301

Arnold R (1826) Dissertatione de parte cephalica nervi sympathici in homine. University of Heidelberg

Crosby EC, Humphrey T, Lauer EW (1962) Correlative anatomy of the nervous system. Macmillan, New York

Friedrich VL, Mugnaini E (1981) Preparation of neural tissue for electron microscopy. In: Heimer L, Robards MJ (eds) Neuroanatomical tract-tracing methods. Plenum, New York, London, pp 345–374

Iggo A (1985) Sensory receptors in the skin of mammals and their sensory functions. Rev Neurol (Paris) 141 : 599–613

Iggo A, Andres KH (1982) Morphology of cutaneous receptors. Annu Rev Neurosci 5 : 1–31

Luschka H von (1850) Die Nerven der harten Hirnhaut. Laupp, Tübingen

Mayberg MR, Zervas NT, Moskowitz MA (1984) Trigeminal projections to supratentorial pial and dural blood vessels in cats demonstrated by horseradish peroxidase histochemistry. J Comp Neurol 223 : 46–56

Penfield W, McNaughton F (1940) Dural headache and innervation of the dura mater. Arch Neurol Psychiatry 44 : 43–75

Ray BS, Wolff HG (1940) Experimental studies on headache. Pain-sensitive structures of the head and their significance in headache. Arch Surg 41 : 813–856

Rhodin JAG (1968) Ultrastructure of mammalian venous capillaries, venules and small collecting veins. J Ultrastruct Res 25 : 452–500

Steiger HJ, Tew JM, Keller JT (1982) The sensory representation of the trigeminal ganglion of the cat. Neurosci Lett 31 : 231-236

Wirth FP, van Buren JM (1971) Referral of pain from dural stimulation in man. J Neurosurg 34 : 630–64

3 The Afferent Innervation of the Rat Mesenteric Vascular Bed

T. M. Scott, J. Robinson, and J. Foote

Introduction

Current theories of cardiovascular control include as part of the afferent system, fibres originating from the heart, from the arch of the aorta and from the baroreceptors located at the bifurcation of the common carotid artery. In addition much of the cardiovascular system has been shown recently to be differentially innervated by fine fibres sensitive to capsaicin (Furness et al. 1982). The cell bodies of these fibres are thought to be located in the trigeminal and dorsal root ganglia (Matsuyama et al. 1984; Liu-Chen et al. 1986; Wanaka et al. 1986). While information concerning the distribution of this presumptive afferent system has been gathered, there is little information concerning its function or role in the integration of cardiovascular control.

We have shown that treatment of adult spontaneously hypertensive rats with capsaicin lowers arterial pressure from hypertensive to normotensive levels, and further that treatment of neonatal SHR prevents the development of hypertension, suggesting that substance P-containing systems are involved in the development of hypertension in this animal model of human essential hypertension (Scott and Pang 1983). In this study we have examined and compared the substance P-like immunoreactive (SPLI) innervation of the mesenteric vascular bed in normotensive and hypertensive rats to determine whether or not a difference in this system exists.

Materials and Methods

Twelve-week-old normotensive Sprague-Dawley (SD) and Wistar Kyoto (WKY) rats and hypertensive Spontaneously Hypertensive Rats (SHR) were anesthetised and perfused through the heart with Zamboni's fixative. The superior mesenteric artery and vein and their major branches were removed and incubated for 2 days in phosphate-buffered saline containing rabbit anti-substance P antibody (Immunonuclear), followed by goat anti-rabbit linking antibody, then peroxidase anti-peroxidase complex raised in rabbit. Diaminobenzidine was used to produce the final product. The vessels were mounted on slides as whole mounts and the SPLI plexus examined and drawn using a camera lucida. The extent of the plexus on each vessel was determined from the drawings by stereology (Weibel 1980), using a superimposed test line.

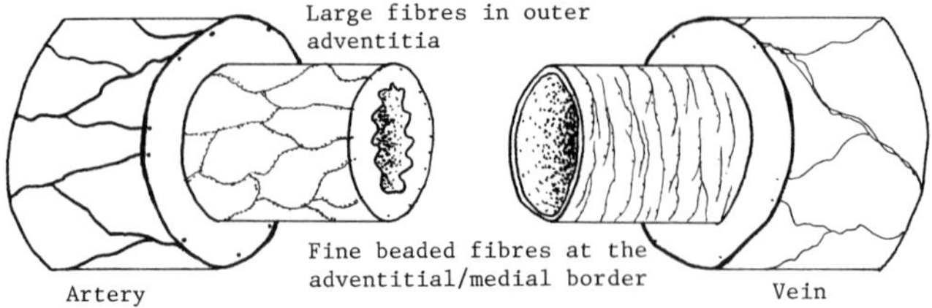

Fig. 1. A diagrammatic representation of the superficial and deep plexuses of the mesenteric arteries and veins

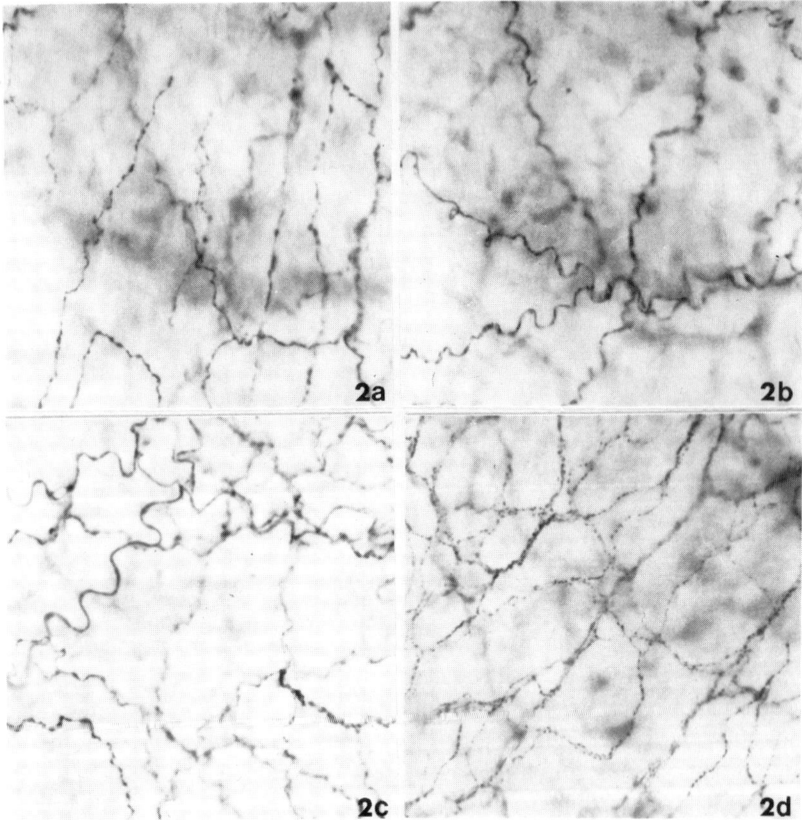

Fig. 2 A. The SPLI plexus at the adventitial medial border of a mesenteric vein from a WKY rat. **B** The same field as **A** but a more superficial focus, showing the fibres of the SPLI plexus in the outer adventitia. **C** The SPLI plexus of a jejunal artery of an SD rat. **D** The beaded fibres of the SPLI plexus of the superior mesenteric artery of a hypertensive rat

Results

As shown diagrammatically in Fig. 1, the SPLI plexus innervating the mesenteric vascular bed was disposed in two planes. Large-diameter fibres, generally with a smooth surface, formed a plexus in the outer adventitia. At the adventitial/medial border a second layer of finer beaded fibres was present. In the arteries this deep layer appeared to run in all directions (Fig. 2c,d), while in the veins the fibres had a predominantly circular orientation (Fig.2a). In all three strains examined the plexus was extensive on both arteries and veins but was particularly heavy on jejunal arteries. No difference in either the form or extent of the plexus was seen when normotensive and hypertensive vessels were compared (Table 1). In both normotensive (Fig. 2b,c) and hypertensive (Fig. 2d) strains the plexus was formed of fibres taking an irregular course, branching and rejoining bundles frequently.

Table 1. A comparison of the extent of the SPLI plexus of the superior mesenteric artery and vein and jejunal artery in normotensive SD and WKY rats and hypertensive SHR

Strain of rat	Plexus length ($\mu m/1 \times 10^5\ \mu m^2$) Superior mesenteric artery	Jejunal artery	Superior mesenteric vein
SD (normotensive)	274 ± 54	570 ± 121	304 ± 73
WKY (normotensive)	299 ± 54	491 ± 68	359 ± 86
SHR (hypertensive)	263 ± 60	534 ± 61	285 ± 61

A significant difference was found between the jejunal arteries and all other vessels ($p < 0.01$), but no differences were detected between strains for any vessel

Discussion

The vessels of the mesenteric vascular bed have an extensive SPLI innervation. Although at 12 weeks of age SHR have a significantly elevated arterial pressure (Pang and Scott 1981), no difference in either the form or the extent of the SPLI plexus was detected when vessels from normotensive and hypertensive rats were compared.

Although the jejunal arteries showed the highest density of innervation, the superior mesenteric artery and vein are perhaps more remarkable in that a high density of SPLI innervation is present in a situation where the density of sympathetic innervation is low. This suggests that the SPLI plexus is either involved in a local response or may be the afferent limb of a system which brings about changes in other parts of the cardiovascular system. Substance P release from peripheral nerves has been shown to be accompanied by increased vascular permeability (Lembeck and Holzer 1979) and might represent a local response to the presence of a vasoactive agent in the vessel wall. The substance P-containing fibres of brain pial vessels originate from trigeminal neurons (Liu-Chen et al. 1983), and it has been suggested that the fibres may transmit information of a nociceptive nature from the blood vessels to the central nervous system, and thus be of importance in mechanisms of vascular head pain (Moskowitz 1984).

The range of vessels which have been shown to be innervated by substance P-containing fibres is wide (Furness et al. 1982; Morris et al. 1986), and it may be that they are not all identical in their structure or function. It is certain, however, that this system of fine unmyelinated fibres will receive further attention and that its place in the function of the vasculature will be elucidated.

References

Furness JB, Papka RE, Della NG, Costa M, Eskay RL (1982) Substance P-like immunoreactivity in nerves associated with the vascular system of guinea pigs. Neuroscience 7 : 447–459

Lembeck F, Holzer P (1979) Substance P as a neurogenic mediator of antidromic vasodilatation and neurogenic plasma extravasation. Naunyn Schmiedbergs Arch Pharmacol 310 : 175–193

Liu-Chen L-Y, Mayberg MY, Moskowitz MA (1983) Immunohistochemical evidence for a substance P containing trigeminovascular pathway to pial arteries in cats. Brain Res 268 : 162–166

Liu-Chen L-Y, Liszczak TM, King JC, Moskowitz MA (1986) Immunoelectron microscopic study of substance P-containing fibers in feline cerebral arteries. Brain Res 369 : 12–20

Matsuyama T, Matsumoto M, Shiosaka S, Hayakawa T, Yoneda S, Kimura K, Abe H, Tohyama, M (1984) Dual innervation of substance P containing neuron system in the wall of the cerebral arteries. Brain Res 322 : 144–147

Morris JL, Gibbins IL, Campbell G, Murphy R, Furness JB, Costa M (1986) Innervation of the large arteries and heart of the toad **(Bufo marinus)** by adrenergic and peptide-containing neurons. Cell Tissue Res 243 : 171–184

Moskowitz MA (1984) The neurobiology of vascular head pain. Ann Neurol 16 : 157–168

Pang S, Scott TM (1981) Stereological analysis of the tunica media of the aorta and renal artery during the development of hypertension in the spontaneously hypertensive rat. J Anat 133 : 513–526

Scott TM, Pang S (1983) Changes in jejunal arteries in spontaneously hypertensive and normotensive rats following neonatal treatment with capsaicin. Acta Stereol 2 : 127–133

Wanaka A, Matsuyama T, Yoneda S, Kimura K, Kamada T, Girgis S, MacIntyre I, Emson PC, Tohyama M (1986) Origins and distribution of calcitonin gene-related peptide-containing nerves in the wall of the cerebral arteries of the guinea pig with special reference to the coexistence with substance P. Brain Res 369 : 185–192

Weibel ER (1980) Stereological methods, vol 2. Theoretical foundations. Academic Press, London

4 Unmyelinated Axons in Spinal Ventral Roots and Motor Cranial Nerves. Do These Fibres Have a Role in Somatovisceral Sensation?

M. Risling, C. Hildebrand, and C.-J. Dalsgaard

The Law of Magendie

Sensory axons enter the spinal cord through the dorsal root and motor axons leave through the ventral root. This description of the different properties of the spinal roots is usually referred to as "the Law of Bell and Magendie". Although Charles Bell successfully claimed priority of this discovery, it is doubtful if he made a correct interpretation of his own experiments (see Cranefield 1974). In his original (unpublished) text, Bell (1811, cited by Cranefield 1974) described the ventral root as a pathway for both efferent and afferent somatic axons, which were governed by the will, while the dorsal root was concerned with the internal organs, i.e. contained both efferent and afferent visceral fibres. In Bell's view, the dorsal root was connected to the cerebellum and the ventral root was an extension of the cerebrum. Magendie (1822a), on the other hand, reported that the dorsal roots "appear more particularly destined for sensibility, while the anterior seem more specially connected with movement". In contrast to Bell, Magendie based his conclusions on rhizotomies in living animals. In addition, Magendie was one of the first researchers ever to use drugs for physiological experiments. He induced tetanic muscular contractions with strychnine (nux vomica) and noted that such convulsions were absent in a leg if its contributing ventral roots had been divided (Magendie 1822b). After dorsal root section, instead, he observed the animal to "move very apparently, although sensibility was at all the time wholly extinct" (Magendie 1822a).

Recurrent Sensibility

Although sensibility seemed to be dependent on the integrity of the dorsal root, Magendie found that pain reactions could be elicited by stimulation of the ventral root. Such reactions, however, were abolished by dorsal root section (Magendie 1822b). This phenomenon, which has also been shown to occur in man (Frykholm et al. 1953), is usually called "recurrent sensibility".

Sensory Axons in Ventral Roots

Ventral roots in both cat and man contain large numbers of unmyelinated axons (Coggeshall 1980). At thoracic and lower sacral levels many of these represent preganglionic sympathetic or parasympathetic efferents (Coggeshall 1980). About 30 % of the axons in the ventral roots L7 and S1 of the cat are unmyelinated (Coggeshall et al. 1974). The vast majority of these axons appear to enter the roots from the periphery, as judged from ventral root division (Coggeshall et al. 1974). Most of these disappear after dorsal root ganglion excision (Coggeshall at al. 1974). C fibres in these roots can be activated either from abdominal and pelvic visceral receptors or by nociceptive stimulation of cutaneous receptive fields in the hindleg (Coggeshall and Ito 1977). Recent studies show that axons with a substance P-like immunoreactivity occur in lumbosacral ventral roots of the cat (Dalsgaard et al. 1982; Risling et al. 1984a). This indicates that a substantial proportion of sensory axons are present in cat ventral roots.

Horseradish peroxidase (HRP) staining experiments have provided circumstantial evidence that sensory axons might enter the spinal cord directly through the ventral root. Maynard et al. (1977) demonstrated labelled neurons in the dorsal root ganglion after HRP injection into the spinal cord in combination with dorsal rhizotomy. These neurons were, however, few in comparison with the number of unmyelinated axons profiles in the ventral root (Maynard et al. 1977). In another study, Light and Metz (1978) crushed HRP into juxtamedullary fascicles of coccygeal ventral roots. They observed several thin HRP-positive axon profiles coursing between the ventral funiculus and the dorsal horn. These axons were assumed to represent central terminations of ventral root afferents, although the ventral root exit zone could not be examined due to heavy staining. These findings suggest the possibility that the Law of Magendie might be incorrect.

In a study dealing with retrograde effects of sciatic nerve resection in young kittens (see below), it was found that L7 ventral roots in control kittens contained only about 15%

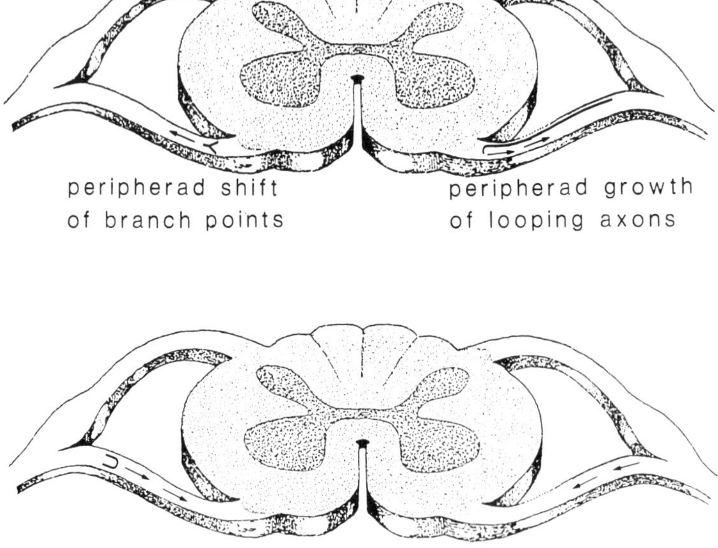

Fig. 1. Schematic drawings illustrating how the content of unmyelinated axon profiles at mid-root level could hypothetically be increased. For explanation see text.

unmyelinated axon profiles (Risling et al. 1980). This should be compared with the previous observation that 30 % of the axons in the L7 ventral root were unmyelinated (Coggeshall et al. 1974). This unexpected finding was confirmed in a study where L7 ventral roots of 25 cats and kittens aged from 3 weeks to 11 years were used (Risling et al. 1981). Sample countings were made in transverse thin sections which were cut at "mid-root level" (halfway between the proximal and distal ends of the roots). In kittens younger than 4 months, the proportion of unmyelinated axon profiles varied around 14.3 %. During months 4-7 a distinct increase took place. In animals older than 7 months, the average proportion of unmyelinated axon profiles was 31.1 % and this figure did not appear to change for at least a decade. The number of myelinated axons in the L7 ventral root was approximately the same in kittens (mean = 5562) and adult cats (mean = 5325). Counts in the C6 ventral root showed that about 20 % of the axon profiles in this root are unmyelinated, both in kittens and adult cats (Risling et al. 1981). Thus, while the average number of unmyelinated axon profiles at mid-root level in the L7 ventral root increased from 926 to 2404 during postnatal development, the number of unmyelinated axons in the C6 root did not appear to change at all.

It was hypothesized that unmyelinated ventral root axons might branch in a manner similar to dorsal root axons (cf. Langford and Coggeshall 1979) and that the increase in the number of unmyelinated axon profiles at mid-root level might be due to a shift of such branch points from the proximal half to the distal half of the L7 ventral root during its postnatal growth (Fig. 1). Alternatively, it was suggested that unmyelinated axons might loop in the proximal half of the root and then grow back 4-7 months postnatally (Fig. 1). A shift of the central end of hairpin loops from the distal to the proximal half of the root (Fig. 1) could also increase the number of axon profiles at mid-root level. Ingrowth of "new" axons into the L7 ventral root (Fig. 1) during the late postnatal development represents another possibility.

Against this background it was decided to estimate the content of unmyelinated axon profiles at different proximodistal levels of the L7 ventral root in seven adult cats and two kittens (Risling and Hildebrand 1982). In all these animals the proportion of unmyelinated axon profiles was highest distally in the ventral root and decreased as the spinal cord was approached (Risling and Hildebrand 1982; see also Vergara et al. 1986). The same trend was seen in both adult cats and kittens, but the values were clearly higher in adults. This finding appears to exclude the possibility of a distad shift of branch points as an explanation for the postnatal increase in the number of axon profiles. Furthermore, in three of the adult cats, the occurrence of unmyelinated axon profiles was examined in juxtamedullary ventral root fascicles including the CNS/PNS transitional region. It was shown that the content of unmyelinated axon profiles decreases markedly near the PNS/CNS border. Outside the ventral root fascicles tiny bundles of PNS-type unmyelinated and small myelinated axons were observed in the pia mater. These unexpected findings suggested the possibility that unmyelinated ventral root axons, instead of entering the spinal cord, might form hairpin loops or leave the root and enter the pia mater.

To address this issue, the distribution of unmyelinated axons was examined in three juxtamedullary L7 ventral root fascicles at 17 levels separated by even 50-μm intervals (Risling 1983; Risling et al. 1984a). In each of these fascicles the proportion of unmyelinated axon profiles decreased as the spinal cord was approached, and it reached zero before the fascicle merged with the spinal cord. The unmyelinated axon profiles tended to occupy increasingly more superficial positions in the fascicles as the distance to the spinal cord decreased. From another adult cat, a series of 3700 consecutive thin sections were cut from the L7 ventral root CNS/PNS transitional region and examined in the electron microscope (Risling 1983; Risling et al. 1984a). No unmyelinated axons were found to enter the spinal cord through the ventral root. Instead, small groups of unmyelinated axons and occasional small myelinated axons left the ventral root at the ventral root-spinal cord junction and coursed into the pia mater. Other groups of axons had disappeared completely at proximal levels. A close examination showed that these axon bundles formed U-turns composed of two peripheral shanks and a central connecting loop. A few axons were surrounded by astrocytic processes at distal levels in the transitional region, i.e. appeared as unmyelinated CNS axons. At more proximal levels, however, these axons returned to the PNS compartment (cf. Carlstedt 1977). Cat CNS axons tend to be myelinated when their diameters exceed 0.2–0.4 μm (Remahl and Hildebrand 1982). In the L7 ventral root of the cat the diameter of the unmyelinated axons ranges from 0.1 to 1.5 μm (Coggeshall et al. 1974). If these axons reach the CNS, many of them should become myelinated as they enter the ventral root CNS compartment; however, no such small myelinated axons were observed in this region. Immunohistochemical examination of juxtamedullary root fascicles and the pia mater in some additional adult cats showed examples of substance P-immunoreactive axons which passed between the root and the pia mater or formed loops (Risling et al. 1984a).

These findings show that the occurrence of sensory unmyelinated axons in ventral root does not necessarily contradict the Law of Magendie. It is tempting to suggest that both looping axons and ventral root pial axons finally enter the CNS via the dorsal root (Fig. 2). This view is compatible with the "recurrent sensibility" reaction as demonstrated by Magendie (see above) and with recent demonstrations of dorsal root axons and dorsal horn neurons which can be activated from the distal (but not from the proximal) stump of a divided ventral root (Chung et al. 1983, 1985; Kim and Chung 1985).

At least some unmyelinated ventral root axons should represent the peripheral axonal process of spinal ganglion neurons rather than a dorsal root axon counterpart. This hypothesis is supported by the finding of chromatolytic spinal ganglion neurons after ventral root division (Norcio and DeSantis 1976). Spinal ganglion neurons show this response after peripheral axotomy but not after dorsal root division (Cragg 1970).

The demonstration of looping unmyelinated axons in the L7 ventral root indicates that the content of unmyelinated axons in this root has probably been overestimated by

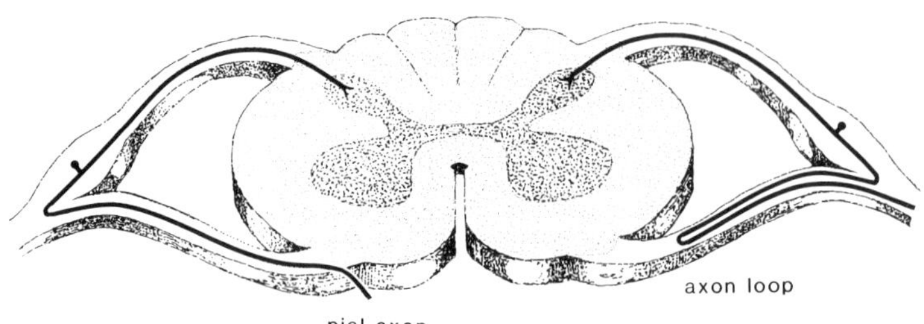

Fig. 2. A schematic drawing showing the suggested anatomical background for the recurrent sensibility reaction

previous countings, since each looping axon will form at least two axon profiles in a cross section. In addition, there is some indirect evidence suggesting that not all unmyelinated axons in the L7 ventral root are sensory. Cathecholaminergic axons occur in all cat ventral roots (Stevens et al. 1983). These axons seem to reach the ventral root and the dorsal root ganglion from the periphery (Stevens et al. 1983). Therefore, axons surviving in the distal stump of a divided ventral root do not necessarily represent sensory axons. In fact, Sherrington (1894) suggested that postganglionic sympathetic axons should account for at least some of the axons that survived in the distal stump after ventral root division. It may be assumed that many of these postganglionic sympathetic ventral root axons are destined for pial blood vessels. This suggestion is supported by the recent demonstration of neuropeptide Y-immunoreactive axons, which are known to be of postganglionic sympathetic origin, in the pia mater near ventral root fascicles (Risling et al. 1985a).

It cannot be excluded that a few unmyelinated axons actually enter the CNS directly through the L7 ventral root (or via other ventral roots), even though no such axons have been detected in the fascicles examined so far. However, in view of the data presented above, these axons should be so few that it appears unlikely that they can play a major role in somatovisceral sensation. If some occasional unmyelinated sensory axons enter the spinal cord directly through the L7 ventral root, these could account for labelling of spinal ganglion neurons after HRP injection into the spinal cord combined with dorsal root division (Maynard et al. 1977). Alternatively, HRP might have been transported to the ganglion by myelinated sensory axons, if such axons enter the spinal cord this way. However, it is also possible that some of the labelled neurons might correspond to pial afferents which have taken up the enzyme and transported it to the ganglion via the ventral root. The failure, so far, to activate dorsal horn neurons from the proximal stump of a divided ventral root (Chung et al. 1983, 1985) supports the view that sensory axons do not enter the spinal cord directly through the ventral root. In contrast, it seems well established that at least some slowly conducting sensory axons course between the ventral root and the dorsal root (Kim and Chung 1985) and finally enter the dorsal horn via the dorsal root (Chung et al. 1983, 1985).

It is likely that unmyelinated ventral root axons have a role in somatovisceral sensation, even though they do not seem to enter the spinal cord directly through the L7 ventral root. According to clinical reports, the ventral part of the spinal pia mater is pain-sensitive (White and Sweet 1955). It appears likely that this pain reaction is transmitted to the CNS via the pia mater-ventral root-dorsal root pathway. In addition, it is tempting to suggest that ventral root sensory axons might be involved in cases of sciatic pain. In this context it is of interest that in an autopsy study concerning dorsolateral disk herniation (Lindblom and Rexed 1948), it was observed that the ventral root was often severely affected by compression, while the dorsal root showed no signs of degeneration.

Ingrowth of Unmyelinated Axons into the L7 Ventral Root

During postnatal development the proportion of unmyelinated axon profiles increases at all proximodistal levels along the L7 ventral root (see above). At least in part this increase appears to reflect a true ingrowth of "new" axons into the ventral root and it is followed by an increase in the content of unmyelinated axons in the pia mater (Risling et al. 1984a).

A more dramatic increase in the content of unmyelinated axon profiles in the L7 ventral root is seen after sciatic nerve resection in young kittens (Ramon Y Cajal 1928; Risling et al. 1980). The proportion of unmyelinated axon profiles in ventral roots connected to sciatic neuromas may exceed 80 % (Risling et al. 1980, 1984b) to be compared with 15 % at mid-root level in normal kittens, i.e. the number of unmyelinated axon profiles is increased from about 900 to more than 20 000. A large proportion of these new unmyelinated axons represent sprouts which enter the ventral root by recurrent growth from the neuroma. Many of these sprouts reach the PNS/CNS transitional region, where they leave the root and course into the pia mater (Fig. 3) (Risling et al. 1984b). A large proportion of these axons are substance P-immunoreactive (Risling et al. 1984c), i.e. they probably originate from injured sensory axons. It therefore appeared worthwhile to assess whether some of them enter the spinal cord and thereby contradict the Law of Magendie. Ongoing studies show that a proportion of the sprouts do indeed enter the ventral root CNS compartment but either end blindly or return to the PNS and reach the pia mater. Thus, the Law of Magendie seems to be valid even if the ventral root is invaded by large numbers of sensory sprouts. It is possible that such sprouts may be involved in the chronic pain syndromes that sometimes occur after peripheral nerve injury.

In one 10-year-old cat with an abdominal neoplasm the L7 ventral roots were quite unexpectedly found to contain 50 % unmyelinated axon profiles at "mid-root level" (Risling and Hildebrand 1981), while the number of myelinated axons was within the normal range (mean = 5179). The origin of these supernumerary unmyelinated axons is obscure. It is

RECURRENT SPROUTING

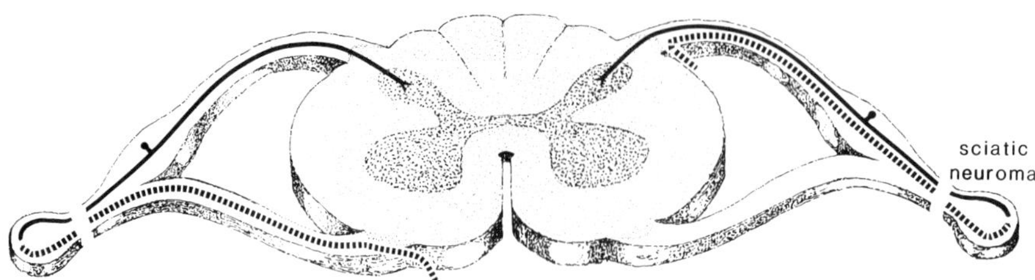

Fig. 3. A schematic drawing illustrating how the ventral and dorsal roots L7 are invaded by sensory axon sprouts originating from the neuroma after sciatic nerve resection in kittens. Axon sprouts are represented by dotted lines. Note that these sprouts do not enter the CNS

known, however, that certain neoplasms may elicit axon outgrowth at sites far away from the tumor (Waddell et al. 1972).

In these examples of axon ingrowth into the L7 ventral root, the ventral root PNS/CNS border seemed to prevent the axons from reaching the spinal cord. Interestingly, the PNS/CNS border does not impede growth in the opposite direction. Thus, many of the axon sprouts that are formed in response to a lesion in the spinal cord ventral funiculus cross the PNS/CNS border and invade the ventral root (Risling et al. 1983).

Unmyelinated Axons in the Spinal Pia Mater

Numerous small bundles of PNS-type axons occur in the spinal pia mater. The majority of these axons are unmyelinated and course along the longitudinal axis of the spinal cord (Clark 1931). There are significantly more axons on the ventral than on the dorsal aspect of the cord (Clark 1931). At least some of the axons reach the "ventral pia mater" from the ventral roots (Clark 1931; Risling et al. 1984a). A population of these axons appear to be of sensory origin and some of them contain substance P-like immunoreactivity (Dalsgaard et al. 1982; Risling et al. 1984a). Some of the pial axons are associated with blood vessels but many seem to lack a vascular relation (Clark 1931; Risling et al. 1984a). In addition to pain perception (White and Sweet 1955), it seems possible that sensory axons in the pia mater might mediate vasodilation (Edvinsson and Uddman 1982). As has been described above, the content of unmyelinated axons in the lumbosacral "ventral pia mater" is increased during postnatal development and following sciatic nerve lesion in kittens.

Unmyelinated Axons in "Motor" Cranial Nerves

The spinal root of the accessory nerve is often considered as a purely motor ventral root counterpart. Recent electron-microscopic studies have revealed that this root contains about 27% unmyelinated axon profiles at the level of the foramen magnum. The proportion of unmyelinated axon profiles is lower in juxtamedullary root fascicles. No unmyelinated axons appear to cross the PNS/CNS border of this root, but several bundles of unmyelinated axons occur in the adjacent pia mater (Risling et al. 1985b). These findings suggest that unmyelinated axons in the spinal root of the accessory nerve contribute to the pial vasomotor and/or sensory innervation. Ongoing studies suggest a similar arrangement in the trochlear, abducens and hypoglossal nerves (cf. Stöhr 1922).

Proximal to the semilunar ganglion the trigeminal nerve splits into two nerve roots, the sensory root (portio major) and the motor root (portio minor), which emerge separately from the pons. The motor root appears to contain all the motor axons distributed by the trigeminal nerve and a population of myelinated proprioceptive sensory axons. In addition, it has been shown that about 10 % of the axon profiles in the motor root of the cat, i.e. about 300 axons, are unmyelinated (Young 1978; Risling et al. 1986). It has been suggested that these axons might represent an additional pathway for trigeminal pain (Young 1978). A recent electron-microscopic study of the PNS/CNS transitional region of the motor root showed that small groups of unmyelinated axons occur on both sides of the PNS/CNS border, in the surrounding pia mater and in perivascular spaces of the CNS compartment. Examination of serial sections showed that some unmyelinated axons actually cross the PNS/CNS border. However, it is not known whether these axons are sensory or whether they finally reach the pons. Thus, the functional significance of these axons remains unknown.

References

Carlstedt T (1977) Observations on the morphology at the transition between the peripheral and the central nervous system in the cat. IV. Unmyelinated fibres in S1 dorsal rootlets. Acta Physiol Scand [Suppl] 446 : 61–71

Chung JM, Lee KH, Endo K, Coggeshall RE (1983) Activation of central neurons by ventral root afferents. Science 222 : 934–935

Chung JM, Lee KH, Kim J, Coggeshall RE (1985) Activation of dorsal horn cells by ventral root stimulation in the cat. J Neurophysiol 54 : 261–272

Clark SL (1931) Innervation of the pia mater of the spinal cord and the medulla. J Comp Neurol 53 : 129–145

Coggeshall RE (1980) Law of separation of function of the spinal roots. Physiol Rev 60 : 716–755

Coggeshall RE, Ito H (1977) Sensory fibres in the ventral roots L7 and S1 in the cat. J Physiol (Lond) 267 : 215–235

Coggeshall RE, Coulter JD, Willis WD (1974) Unmyelinated axons in the ventral roots of the cat lumbosacral enlargement. J Comp Neurol 153 : 39–58

Cragg BG (1970) What is the signal for chromatolysis? Brain Res 23 : 1–21

Cranefield PF (1974) The way in and the way out. Futura, New York

Dalsgaard C-J, Risling M, Cuello AC (1982) Immunohistochemical localization of substance P in the lumbosacral pia mater and ventral roots of the cat. Brain Res 246 : 168–171

Edvinsson L, Uddman R (1982) Immunohistochemical localization and dilatory effect of substance P on human cerebral vessels. Brain Res 232 : 466–471

Frykholm R, Hyde J, Norlén G, Skoglund CR (1953) On pain sensations produced by stimulation of ventral roots in man. Acta Physiol Scand [Suppl 106] 29 : 455–469

Kim J, Chung JM (1985) Electrophysiological evidence for the presence of fibers in continuity between dorsal and ventral roots in the cat. Brain Res 338 : 355–359

Langford LA, Coggeshall RE (1979) Branching of sensory axons in the dorsal root and evidence for the absence of dorsal root efferent fibers. J Comp Neurol 184 : 193–204

Light AR, Metz CB (1978) The morphology of the spinal cord efferent and afferent neurons contributing to the ventral roots of the cat. J Comp Neurol 179 : 501–516

Lindblom K, Rexed B (1948) Spinal nerve injury in dorso-lateral protrusions of lumbar disks. J Neurosurg 5 : 413–432

Magendie F (1822a) Expériences sur les fonctions des racines des nerfs rachidiens. J Physiol Exp Pathol 2 : 276–279 (reprinted in Cranefield 1974)

Magendie F (1822b) Expériences sur les fonctions des racines des nerfs qui naissent de la moelle épiniere. J Physiol Exp Pathol 2 : 366–371 (reprinted in Cranefield 1974)

Maynard CW, Leonard RB, Coulter JD, Coggeshall RE (1977) Central connections of ventral root afferents as demonstrated by the HRP method. J Comp Neurol 172 : 601–608

Norcio R, DeSantis M (1976) The organization of neuronal somata in the first sacral spinal ganglion of the cat. Exp Neurol 50 : 246–258

Ramon y Cajal S (1928) Degeneration and regeneration of the nervous system. Hafner, New York (reprinted 1959)

Remahl S, Hildebrand C (1982) Changing relation between onset of myelination and axon diameter range in developing feline white matter. J Neurol Sci 54 : 33–45

Risling M, Remahl S, Hildebrand C, Aldskogius H (1980) Structural changes in kittens' ventral and dorsal roots L7 after early postnatal sciatic nerve transection. Exp Neurol 67 : 265–279

Risling M, Hildebrand C (1981) Abnormally high content of unmyelinated axon profiles in the ventral root L7 of a cat with and abdominal neoplasm. Acta Neuropathol (Berl) 54 : 169–172

Risling M, Hildebrand C, Aldskogius H (1981) Postnatal increase of unmyelinated axon profiles in the feline ventral root L7. J Comp Neurol 201 : 243–351

Risling M, Hildebrand C (1982) Occurrence of unmyelinated axon profiles at distal, middle and proximal levels in the ventral root L7 of cats and kittens. J Neurol Sci 56 : 219–231

Risling M (1983) Population changes in cat spinal roots following nerve injury and during normal development. Thesis, Karolinska Institutet, Stockholm

Risling M, Cullheim S, Hildebrand C (1983) Reinnervation of the ventral root L7 from ventral horn neurons following intramedullary axotomy in adult cats. Brain Res 280 : 15–23

Risling M, Dalsgaard C-J, Cukierman A, Cuello AC (1984a) Electron microscopic and immunohistochemical evidence that unmyelinated ventral root axons make U-turns or enter the spinal pia mater. J Comp Neurol 225 : 53–63

Risling M, Hildebrand C, Cullheim S (1984b) Invasion of the L7 ventral root and spinal pia mater by new axons after sciatic nerve division in kittens. Exp Neurol 83 : 84–97

Risling M, Dalsgaard C-J, Cuello AC (1984c) Invasion of lumbosacral ventral roots and spinal pia mater by substance P-immunoreactive axons after sciatic nerve lesion in kittens. Brain Res 307 : 351–354

Risling M, Dalsgaard C-J, Terenius L (1985a) Neuropeptide Y-like immunoreactivity in the lumbosacral pia mater in normal cats and after sciatic neuroma formation. Brain Res 358 : 372–375

RISLING M, HILDEBRAND C, UHLER G (1985b) Presence of unmyelinated axons in the spinal root of the feline accessory nerve. Brain Res 342 : 374–378

RISLING M, FRIED K, HILDEBRAND C, CUKIERMAN A (1986) Unmyelinated axons in the feline trigeminal root. Anat Rec 214 : 198–203

SHERRINGTON CS (1894) On the anatomical constitution of nerves of skeletal muscles; with remarks on recurrent fibres in the ventral spinal nerve-root. J Physiol (Lond) 17 : 211–258

STEVENS RT, HODGE CJ, APKARIAN AV (1983) Catecholamine varicosities in cat dorsal root ganglion and spinal ventral roots. Brain Res 261 : 151–154

STÖHR P (1922) Über die Innervation der Pia mater und des Plexus chorioideus des Menschen. Z Anat Entwicklungsgesch 63 : 562–607

VERGARA I, OBERPAUR B, ALVAREZ J (1986) Ventral root nonmedullated fibers: Proportion, calibers and microtubular content. J Comp Neurol 248 : 550–554

WADELL WR, BRADSHAW RA, GOLDSTEIN MN, KIRSCH WM (1972) Production of human nerve-growth factor in a patient with a liposarcoma. Lancet 1 : 1365–1367

WHITE JC, SWEET WH (1955) Pain – its mechanisms and neurosurgical control. Thomas, Springfield

YOUNG RF (1978) Unmyelinated fibers in the trigeminal motor root. Possible relationship to the results of trigeminal rhizotomy. J Neurosurg 49 : 538–543

5 The Location of Unmyelinated Primary Afferent Fibers in Spinal White Matter

R. E. Coggeshall and K. Chung

Introduction

This symposium is concerned with the role of fine afferent nerve fibers in somatovisceral sensation. The location of these fibers in the spinal white matter as they carry sensory information toward central synaptic areas is of obvious importance in this regard. A key method for determining these pathways has been to trace these fibers from the dorsal root, where they are gathered into a single anatomical structure, to their destinations in the gray matter of the spinal cord or in certain nuclei in the brain stem (e.g., Ramon y Cajal 1909). From this work comes the commonly accepted generalization that the large or coarse myelinated primary afferent fibers enter the dorsal funiculus, whereas the fine myelinated and unmyelinated primary afferent fibers enter the dorsolateral fasciculus or tract of Lissauer (Ramon y Cajal 1909). A possible difficulty with this generalization is that the fine fibers, the unmyelinated fibers in particular, are beyond the resolution of the light microscope, which was the major morphological tool used when the primary afferent pathways were first described. In addition, the death of fine fibers, particularly unmyelinated fibers, leaves relatively little debris, so techniques based on recognizing degenerating myelin or axoplasm are not very useful for these axons. Thus it seemed desirable to reexamine the white matter of the spinal cord with the electron microscope to see whether these regions of the central nervous system contain a significant number of previously unrecognized unmyelinated axons. To our surprise, at least for sacral segments in the rat and cat, the data indicated that there are large numbers of unmyelinated axons in the white matter (Chung et al. 1979, 1985; Langford and Coggeshall 1981; Chung and Coggeshall 1983). The next obvious question was whether any of these unmyelinated fibers are primary afferents. One way to determine this is to cut one or several consecutive dorsal roots and see if this results in the death of axons on the operated side. The purpose of the present communication is to describe the results of experiments where this was done. The data indicate that unmyelinated primary afferent axons are more widely distributed in spinal white matter than was previously recognized.

Materials and Methods

Adult cats or rats of either sex were used. Anesthesia was with sodium pentobarbital (Nembutal 40 mg/kg). When anesthesia was deep, 5–8 consecutive dorsal roots (usually L6–Caudal 2 in the cat and L6–Caudal 3 in the rat) were cut midway between cord and dorsal root ganglion. In all cases recovery was uneventful and there were no signs of discomfort such as biting or scratching the denervated area. After 1 week the animals were reanesthetized as above. When anesthesia was deep, the animals were perfused and sections were embedded for electron microscopy as detailed in various publications (Chung et al. 1979; Chung and Coggeshall 1979, 1985). Myelinated and unmyelinated axons were counted in the three major funiculi (dorsal, lateral, and ventral) and in the smaller tract of Lissauer in the S2 segments on both the operated and unoperated sides. All axons were counted.

The two critical areas of spinal cord for this study are the dorsal and dorsolateral funiculi. The dorsal funiculi are clearly bounded, so that there is no question as to the areas to count. The dorsolateral funiculi are more difficult. The dorsal, medial and lateral boundaries (the tract of Lissauer, dorsal horn, and pial surface of the cord) are clear, but the ventral border does not have a normal anatomical landmark. To get a reproducible ventral border, therefore, we drew a line directly laterally from the curve in the gray matter that indicated the junction of the dorsal and ventral horns. This gave a relatively clear and repeatable ventral boundary of the dorsolateral funiculi on both the operated and normal sides of the animal.

Results

Light-microscopic examination of the S2 rat and cat spinal cord contralateral to the dorsal rhizotomies reveals normal-appearing dorsal and lateral funiculi, with the predominant cytologic features being large myelinated axons, glial nuclei, and blood vessels. Electron-microscopic examination reveals these structures with greater clarity. In addition, unmyelinated axons are seen in the interstices between the other elements (Fig. 1). Cross sections

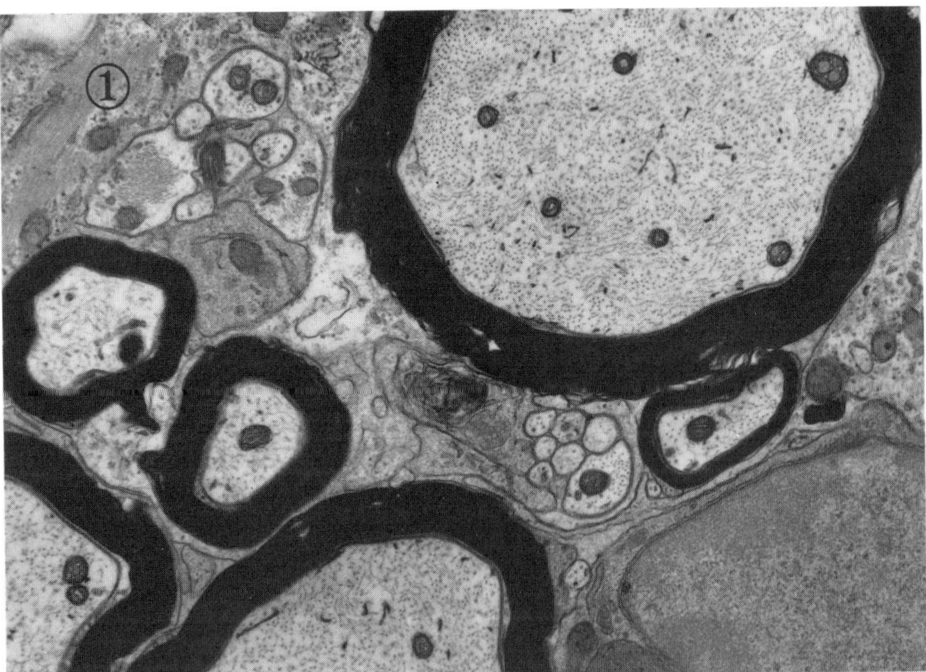

Fig. 1. A view of myelinated and unmyelinated axons in the rat dorsal funiculus. Note that the unmyelinated axons are round or oval on cross section and that their organelles consist of filaments, tubules, and mitochondria. Magnification x 22 000

Table 1. Number of axons in rat and cat dorsal funiculus and rat dorsolateral funiculus contralateral (normal side) and ipsilateral (operated side) to unilateral dorsal rhizotomies

	Normal side		Operated side	
	MY	UN	MY	UN
Rat dorsal funiculus n = 5	6750	3450	2050	2000
Rat dorsolateral funiculus n = 3	7800	50500	7900	37900
Cat dorsal funiculus n = 3	22500	8500	11500	3700

Note the reduction in number of axons on the operated side in all categories except myelinated axons in the dorsolateral funiculus

of these axons show roughly circular or oval profiles, but many indent each other. They range from 0.1 to 1.0 μm in diameter. The organelles in these axons consist of microtubules, neurofilaments, mitochondria, and occasional cisternae of the agranular endoplasmic reticulum. They can be distinguished from astrocytic processes because of the large number of closely packed glial filaments in the latter. The unmyelinated fibers, as noted earlier (Chung et al. 1985), are most numerous in the dorsal and lateral part of the lateral funiculus and the tract of Lissauer but are scattered throughout the white matter.

On the side of the animal where the rhizotomies were performed, large numbers of degenerated myelinated axons are seen in the dorsal funiculi. There are few degenerated myelinated axons elsewhere in the white matter. At the level of the electron microscope, the above can be seen with greater clarity. In addition, unmyelinated axons can also be seen, although there are fewer on the operated side in the dorsal and dorsolateral funiculi. Although histograms have not been prepared, it is apparent that the majority of large myelinated axons are removed by dorsal rhizotomy in the dorsal funiculi.

Counts of myelinated and unmyelinated axons in the dorsal and dorsolateral funiculi of the S2 segment of cat and rat spinal cord contralateral and ipsilateral to the dorsal rhizotomies are presented in Table 1. The figures have been rounded off to the nearest 50 for clarification. If the counts in Table 1 are expressed in percentages, the S2 dorsal funiculus on the operated side of the rat has 30 % as many myelinated and 58 % as many unmyelinated axons as on the normal side, the S2 dorsal funiculus of the cat has 51 % as many myelinated and 44 % as many unmyelinated axons as on the normal side, and the S2 dorsolateral funiculus of the rat has 101 % as many myelinated and 75 % as many unmyelinated axons as on the normal side. If one combines the counts with previously published data on the tract of Lissauer in the rat (Chung et al. 1979), there are approximately 1400 unmyelinated sensory axons in the posterior funiculus, 3200 unmyelinated sensory axons in the tract of Lissauer, and 12 600 unmyelinated sensory axons in the dorsolateral funiculus for the S2 segment of the rat. By comparison, there are 4700 myelinated dorsal root axons in the dorsal funiculus and 950 myelinated dorsal root axons in the tract of Lissauer for this same segment of rat spinal cord.

Discussion

The present study provides evidence that there are fewer unmyelinated fibers ipsilateral than there are contralateral to unilateral dorsal rhizotomies in the S2 dorsal and dorsolateral funiculi of rat and cat spinal cord. Since it is accepted that dorsal roots contain only processes of dorsal root ganglion cells, and that mammalian axons die when separated from their cell bodies (Waller 1852), we conclude that the discrepancy in axon numbers is due to the presence of significant numbers of unmyelinated dorsal root ganglion cell axons in the dorsal and dorsolateral funiculi. Since the processes of dorsal root ganglion cells are primary afferent axons, this presumably implies that unmyelinated primary afferent fibers are found in significant numbers in the dorsal and dorsolateral funiculi, as well as in the tract of Lissauer, where they are already known to exist.

Given that the above reasoning is accepted, previous data show that there are approximately 11 000 myelinated and 4600 unmyelinated primary afferent axons in the dorsal funiculi of the cat (Chung and Coggeshall 1985). Thus approximatelly 30% of primary afferent axons in cat S2 dorsal funiculus are unmyelinated. The functions of these unmyelinated sensory fibers are not yet known, but they should be remembered when the fibers of the dorsal column are discussed. We can make a more complete estimate of dorsal root axon numbers in the spinal cord of the rat. Our data indicate that there are approximately 4700 myelinated and 1400 unmyelinated dorsal root axons in the S2 dorsal funiculus, 12 600 unmyelinated dorsal root axons in the S2 dorsolateral funiculus, and 950 myelinated and 3200 unmyelinated dorsal root axons in the S2 tract of Lissauer (Chung et al. 1979). The conclusions are that for the white matter of the S2 segment of rat spinal cord (1) there are approximately 3 times as many unmyelinated as myelinated sensory axons, (2) the majority of unmyelinated sensory axons and the largest total numbers of sensory axons are in the dorsolateral funiculus, and (3) there are a significant number of unmyelinated sensory axons in the dorsal funiculus. These last two conclusions are relatively unexpected.

Before proceeding to brief speculations about function related to the presence of unmyelinated primary afferent fibers in the dorsal and dorsolateral funiculi, it is worthwhile considering whether the above conclusions are correct. Possible difficulties are (1) that we misidentified the fine fibers, so the counts are not accurate, and (2) that we infarcted the dorsal horn and killed some intrinsic neurons when we cut the roots and that the observed decrease in axons reflects this rather than loss of sensory axons. As to the question of identifying the fibers, the criteria for identifying unmyelinated axons are fairly clear (Peters et al. 1976), and the only likely candidates for confusion among non-neural cells are astrocyte processes. These, however, are generally larger than unmyelinated axons, do not by and large travel in a strictly craniocaudal direction, and contain large quantities of glial filaments, so the distinction is not difficult. Furthermore, a significant number of the presumptive axons disappear following dorsal rhizotomy. Dendrites from dorsal horn neurons also enter the white matter of the dorsal and dorsolateral funiculi (Lima and Coimbra 1986; Meyers and Snow 1982; Sedivec et al. 1986). These might be confused with axons, but are larger, do not usually run in a strictly craniocaudal direction, and have synaptic endings on them, and thus should not be a significant source of confusion. As to the possibility of infarction of the dorsal horn caused by dorsal rhizotomies, there are no histological signs of damage except for the death of myelinated and unmyelinated axons and the glial reactions to this, neurons are not lost in the dorsal horn (Coggeshall et al. 1981), and there are no signs of chromatolysis. For these reasons we do not consider that an interference with blood supply influences our results. We feel our counts are correct and reflect loss of axons caused by severance of the dorsal root.

One disturbing feature of our conclusions, however, is that there is as yet little corroborating evidence for fine sensory axons in either the dorsal or dorsolateral funiculi. It is true that Ranson (1913) mentioned that some sensory axons could be found lateral to the tract of Lissauer, but there seem to be no reports of labeling of fine sensory axons in this location after retrograde transport of such markers as HRP or after immunocytochemical localizations. This may, of course, be a result of the fact that they have not been searched for, but until such corroborative evidence becomes available, our conclusions must remain somewhat tentative.

Finally, if we assume that the loss of axons described above does indicate large numbers of unmyelinated sensory axons in the dorsal and dorsolateral funiculi, then what could their functions be? We do not have a specific answer, but one possibility is that there is no areal specialization and that they represent the same type of fibers as seen in the dorsal root and tract of Lissauer. Another possibility, however, is that they are specialized and that different groups of these fibers carry different kinds of information. Perhaps the major point to make at present is that the very large concentration of axons in the dorsolateral funiculus might be remembered when evaluating surgical procedures for the relief of pain that involve selective damage in these areas (e.g., Ranson and von Hess 1916).

Acknowledgements. This work was supported by NIH grants NS 10161 and NS 17039, the Texas Neurofibromatosis Foundation, and the Muscular Dystrophy Association of America.

References

Chung K, Coggeshall RE (1979) Primary afferent axons in the tract of Lissauer in the cat. J Comp Neurol 186:451–463

Chung K, Coggeshall RE (1983) Numbers of axons in the lateral and ventral funiculi of rat sacral spinal cord. J Comp Neurol 214:72–78

Chung K, Coggeshall RE (1985) Unmyelinated primary afferent fibers in dorsal funiculi of cat sacral spinal cord. J Comp Neurol 238:365–369

Chung K, Langford LA, Applebaum AE, Coggeshall RE (1979) Primary afferent fibers in the tract of Lissauer in the rat. J Comp Neurol 184:587–598

Chung K, Sharma J, Coggeshall RE (1985) Numbers of myelinated and unmyelinated axons in the dorsal, lateral, and ventral funiculi of the white matter of the S2 segment of cat spinal cord. J Comp Neurol 234:117–121

Coggeshall RE, Chung K, Chung JM, Langford LA (1981) Primary afferent axons in the tract of Lissauer in the monkey. J Comp Neurol 196:431–442

Langford LA, Coggeshall RE (1981) Unmyelinated axons in the posterior funiculi. Science 211:176–177

Lima D, Coimbra A (1986) A Golgi study of the neuronal population of the marginal zone (lamina I) of the rat spinal cord. J Comp Neurol 244:53–71

Meyers DER, Snow, PJ (1982) The morphology of physiologically identified deep spinothalamic tract cells in the lumbar spinal cord of the cat. J Physiol (Lond) 329:373–388

Peters A, Palay SL, Webster HdeF (1976) The fine structure of the nervous system. Saunders, Philadelphia

Ramon y Cajal S (1909) Histologie du système nerveux de l'homme et des vertébrés. Maloine, Paris

Ranson SW (1913) The course within the spinal cord of the non-medullated fibers in the dorsal roots. A study of Lissauer's tract in the cat. J Comp Neurol 23:250–281

Ranson SW, von Hess CL (1916) The conduction within the spinal cord of the afferent impulses producing pain and the vasomotor reflexes. Am J Physiol 38:128–152

Sedivec MJ, Copowski JJ, Mendell LM (1986) Morphology of HRP-injected spinocervical tract neurons: effect of dorsal rhizotomy. J Neurosci 6:661–672

Waller A (1852) A new method for the study of the nervous system. Lond J Med 4:609–625

6 The Functional Development of C Fibers and Their Central Connections

M. Fitzgerald

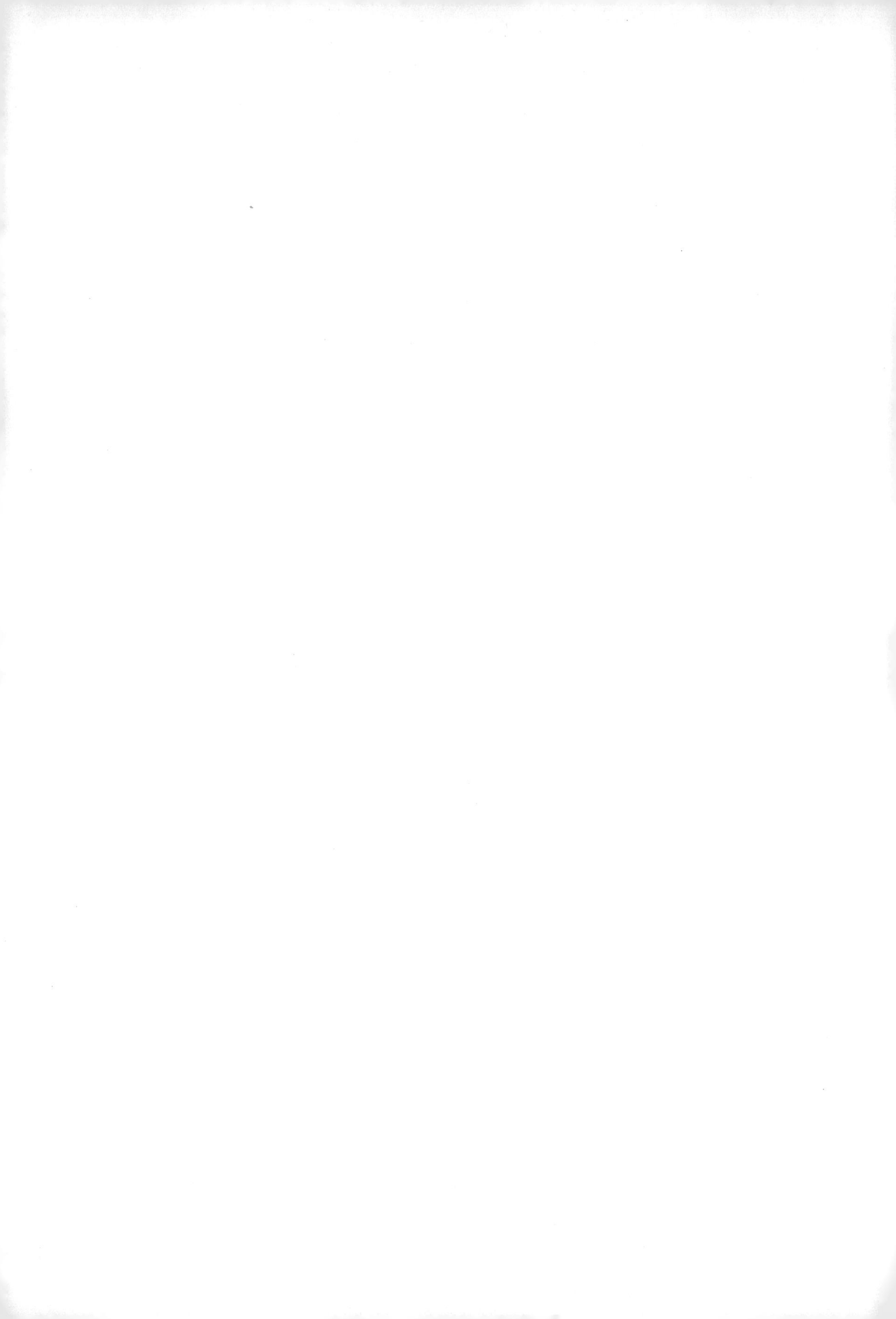

The special fascination that unmyelinated C sensory afferents hold for somatosensory physiologists is evident from the chapters in this book. While more is discovered about the roles and properties of C fibers in the adult nervous system, one aspect of these afferents has remained unexamined; their development and their functional role in the immature somatosensory system. This chapter will report on our investigations into this problem.

Development of Peripheral C Fiber Nociceptors

Conduction Velocities

Peripheral nerve does not begin to myelinate until after birth in the rat, so the separation of developing C fibers by conduction velocity is not possible. Figure 1 shows that up until postnatal day (PD) 3, all primary afferents conduct at less than 1.0 $m.s^{-1}$, but that beginning on day 1 and apparent by day 3, a bimodal distribution of conduction velocities emerges, apparently representing early myelinating A and remaining C fiber groups. The velocity of the fast group of afferents then increases considerably with age, while a slowly conducting group remains at less than 1.0 $m.s^{-1}$ (Fitzgerald 1986).

Physiological Properties

Despite uniform conduction velocities, polymodal nociceptors can be isolated as a functional group in hindlimb skin from the day of birth. Strikingly, their receptor properties are exactly as found in the adult. They respond to high-intensity mechanical stimulation ($>$ 0.3 g), noxious heating of the skin and application of noxious chemicals, and their receptive fields are small. Repeated stimulation causes a slow build-up of background firing to develop. There is no obvious postnatal alteration in these properties. Examples are shown in Fig. 2. This is in marked contrast to low-threshold mechanoreceptors and other receptor types destined to have A afferent fibers (Fitzgerald 1986).

Prenatal Development

Clearly, then, C fiber polymodal nociceptors develop as an afferent subgroup prenatally. Dorsal root ganglion (DRG) cells are born over embryonic days (ED) 12–15 (Altman and Bayer 1984) and peripheral sensory fibers grow out into the limb bud on ED 14. Therefore, potentially, these and other receptor types may be identifiable from the time they make contact with the skin. To investigate this, "in vivo" recordings have begun in the DRG of foetal rats over ED 17–21 (birth). The foetuses are removed from the uterus but kept in contact with the maternal circulation through the umbilical cord (Fitzgerald, in preparation). In 31 single afferents recorded on ED 18–19, over 20 % have properties that resemble C fiber polymodal nociceptors, with slowly adapting responses to pinching and (where tested) heating and mustard oil application. Background firing was a prominent feature of these units.

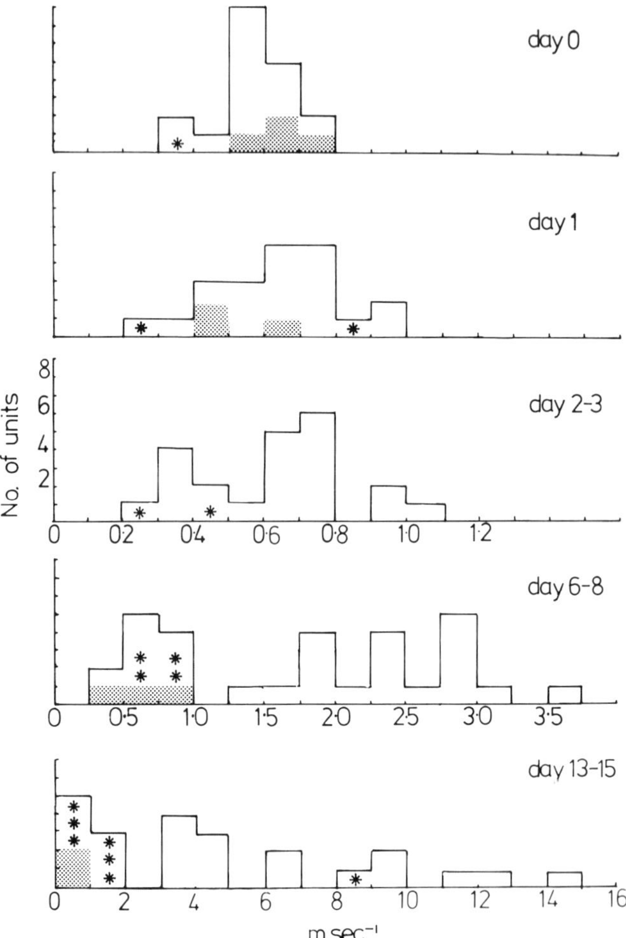

Fig. 1. The distribution of conduction velocities of primary afferent units recorded from the L4 dorsal root ganglion using tungsten microelectrodes on postnatal days 0, 1, 2–3, 6–8, 13–15. Note the change of scale with increasing age. The shaded areas represent polymodal nociceptor units and the stars represent high-threshold mechanoreceptor (HTM) units that did not respond to heating or chemical stimulation of the skin. The majority of HTM units will have small myelinated Aδ fibers in the adult. Anesthesia was lg/kg urethane i.p. For further details see text and Fitzgerald (1987)

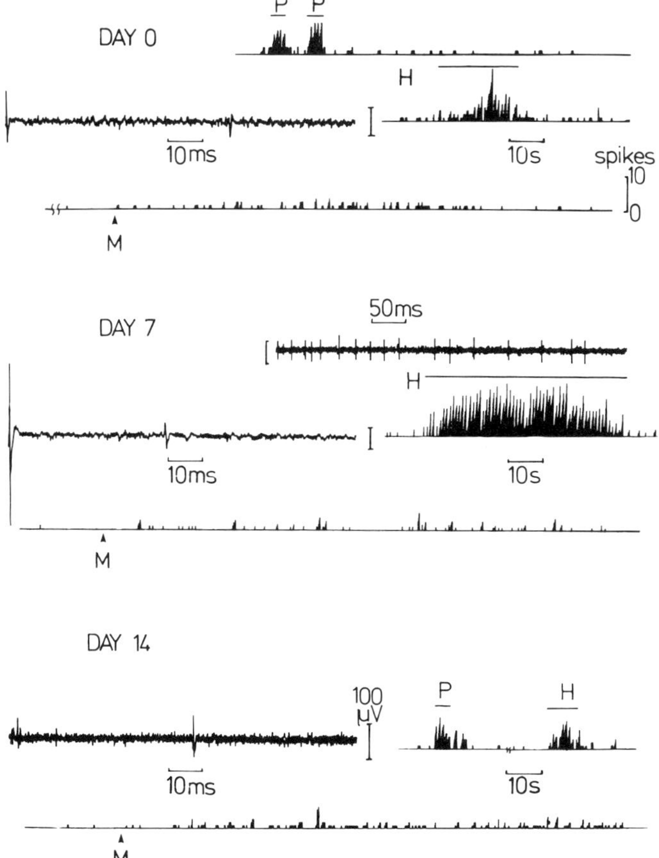

Fig. 2. Typical responses of polymodal nociceptors recorded on day 0, day 7 and day 14. For each unit there is a raw trace on the left which shows the evoked action potential from electrical stimulation of the receptive field. Scale: 100 μV. For each unit there are also examples of their responses to nocious skin stimulation. Day 0: The ratemeter records show the pattern and frequency of the evoked response to pinching (P), heating to 50 °C (H) and applcation of mustard oil (M) to the receptive field. Day 7: Ratemeter records show the evoked response to heating and mustard oil and the raw trace on the top right is a sample of the firing pattern during the displayed heating stimulus. Day 14 : the ratemeter records of pinch, heat and mustard oil evoked responses show their similarity to the polymodal nociceptor recorded on day 0. (From Fitzgerald 1987)

Neurogenic Oedema

Neurogenic oedema in neonatal rat pups was measured following intravenous injection of Evans blue dye into urethane-anaesthetized rat pups. The concentration of Evans blue dye extracted from the hindfoot skin following application of mustard oil or sciatic nerve stimulation (5 mA, 500 μs, 0.5 Hz for 10 min) was measured. No neurogenic oedema could be measured until postnatal day 11 (Fitzgerald and Gibson 1984). This was not due to lack of "leakiness" of neonatal blood vessels. On the contrary, nonspecific Evans blue dye release is more easily evoked by tissue damage in neonates than in the adult.

Peptide and FRAP Content

Substance P (SP) can be observed in small DRG cells on ED 17 (Semba et al. 1982) and FRAP (fluoride resistant acid phosphatase) much earlier on ED 15, almost as soon as they are born (Schoenen 1978). In postnatal studies, we have observed SP and FRAP in peripheral nerve and skin on PD 1 (Fitzgerald and Gibson 1984) and it may well be in these regions before then.

Development of C Fiber Connections in the Dorsal Horn

The Growth of C Fibers into the Dorsal Horn

Early silver stains (Windle and Baxter 1936) and more recent horseradish peroxidase (HRP) tracer studies (Smith 1983) have demonstrated that the lumbar dorsal roots first penetrate the cord at ED 16 and the grey matter a day later on ED 17.

To find when C fibers grow into the cord we have exploited the preferential labelling of C fibers that occurs when WGA-HRP (wheatgerm agglutinin-horseradish peroxidase) is applied to a peripheral nerve and retrogradely transported transganglionically to central terminals in the spinal cord (Robertson and Grant 1985). Foetuses aged ED 18, 19 and 20 were briefly exposed under barbiturate anesthesia, and 7% WGA-HRP dissolved in Tween 80 was injected into one sciatic nerve. The foetuses were then replaced in the uterus and allowed to recover. The foetal cords were removed and histologically processed using the TMB staining procedure 24 h later. In the case of injections on ED 20, the pups were born naturally in this intervening period. The results show that C fibers grow in through the dorsal roots and penetrate the superficial dorsal horn on ED 19. By ED 21/PD 0 they have penetrated the whole depth of substantia gelatinosa (SG) but density of terminals is still sparse (Fitzgerald 1987). Postnatal WGA-HRP labelling shows that by PD 1 the density of C fiber terminals has greatly increased and at PD 2 it resembles that in the adult.

Specificity of C Fiber Connections

In the adult, the central terminals of each peripheral nerve have a precise field of termination in the dorsal horn with no overlap with terminal feids of other afferents (Swett and Woolf 1985). Anatomical mapping of C fiber terminals of specific nerves in the neonatal dorsal horn has demonstrated that this somatotopy is present from the time C fibers first grow into the cord (Fitzgerald and Swett 1983). The same specificity of connections is also demonstrated in afferents growing into deep dorsal horn and ventral horn (Smith 1983). This precision can be disrupted, however, if a peripheral nerve is sectioned in the early neonatal period (Fitzgerald 1985b).

Peptides and FRAP in Central C Fiber Terminals

Substance P and FRAP in C fiber terminals in the dorsal horn develop quite differently from one another. SP is apparently already in the growing C fiber dorsal roots as they enter the spinal cord, since it can be observed in the roots and dorsolateral white matter on ED 20 (Semba et al. 1982), although the amount of SP in the terminals in SG is very sparse on PD 1 (Fitzgerald and Gibson 1984) and does not reach adult density until the 2nd postnatal week. FRAP, on the other hand, is not present in the spinal cord at all until 12 h after birth and then makes its first appearance as a complete band in lamina II, albeit a low-intensity one, rather than gradually growing in dorsoventrally (Fitzgerald and Gibson 1984). The full density of FRAP staining is not observed until PD 5–6. These differences may reflect differential central growth of SP- and FRAP-containing C fiber afferents, but more likely reflects the different transport and metabolism of the peptides and FRAP.

The Development of C Fiber Evoked Activity in the Spinal Cord

Activity Evoked by Electrical Stimulation of the Skin

Because of the slow conduction in all afferents in the newborn rat it is not possible to pick out a high-threshold long-latency burst of evoked activity which can be unequivocally attributed to C fibers and distinguished from low-threshold short-latency A fiber evoked activity. Nevertheless, when recording from cells in SG it was possible from PD 1 to evoke one spike at a mean latency of 41 ± 3 ms and a second higher threshold one at 55 ± 4 ms (Fitzge-

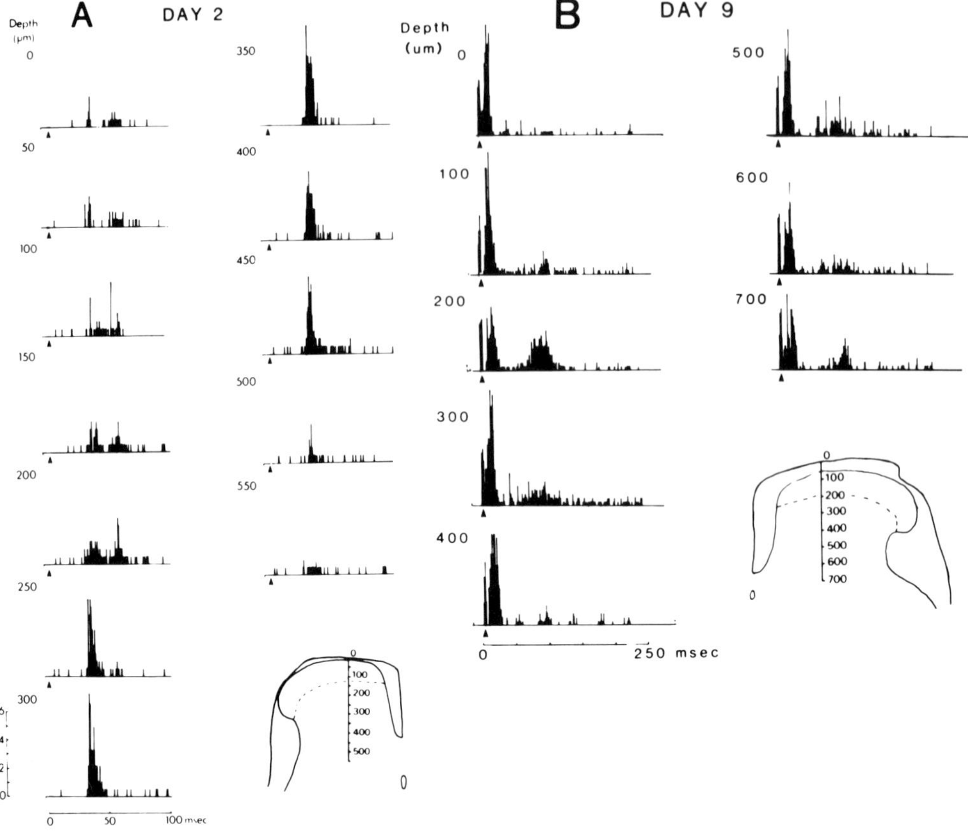

Fig. 3 A, B. Depth profiles of dorsal horn multiunit activity evoked by electrical stimulation of the hind-foot skin recording at 50- or 100 μm steps through the L4 dorsal horn with a tungsten microelectrode. The responses are displayed as poststimulus time histograms, bin width 6.4 ms. Anesthesia was 1 g/kg urethane. A. On PD 2, the latency of the first evoked burst in the dorsal horn is very long at 25–30 ms. In the superficial dorsal horn two peaks are observed, but in the deep laminae only the first, A fiber-like response is evoked. B. On PD 9 there is a considerable decrease in latency of the first evoked burst. Now in both superficial and deep laminae there are two peaks, an early A fiber-like response and a later C fiber-like response

rald 1985a). With increasing age, the first response consisted of more spikes and was evoked at much shorter latencies (14 ± 3 ms on PD 7) while the second response remained at long latencies (60 ± 1.5 ms on PD 7). It seems reasonable to suppose that in the newborn cord, the second long latency response is evoked at least in part by C fibers, but this is not necessarily so. The situation is completely different for cells recorded deep in the dorsal horn in laminae III–VI. These cells only ever showed an early short-latency response (shorter than in SG, at 35 ± 1 ms on PD 1 and 10 ± 0.5 ms on PD 7) up until PD 7. After this time, long-latency, C fiber evoked responses at latencies of 75 ms were observed. This difference in the development of electrically evoked activity in superficial and deep laminae of the dorsal horn is illustrated in Fig. 3.

Activity Evoked by Natural Skin Stimulation

The receptive field properties were mapped using light brushing, touching and pinching of the skin (Fitzgerald 1985a). In the immediate postnatal period over 50 % of all dorsal horn cells respond only to high-intensity mechanical stimuli (75 % in SG) although the numbers of cells responding to low-intensity mechanical stimulation of the skin or to a combination of both increases with age. The requirement for intense stimulation to evoke a response is likely to reflect the weak synaptic linkage between primary afferents and dorsal horn cells rather than any differential capacity of low- and high-threshold afferents to excite cells. Several properties of dorsal horn cells differ considerably from those in the adult. Mean receptive fields are large in the neonate. The mean area was 14.2 % of total hindlimb area at birth, whereas by PD 15 it was 3.6 % (Fig. 4). It is possible to find cells with small receptive fields on PD 0–1, but many cover several nerve territories and dermatomes. Nevertheless their receptive fields have clear boundaries, and somatotopic organization within the dorsal horn was clear. A further striking feature of neonatal dorsal horn cells is that the initial low-frequency response to skin stimulation was followed, in 37 % of cases, by long periods of afterdischarge lasting 30–60 s. In half these cells, the frequency of firing in the afterdischarge was equal to or greater than that of the initial response. It declined with age, and by PD 15, 28 % of cells still showed some kind of afterdischarge but only for up to 7 s and much lower frequencies than the initial responses.

The Development of C Fiber Evoked Reflexes

Pinching or heating the skin of the hindlimb of a newborn rat results in a flexion reflex which is exaggerated compared to that in the adult (Fitzgerald and Gibson 1984). Repeated stimuli result in "wind-up" of the reflex, chronic flexion and recruitment of other parts of the body in the response. This is not an effect attributable to the afferent input (Fitzgerald 1986) or to the muscle, since it is observed when recorded from flexor motor axons. The responses become greatly attenuated by the end of the 1st postnatal week and are similar to those in the adult by PD 14. These exaggerated reflexes may be a reflection of the unusual dorsal horn properties described above and result from the same underlying mechanisms.

Despite the exaggerated nature of the flexion reflex no response at all can be evoked by skin application of mustard oil, a specific C fiber chemical stimulus, until PD 10 (Fig. 5). The onset of the chemically-evoked reflex exactly parallels the development of neurogenic oedema (discussed in the subsection "Neurogenic Oedema" above). Cutaneous C fibers respond to mustard oil from birth (Fitzgerald 1986), and so the answer must lie in the central connections.

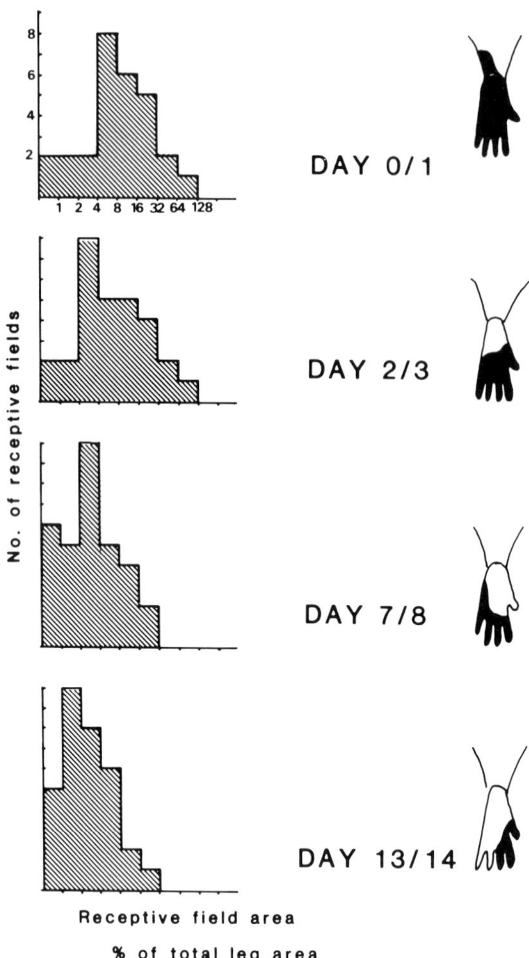

Fig. 4. Histograms of the distribution of receptive field areas of dorsal horn cells in neonatal spinal cord at various postnatal ages with typical fields illustrated beside them. Recordings were made under the same conditions as in Fig. 3. The receptive field areas are expressed as a percentage of total hindlimb skin area. Note the logarithmic scale. (From Fitzgerald 1985a)

Conclusions

The various properties of C fiber polymodal nociceptors develop over different time periods. Histochemical differentiation occurs early, with SP and FRAP expression occurring well before birth. The physiological receptor properties of mechanosensitivity, thermosensitivity and chemosensitivity are fully developed at birth, and foetal recordings indicate that these receptors are functional and very active in the prenatal period. In contrast to this, the ability of C fibers to produce neurogenic oedema develops remarkably late, in the 2nd post-

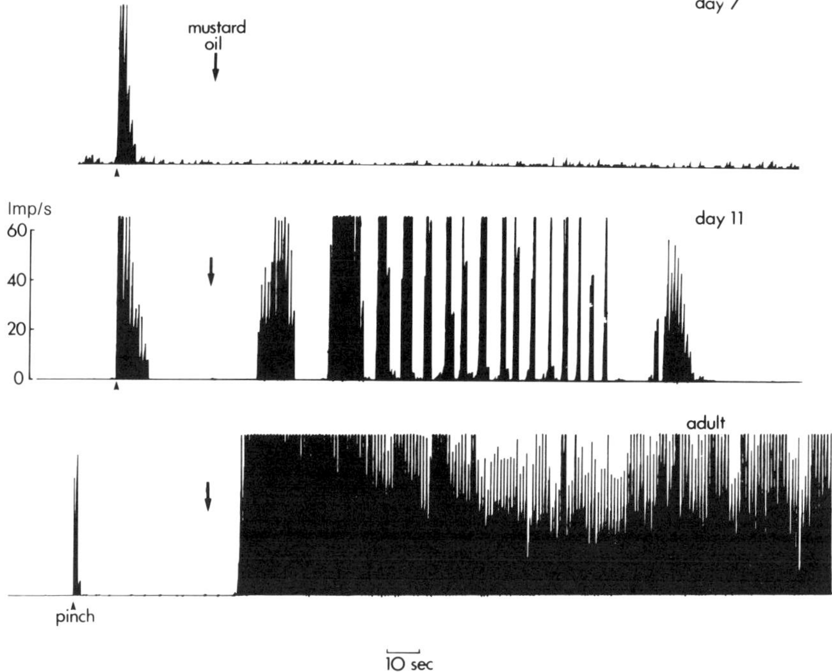

Fig. 5. Application of the irritant chemical mustard oil to skin of the lateral foot produces a profound and long reflex-withdrawal response in the adult rat lightly anesthetized with urethane 1g/kg). The bottom trace illustrates this from ratemeter records of the multiunit hamstring muscle EMG (bin size 1 s). The response lasts for up to 10 min. On the top trace it can be seen that the 7-day-old rat pup at the same anesthetic dose shows no response at all to application of mustard oil. Sensitivity begins on PD 10–11 (middle trace) and at this stage is weak, short-lived and consists of rhythmic bursts of activity. (From Fitzgerald and Gibson 1984)

natal week. This may reflect a slow maturation of the levels of the chemical mediator involved or its pharmacological receptors.

The first C fibers penetrate the lumbar dorsal horn 48 h before birth, some 3 days later than future A fibers (Fitzgerald 1987). The terminals continue to grow and elaborate over the early postnatal periods. Their growth is precise, restricted to SG and somatotopically specific. C fibers from a particular peripheral nerve grow into a particular part of the cord.

Dorsal horn cells in the superficial laminae (SG) respond to both fast-conducting and slowly conducting afferents from PD 0, whereas cells in deeper laminae only respond to fast A fiber type volleys until PD 7–8. After this time, the second late C fiber evoked response slowly emerges in the deep dorsal horn. This may be a result of slow maturation of interneuronal connections responsible for relaying C fiber input to deeper laminae or perhaps insufficient dendritic growth in deep dorsal horn cells. There is anatomical evidence for postnatal maturation of SG interneurones as opposed to prenatal maturation of projection cells (Bicknell and Beal 1984).

Over this period, receptive fields slowly shrink and the long afterdischarges observed in newborn cells are reduced. This change in dorsal horn cell properties may also be the result of immature interneuronal function involved in local or descending controls (Fitzgerald and Koltzenberg 1986). Alternatively, they may reflect the maturation of the intrinsic membrane properties of dorsal horn neurones.

To what extent C fiber terminals growing into SG and forming new connections over the early postnatal period influence these events is not yet clear. Destruction of C fibers with neonatal capsaicin results in adult dorsal horn cells with unusually large receptive fields (Wall et al. 1982) and reduced descending inhibition (Cervero and Plenderleith 1985). Both these effects point to an arrest of normal maturation of dorsal horn circuitry in the absence of C fiber input.

Chemically evoked reflexes, tested with the specific C fiber irritant, mustard oil, develop long after noxious thermal and mechanically evoked reflexes. This could simply be due to the fact that C fibers do not activate the central reflex pathways until this time, either through immature connections or through lack of neurotransmitter. Another possibility is that the central processing of chemoreceptive information requires its own transmitter or central circuitry. The factor involved could be the same one that produces neurogenic oedema in the periphery. There is some evidence for this in the adult. Blockade of axon transport in C fibers with vinblastine leaves noxious mechanical and thermal reflexes intact while blocking chemically evoked reflexes and neurogenic oedema (Fitzgerald et al. 1984).

The first postnatal weeks are a time of great importance in the maturation of C fibers and their central connections. We have examined the development of their peripheral receptor properties, their growth into the dorsal horn, their neurochemistry, their first functional connections with dorsal horn cells and the reflexes they evoke. Much can be learnt about the role of C fibers in development and also in the adult from such studies.

References

Altman J, Bayer SA (1984) The development of the rat spinal cord. Adv Anat Embryol Cell Biol 85 : 1-166

Bicknell HR, Beal JA (1984) Axonal and dendritic development of substantia gelatinosa neurons in the lumbosacral spinal cord of the rat. J Comp Neurol 226 : 508–522

Cervero F, Plenderleith MB (1985) C fiber excitation and tonic descending inhibition of dorsal horn neurones in adult rats treated at birth with capsaicin. J Physiol (Lond) 365 : 223–237

Fitzgerald M (1985a) The postnatal development of cutaneous afferent input and receptive field organization in the rat dorsal horn. J Physiol (Lond) 364 : 1–8

Fitzgerald M (1985b) The sprouting of saphenous nerve terminals in the spinal cord following early postnatal sciatic nerve section in the rat. J Comp Neurol 240 : 407–413

Fitzgerald M (1987) Cutaneous primary afferent properties in the hindlimb of the neonatal rat. J Physiol (Lond) 383 : 79–92

Fitzgerald M (1987) The prenatal growth of fine diameter primary afferents into the rat spinal cord: a transganglionic tracer study. J Comp Neurol (in press)

FITZGERALD M, GIBSON S (1984) The postnatal physiological and neurochemical development of peripheral sensory C fibers. Neuroscience 13 : 933–944

FITZGERALD M, KOLTZENBERG M (1986) The functional development of descending inhibitory pathways in the dorsolateral funiculus of the newborn rat spinal cord. Dev Brain Res 24 : 261–270

FITZGERALD M, SWETT J (1983) The termination pattern of sciatic nerve afferents in the substantia gelatinosa of neonatal rats. Neurosci Lett 43 : 149–154

FITZGERALD M, WOOLF CJ, GIBSON SJ, MALLABURN PS (1984) Alterations in the structure, function and chemistry of C fibers following local application of vinblastine to the sciatic nerve of the rat. J Neurosci 4 : 430–441

ROBERTSON B, GRANT G (1985) A comparison between wheatgerm agglutinin and choleragenois-horseradish peroxidase as anterogradely transported markers in central branches of primary sensory neurones in the rat with some observations in the cat. Neuroscience 14 : 895–905

SCHOENEN J (1978) Histochemistry of developing rat spinal cord. Neuropathol Appl Neurobiol 4 : 37–46

SEMBA E, SHIOSAKA S, HARA Y, INAGAKI S, SAKANAKA M, TAKATSUKI K, KAWAI Y, TOHYAMA M (1982) Ontogeny of the peptidergic system in the rat spinal cord: immunohistochemical analysis. J Comp Neurol 208 : 54–66

SMITH CL (1983) The development and postnatal organization of primary afferent projections to the rat thoracic spinal cord. J Comp Neurol 220 : 29–43

SWETT JE, WOOLF CJ (1985) The somatotopic organization of primary afferent terminals in the superficial laminae of the dorsal horn of the rat spinal cord. J Comp Neurol 231 : 66–77

WALL PD, FITZGERALD M, NUSSBAUMER JC, VAN DER LOOS H, DEVOR M (1982) Somatotopic maps are disorganized in adult rodents treated with capsaicin as neonates. Nature 295 :691–693

WINDLE WF, BAXTER RE (1936) Development of reflex mechanisms in the spinal cord of albino rat embryos. Correlation between structure and function and comparisons with the cat and the chick. J Comp Neurol 63 : 189–209

7 Identification of C Fiber Primary Afferent Endings in the Substantia Gelatinosa of the Newborn Rat: An Electron-Microscopic Study

D. Pignatelli, A. Coimbra, and W. Zieglgänsberger

It is known that cutaneous unmyelinated (C fiber) primary afferents mainly terminate in the substantia gelatinosa (lamina II) of the spinal cord dorsal horn (Light and Perl 1979). In the adult rat, electron-microscopic (EM) cytochemical studies (Coimbra et al. 1974; Ribeiro-da-Silva et al. 1986) showed the inner region of lamina II (lamina IIi) to contain FRAP (fluoride-resistant acid phosphatase)-reactive dark scalloped central terminals of synaptic glomeruli in its dorsal part, while in the ventral part similar dark endings without FRAP occurred along with large clear central endings. Neonatal systemic administration of capsaicin resulted in the disappearance of all dark scalloped central endings of glomeruli in the adult animals and left the large clear central endings intact (Ribeiro-da-Silva and Coimbra 1984); thus the former, whether or not they contained FRAP, were thought to represent the terminations of nociceptive C fiber afferents in the substantia gelatinosa and the latter to be those of large myelinated fibers (Ribeiro-da-Silva and Coimbra 1984). The cellular population of the substantia gelatinosa is predominantly formed by interneurons containing synaptic transmitters and/or peptides (Hunt et al. 1981), which are thought to modulate nociceptive inputs through axoaxonic and dendroaxonic contacts in synaptic glomeruli (Ribeiro-da-Silva and Coimbra 1982). Curiously, the maturation of local interneurons and the arrival of C fiber afferents in the substantia gelatinosa occur during the early postnatal period. While second-order projection and propriospinal neurons develop their processes in the prenatal stage (Bicknell and Beal 1984), the more abundant intrinsic nonprojection neurons form their specific processes postnatally, which involves the transformation of early dendrites and the sprouting of an axon (Bicknell and Beal 1984). Fine primary afferent fibers have only been detected 24 h after parturition with HRP labelling (Smith 1983), although WGA-HRP labelling has recently identified them in the substantia gelatinosa just before birth (Fitzgerald, this volume). The FRAP band, which indicates the presence of the FRAP-reactive subpopulation of fine afferents (Ribeiro-da-Silva et al. 1986), only appears at postnatal day 1 (P1) and becomes distinct at P5–6 (Fitzgerald and Swett 1983; Mattio et al. 1981). The postnatal stage of development is thus an excellent model from which to investigate the establishment of connections between incoming C fiber afferents and gelatinosa cells, with the consequent onset of pain-modulation phenomena. However, synaptic glomeruli are rare in the newborn animal, so it is very difficult to recognize primary afferent endings with the EM. The aim of this work was to identify C fiber primary endings in the neonatal rat through their fine structural features and acute susceptibility to capsaicin administration (Jancsó et al. 1977).

Methods

Pregnant rats from the Sprague-Dawley-derived colony of the Gulbenkian Institute of Science, Oeiras, were used.

Morphological Studies of the Normal Spinal Cord. Pups were anesthetized with ether at postnatal days PO (day of birth), P1, P2, and P5 and perfused through the left ventricle with a mixture of 1% paraformaldehyde and 1% glutaraldehyde in 0.12 M phosphate buffer containing calcium chloride 0.02 mM. The cervical spinal cord segment between C4 and C6 was transversely sectioned at 50- and 100-µm intervals using a Vibratome (Lancer, St. Louis, U.S.A.). The 100-µm-thick sections were immersed in 1.5 % aqueous uranyl acetate for 45 min followed by 1 % OsO_4 for 2 h in the same buffer containing 0.02 mM $CaCl_2$ and embedded in Epon. The larger and smaller diameters of each synaptic vesicle were measured in the axon terminals and the mean value expressed as the synaptic vesicle diameter. Some

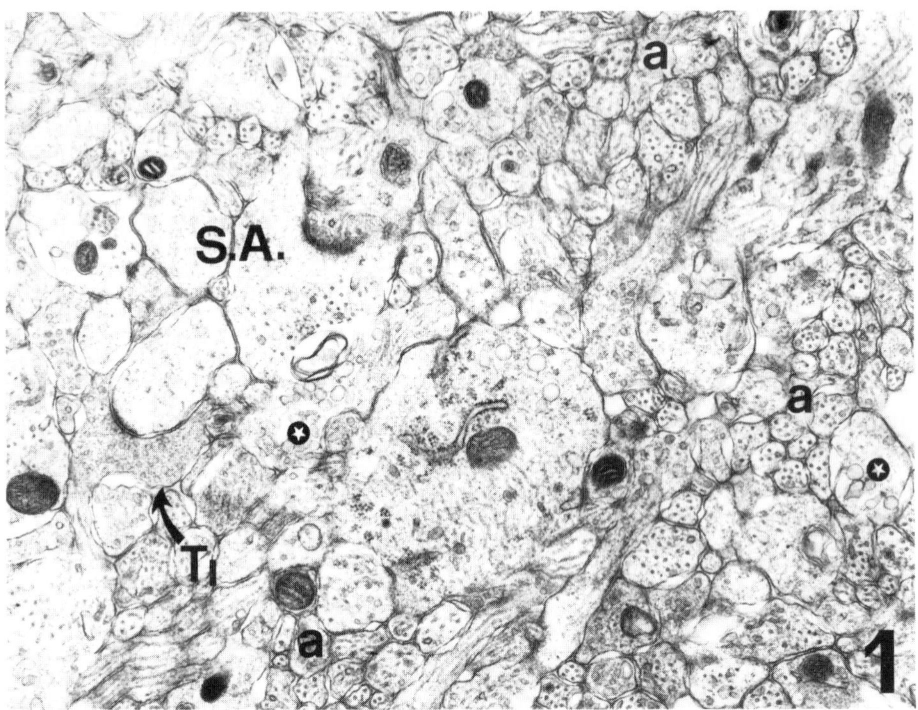

Fig. 1. Survey picture of the substantia gelatinosa neuropil in a P2 pup. Note the axon fields (a) and one synaptic area (S.A.) showing one small dark sinuous terminal (Tl). Dendritic profiles with addition vesicles (*) (Falls and Gobel 1979) are common. Magnification x 18 480

50-µm sections were stained with toluidine blue according to Rexed (Coimbra et al. 1986).

Study of the Effects of Capsaicin. Other pups were injected subcutaneously 24–48 h after parturition with 50 mg/kg capsaicin (Sigma Chemical Co.) and perfused 4 and 6 h later (four pups at each time). Two additional animals received 0.15 ml of vehicle (10 % Tween 80 and 10 % ethanol in 0.9 % saline) and, like those injected with capsaicin, were perfused and the spinal cords processed for Epon embedding.

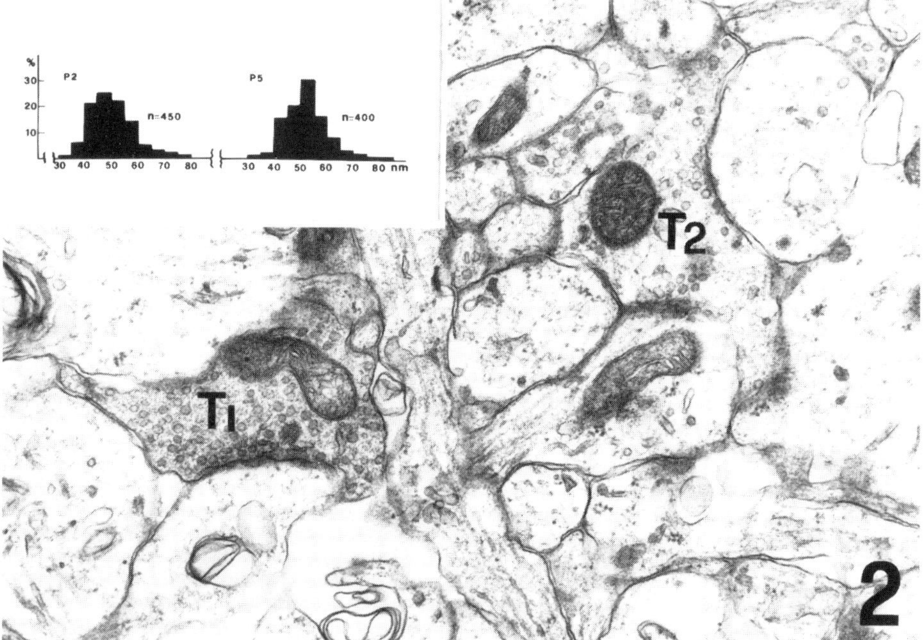

Fig. 2. At higher power at PO, one small dark sinuous terminal (T1) and one clear terminal (T2). Magnification x 23 760. In the inset, size-frequency diagrams of synaptic vesicle diameters in the small sinuous terminals at P2 and in the dark scalloped central endings at P5

Results

Morphological Observations in Normal Animals

Lamina II showed a similar ultrastructural appearance at PO through to P2. Throughout the lamina, the neuropil among the round perikarya showed groups of cross-sectioned small axons rich in neurotubules alternating with synaptic areas including profiles with synaptic vesicles and dendritic profiles (Fig. 1). Synaptic contacts in these areas were much less abundant than in the adult. Typical dark scalloped central terminals of glomeruli were absent, and instead, small dark sinuous terminals full of round or oval synaptic vesicles having one or two axodendritic synapses were frequent (Figs. 1, 2). These endings occurred in clusters and were interconnected by thin dark axons (Fig. 3). Synaptic vesicle diameters ranged from 30 to 80 nm, with the size frequency distribution peaking at 45–50 nm (Fig. 2, inset). In the ventral half of lamina IIi some nonsinuous, sometimes large, terminals occurred with light background cytoplasm, containing round vesicles which were less numerous than in the dark terminals (Fig. 2). These terminals were often presynaptic to two or three plain

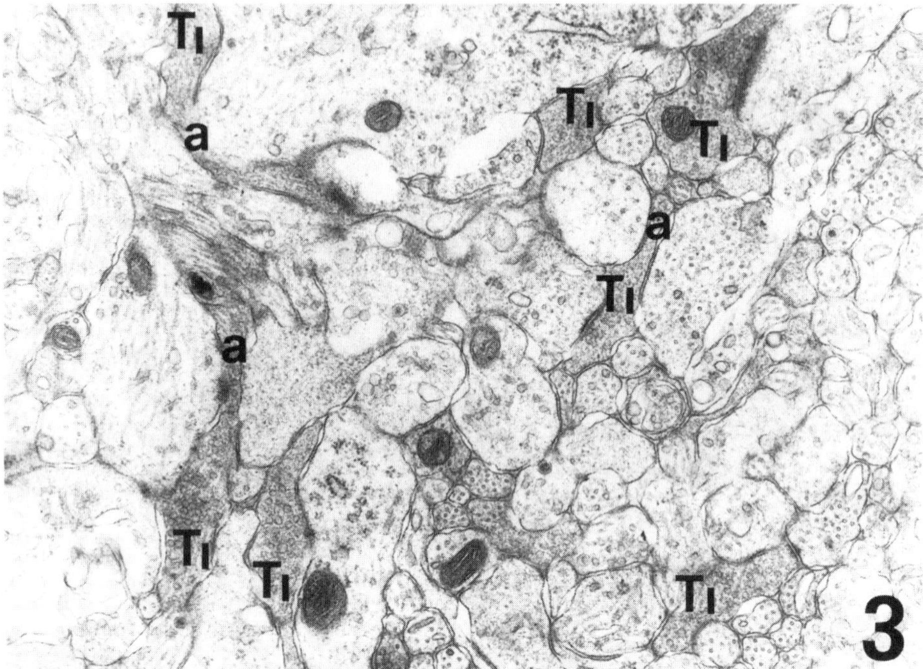

Fig. 3. A cluster of small sinuous terminals at P2 (T1) with the interconnecting dark axons (a). Magnification x 19 800

dendrites and to one dendrite with synaptic vesicles. Although these two types of presynaptic endings were the most numerous, other small clear profiles with small round vesicles clustered against the synaptic cleft were presynaptic to one dendritic profile. At day P5, some typical glomeruli were present in the synaptic areas, each centered by a dark scalloped central terminal (C_1 terminals) or by a large clear round terminal (C_2 terminals), either with or without neurofilaments (Ribeiro-da-Silva and Coimbra 1982). The size-frequency distribution of the synaptic vesicles in the dark scalloped central terminals at P5 was very similar to that of small sinuous terminals at P2 (Fig. 2, inset).

Effects of Capsaicin

The fine morphology of control animals injected with the vehicle did not differ from that in noninjected rats. After capsaicin administration, very dark, shrunken terminals occurred in clusters in the synaptic areas of lamina II (Fig. 4). At 4 h it was sometimes possible to recognize a few round synaptic vesicles in them, as well as one to two axodendritic synapses (Fig. 4, inset). The clear endings looked normal. Some dark degenerated endings were engulfed in glial cells (Fig. 4). Very few normal small sinuous endings were present at 4 and 6 h.

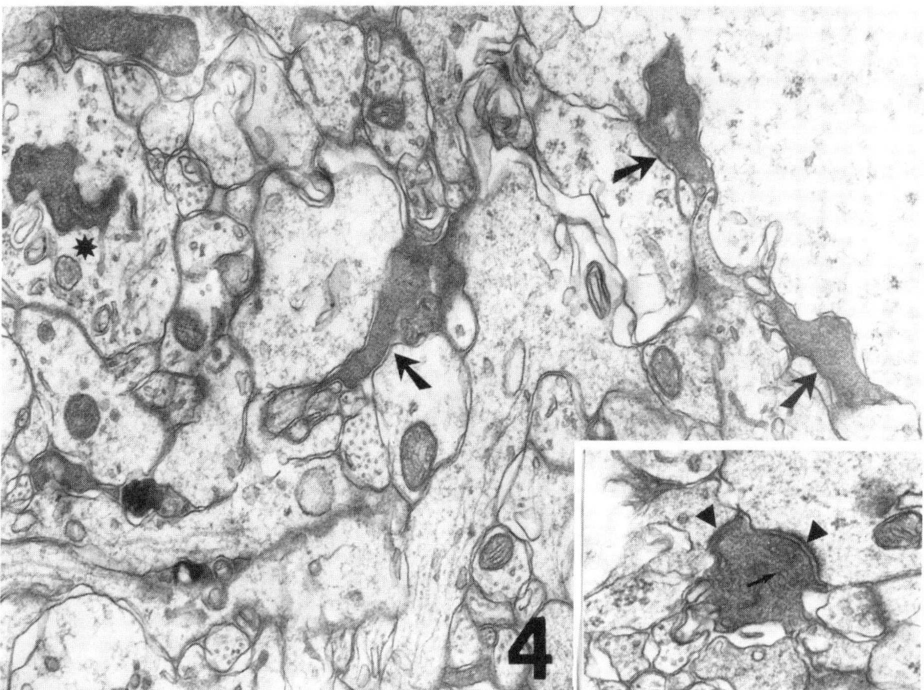

Fig. 4. Following a capsaicin injection (6 h), the small sinuous terminals are degenerated (arrows). One changed ending is phagocytosed by glia (*). Magnification x 23 760. In the inset, detail of a degenerated terminal at 4 h showing some synaptic vesicles (arrow) and two axodendritic synapses (arrowheads). Magnification x 31 680

Comments

These findings suggest that the nonglomerular small sinuous endings which occur throughout the substantia gelatinosa arise from C fiber primary afferents. First, they display great similarity regarding contour, background cytoplasm density, and size-frequency distribution of the synaptic vesicles with the dark scalloped central terminals of typical adult glomeruli which start to appear at P5. In the adult, these central terminals are mainly located in dorsal lamina II (Ribeiro-da-Silva and Coimbra 1982) where most HRP-labelled fine fibers are present (Light and Perl 1979). They were absent in rats that had received a neonatal systemic injection of capsaicin (Ribeiro-da-Silva and Coimbra 1984), which also destroys most unmyelinated dorsal root fibers (Nagy et al. 1981). Second, the small sinuous endings showed intense dark degeneration upon short-term capsaicin treatment. This conclusion was based on the fact that the degenerated profiles had the same location in the neuropil and the same synaptic contacts as the small sinuous endings of untreated animals, and furthermore also occurred in clusters. In the newborn rat, subcutaneous injections of the drug have previously been shown to provoke the acute appearance of degenerated terminals in the substantia gelatinosa (Jancsó et al. 1977; Nagy et al. 1980), as well as the degeneration of many unmyelinated fibers in dorsal roots (Jancsó et al. 1977). However, the normal appearance of the degenerated endings was not disclosed. It should be noted that we have recently observed a faint acid phosphatase reaction in the small sinuous endings of normal pups at day P2, which became strong and typically situated in the dark scalloped central terminals at day P5 (unpublished observations). Since the enzyme has been exclusively detected in these types of endings in the substantia gelatinosa of the adult rat (Ribeiro-da-Silva et al. 1986) which are presumed to represent the spinal cord projections of FRAP-positive dorsal root ganglion cells (Dodd et al. 1984; Nagy and Hunt 1982), it may be concluded that at least some of the endings studied here correspond to this population in newborn animals.

The exclusive axodendritic contacts of the small sinuous endings are suggestive of an excitatory role for these boutons on postsynaptic dendrites of second-order projection neurons, which are known to have developed their processes in the prenatal stage (Bicknell and Beal 1984). The appearance of the first synaptic glomeruli at day P5, in which dark scalloped central terminals may be postsynaptic to a postsynaptic dendrite, is highly suggestive of the establishment at this period of contacts with local interneurons which are undergoing their postnatal maturation (Bicknell and Beal 1984; Falls and Gobel 1979). Such presynaptic dendrites found in the first synaptic glomeruli of the rat at P5 may convey the first modulatory influences exerted by the developing interneurons on the incoming nociceptive afferents. It may be added that axoaxonic synapses were only observed in this type of glomeruli on day P15 (unpublished observations), which indicates the later establishment of inhibition of C fiber primary afferents by axons of cord cells and/or by descending fibers, as suggested by the onset of descending inhibition from the brain stem onto the dorsal horn at about the same age (Fitzgerald and Koltzenburg 1986).

Acknowledgements. This work was supported by a grant from the Stiftung Volkswagenwerk and by grant 48/85 from Oporto University.

References

Bicknell HR, Beal JA (1984) Axonal dendritic development of substantia gelatinosa neurons in the lumbosacral spinal cord of the rat. J Comp Neurol 226 : 508–522

Coimbra A, Sodré-Borges BP, Magalhães MM (1974) The substantia gelatinosa Rolandi of the rat. Fine structural cytochemistry (acid phosphatase) and changes after dorsal root section. J Neurocytol 3 : 199–217

Coimbra A, Ribeiro-da-Silva A, Pignatelli D (1986) Rexed's laminae and the acid phosphatase (FRAP)-band in the spinal cord superficial dorsal horn of the neonatal rat. Neurosci Lett 71 : 131–136

Dood J, Jahr CE, Jessel T (1984) Neurotransmitters and neuronal markers at sensory synapses in the dorsal horn. Adv Pain Res Ther 6 : 105–121

FALLS W, GOBEL S (1979) Golgi and EM studies of the formation of dendritic and axonal arbors: The interneurons of the substantia gelatinosa of Rolando in newborn kittens. J Comp Neurol 187 : 1–18

FITZGERALD M, KOLTZENBURG M (1986) The functional development of descending inhibitory pathways in the dorsolateral funiculus of the newborn rat spinal cord. Dev Brain Res 24 : 261–270

FITZGERALD M, SWETT J (1983) The termination pattern of sciatic nerve afferents in the substantia gelatinosa of neonatal rats. Neurosci Lett 43 : 149–154

HUNT SP, KELLY JS, EMSON PC, KIMMEL JR, MILLER RJ, WU J-Y (1981) An immunohistochemical study of neuronal populations containing neuropeptides or gamma-aminobutyrate within the superficial layers of the rat dorsal horn. Neuroscience 6 : 1883–1898

JANCSÓ G, KIRALY E, JANCSÓ-GABOR A (1977) Pharmacologically induced selective degeneration of chemosensitive primary sensory neurones. Nature 270 : 741–743

LIGHT AR, PERL ER (1979) Reexamination of the dorsal root projection to the spinal dorsal horn including observations on the differential terminations of coarse and fine fibers. J Comp Neurol 186 : 117–132

MATTIO TG, ROSENQUIST TH, KIRBY ML (1981) Appearance of acid phosphatase in neonatal rat substantia gelatinosa. Exp Brain Res 41 : 411–413

NAGY JI, HUNT SP (1982) Fluoride-resistant acid phosphatase-containing neurones in dorsal root ganglia are separate from those containing substance P or somatostatin. Neuroscience 7 : 89–97

NAGY JI, VICENT SR, STAINES WA, FIBIGER HC, REISINE TD, YAMAMURA HI (1980) Neurotoxic action of capsaicin on spinal substance P neurons. Brain Res 186 : 435–444

NAGY JI, HUNT SP, IVERSEN LL, EMSON PC (1981) Biochemical and anatomical observations on the degeneration of peptide-containing primary afferent neurons after neonatal capsaicin. Neuroscience 6 : 1923–1934

RIBEIRO-DA-SILVA A, COIMBRA A (1982) Two types of synaptic glomeruli and their distribution in laminae I–III of the rat spinal cord. J Comp Neurol 209 : 176–186

RIBEIRO-DA-SILVA A, COIMBRA A (1984) Capsaicin causes selective damage to type I synaptic glomeruli in rat substantia gelatinosa. Brain Res 290 : 380–383

RIBEIRO-DA-SILVA A, CASTRO-LOPES JM, COIMBRA A (1986) Distribution of glomeruli with FRAP-containing terminals in the substantia gelatinosa of the rat. Brain Res 377 : 322–329

SMITH CL (1983) The development and postnatal organization of primary afferent projections to the rat thoracic spinal cord. J Comp Neurol 220 : 29–43

8 Glutamic Acid Coexists with Substance P in Some Primary Sensory Neurons

G. Battaglia, A. Rustioni, R.A. Altschuler, and P. Petrusz

Glutamic acid (GA) and substance P (SP) appear to meet some of the criteria necessary for consideration as candidate chemical mediators in the dorsal root ganglia (DRG) neurons (Salt and Hill 1983). GA is highly concentrated in the dorsal root ganglia, dorsal roots, and dorsal horn of the spinal cord (Johnson and Aprison 1970).

GA may be the synaptic mediator in small DRG neurons, as most dorsal horn neurons excited by C-fiber stimulation are also excited by GA (Schneider and Perl 1985). Glutamine is selectively taken up by small lumbar DRG neurons of rats and mice (Duce and Keen 1983), and antisera raised against phosphate-dependent glutaminase (GLN), an enzyme of the glutamine cycle involved in the synthesis of glutamate, label a fraction of small DRG neurons (Cangro et al. 1985). On the other hand, only large DRG neurons are labeled by the retrograde transport of ^{3}H–D–aspartate (^{3}H–D–Asp) (Barbaresi et al. 1985), which is believed to be taken up selectively by putative glutaminergic neurons. Substance P is present in a subpopulation of small DRG neurons, and is predominantly located in lamina I and the outer layer of lamina II of the spinal cord (Hökfelt et al. 1975). It is released from spinal cord slices upon depolarization, and when applied to spinal neurons causes progressive depolarization (Henry 1976).

An immunocytochemical probe for GA has been employed in this study to obtain more direct information about possible glutaminergic neurons in the DRG. The staining of DRG neurons obtained with this anti-GA serum is compared to that obtained with an antibody against GLN. An antiserum against SP has also been employed to determine whether GA and SP are confined to separate or overlapping populations of DRG neurons. The preparation of antisera against L-GA was similar to that previously described by Storm-Mathisen et al. (1983). GA was made antigenic by a covalent link to keyhole limpet hemocyanin (KLH), using glutaraldehyde as cross-linking agent. Next, 1 ml of 100 μM GA was mixed with 1 ml of a solution containing 12 mg/ml KLH in phosphate buffer 0.1 M at pH 7.3 and with 20 μl of a 50% glutaraldehyde solution. The mixture was then vortexed, dialyzed, and diluted with phosphate-buffered saline pH 7.4 to a final volume of 10 ml. The KLH-conjugated GA was emulsified with complete Freund's adjuvant and then injected subcutaneously into rabbits. The anti-GA serum was characterized by immunocytochemistry and immunoabsorption on sections from rat brain and spinal ganglia. Intense immunostaining of neurons was observed in the cerebral cortex, the hippocampus, the habenula, the cerebellum, and the cochlear nuclei. Only the KLH-GA conjugate was able to block the immunostaining, while similarly prepared conjugates of GABA, L-glutamine, aspartate, β-alanine, α-amino-butyric acid, L-leucine, ε-amino-*n*-caproate, taurine, glycine, γ-amino-β-hydroxy-butyrate, δ-amino-*n*-valerate, δ-amino-levulinate, L-asparagine, succinate, oxalacetate, L-malate, fumarate, *N*-acetyl-L-aspartate, α-ketoglutarate, isoleucine, and L-ornithine were ineffective. A preliminary report on the characterization of the antiserum has been published (Hepler et al. 1985), and a full paper is in preparation.

Adult Sprague-Dawley rats and one monkey (*Macaca fascicularis*) were perfused with either 4% paraformaldehyde or 4% carbodiimide in 0.1 M phosphate buffer at pH 7.3. In some rats the left dorsal horn at C5 to C7 was infiltrated with colchicine (up to 1 μl of a 100 μg/μl solution) 24–48 h prior to perfusion. Cervical DRG were postfixed for 1–3 days, wax-embedded, and cut into consecutive 4-μm-thick sections. After dewaxing and rinsing in Tris-buffered saline (TBS) adjacent sections were incubated with the three different antisera, applied as 30- to 40-μl drops onto the sections. After preincubation with 2% normal goat serum, the sections were incubated in the primary antisera (anti-GA serum diluted 1:10 000; anti-GLN and anti-SP sera diluted 1:3000), then in biotinylated goat anti-rabbit IgG (vector, diluted 1:200), and finally in avidin-biotin complex vector: 10 μl avidin DH and 10 μl biotinylated horseradish peroxidase (HRP) in 1 ml TBS. Peroxidase staining was obtained by incubating the sections in diaminobenzidine (0.1%) and hydrogen peroxide (0.01%) in 50 mM sodium cacodylate buffer pH 5.5. Quantitative data were derived from a series of three consecutive sections taken at 100-μm intervals from C6 and C7 DRG of one rat and from C7 of another rat, and at 250-μm intervals from C6 and C7 of one monkey. By this method neurons containing more than one marker could be identified on adjacent sections reacted with the three different antisera. Only neurons displaying a nucleolus in the middle section were considered in the cell counts and area measurements. neurons are located which, based on experiments using other techniques, have been proposed to use glutamate as synaptic mediator. Furthermore, cytochrome oxidase, a marker of neuronal metabolic activity, stains a population of small and large DRG neurons overlapping but not matching the population labeled by the anti-GA serum (work in progress). The

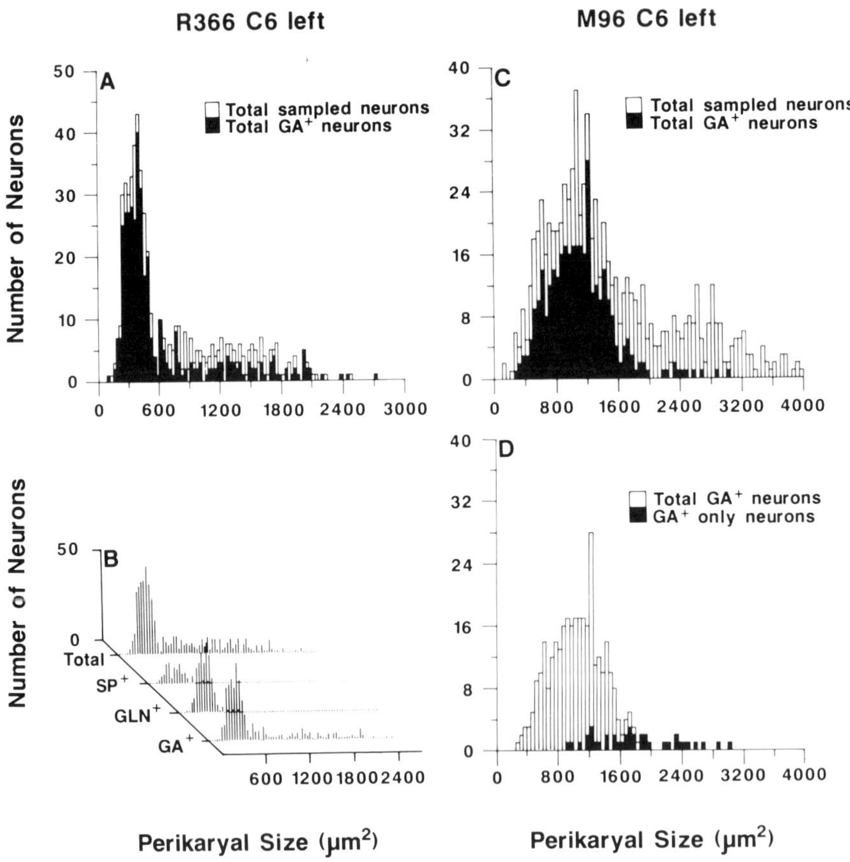

Fig. 1 A–D. Histograms displaying the number and perikaryal size of labeled neurons in left C6 DRG of rat r366 (left), and in left C6 DRG of monkey m96 (right). Comparison between GA+ and total sampled neurons in **A** and **C**; between neurons labeled by the three different antisera and total sampled neurons in **B**; between neurons labeled only by the anti-GA serum and total GA+ neurons in **D**

Table 1. Percentages and mean perikaryal areas (MPA, μm^2) of single-labeled and unlabeled neurons in C6 and C7 of two rats (r366 and r341) and one monkey (m96)

DRG	GA+		GLN+		SP+		Unlabeled	
	%	MPA	%	MPA	%	MPA	%	MPA
r366 C6 (550)	69.63	632	44.00	375	15.64	374	26.00	1080
r366 C7 (503)	65.21	502	40.36	359	13.32	356	32.01	1270
r341 C7 (507)	63.31	480	41.62	335	no colchicine		35.89	1100
m96 C6 (749)	45.13	1114	47.00	963	no colchicine		47.80	1960
m96 C7 (775)	58.84	1105	52.90	966	no colchicine		35.87	1980

The figures in parentheses refer to the number of sampled neurons for each ganglion

Neurons labeled by the anti-GA serum (GA+ cells) represent 60 %–70 % of the rat DRG population (Table 1). They include about 90 % of the small neurons with mean perikaryal area around 300–400 μm^2, and 35 %–50 % of the large neurons with perikaryal area greater than 600 μm^2 (Figs. 1A, 2A). DRG neurons labeled by either the anti-GLN serum (GLN+ cells; Figs. 1B, 2B), or anti-SP serum (SP+ cells; Figs. 1B, 2C) are small (mean area 335 to 375 μm^2 and 356 to 374 μm^2 respectively) and account for approximately 40 % and 15 % of the counted cells respectively (Table 1). The use of colchicine is necessary to visualize SP+ neurons, and it increases the number of large GA+ cells. The percentage of GLN+ cells, on the other hand, is not clearly affected by the pretreatment with colchicine. In the monkey, 45 %–60 % of the DRG neurons are GA+ and are mostly of small size (Table 1, Figs. 1C, 2D). GLN+ neurons, in the same species, account for about 50 % of the DRG population (Table 1) and have perikaryal areas distributed between 200 and 1600 μm^2, with a peak at 800-1200 μm^2 (not shown). None of the cells larger than 2000 μm^2 are GLN+ (Fig. 2E). Table 2 shows the percentages of single-, double-, and triple-labeled perikarya for each of the three categories of labeled neurons. In the rat, about 60 % of GA+ neurons are also GLN+, whereas almost all GLN+ neurons are GA+. Virtually none of the double-labeled cells have a perikaryal area greater than 600 μm^2. In the monkey, the majority of GA+ neurons (81 %–88 %) and GLN+ neurons (85 %–90 %) are double-labeled, i.e., GA+ and GLN+. There is, however, a small population of single-labeled GLN+ and GA+ neurons, with clearly differing mean perikaryal areas (483 and 663 μm^2 vs 1447 and 1792 μm^2 respectively; Table 2, Fig. 1D). In the two ganglia from the colchicine-treated rat the majority of SP+ neurons (58.2 %–67.4 %) are triple-labeled, and the bulk of double-labeled SP+ neurons are GA+. The percentages of SP+ neurons positive for GA are 87.2 % and 88.1 % respectively in C6 and C7. No difference is evident in the size distribution of the single-labeled vs double- or triple-labeled SP+ neurons.

The principal finding of this study is the fact that many but not all small, and some large DRG neurons are immunoreactive to an anti-GA serum. Although with the method used in the present study it is impossible to differentiate the transmitter from the metabolic pool of glutamic acid, some considerations argue against the possibility that the anti-GA serum is only a metabolic marker. Neurons labeled by this antiserum in the somatosensory cortex of rats and monkeys are predominantly seen in layers III and V (Conti et al. 1985), where

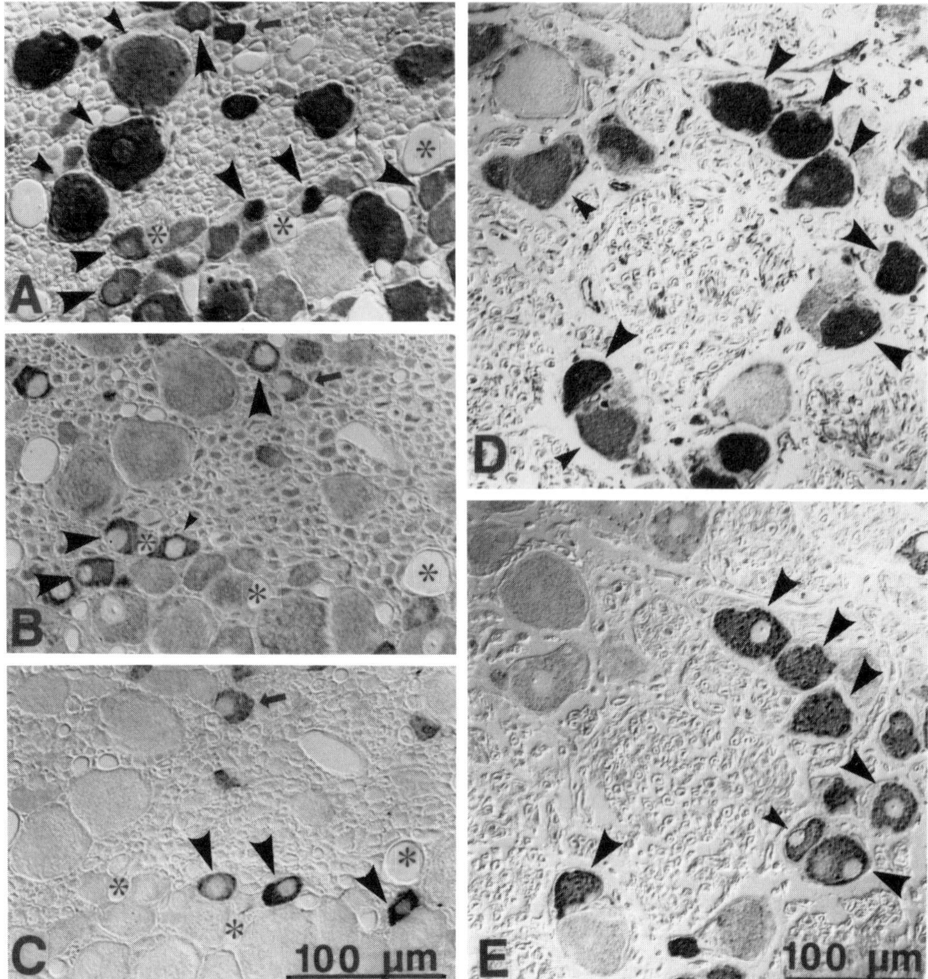

Fig. 2 A–E. Left: three consecutive rat DRG sections reacted with anti-GA (**A**), anti-GLN (**B**), and anti-SP serum (**C**). Right: two consecutive monkey DRG sections reacted with anti-GA (**D**) and anti-GLN serum (**E**). Small arrowheads, large arrowheads, and arrows show single-, double-, and triple-labeled neurons respectively; asterisks mark capillaries as reference points

labeling obtained with the anti-GA serum in the DRG supports the results of Schneider and Perl (1985), who reported excitatory responses to GA for the majority of spinal units excited by C fibers. The present results can be also reconciled with the retrograde labeling of only large DRG neurons after injection of ^{3}H-D-Asp (Barbaresi et al. 1985), if one assumes that small DRG neurons, although using GA as neurotransmitter, do not transport ^{3}H-D-Asp (for a discussion of the interpretation of results with transport of ^{3}H-D-Asp, see Cuénod and Streit 1983). Failure of large GA+ neurons to label with the anti-GLN serum could be explained by metabolic differences in large and small DRG neurons. For instance, large

Table 2. Percentages and mean perikaryal areas (MPA, μm^2) of single-, double-, and triple-labeled perikarya for each of the three categories of labeled neurons in the same ganglia as in Table 1

GA+ labeling	GA+ only %	MPA	GA+, GLN+ %	MPA	GA+, SP+ %	MPA	GA+,GLN+, SP+ %	MPA
r366 C6	36.8	1070	43.6	380	4.4	418	15.2	365
r366 C7	34.1	783	47.9	354	6.1	338	11.9	372
r341 C7	35.5	745	64.5	334	no colchicine		no colchicine	
m96 C6	11.6	1792	88.4	1020	no colchicine		no colchicine	
m96 C7	19.1	1447	80.9	1020	no colchicine		no colchicine	
GLN+ labeling	GLN+ only		GLN+ GA+		GLN+ SP+		GLN+ GA+ SP+	
r366 C6	5.3	376	69.0	380	1.7	275	24.0	365
r366 C7	3.0	402	77.3	354	0.5	242	19.2	372
r366 C7	1.9	380	98.1	334	no colchicine		no colchicine	
m96 C6	15.1	663	84.9	1020	no colchicine		no colchicine	
m96 C7	10.0	483	90.0	1020	no colchicine		no colchicine	
SP+ labeling	SP+ only		SP+ GA+		SP+ GLN+		SP+ GA+ GLN+	
r366 C6	8.1	400	19.8	418	4.7	275	67.4	365
r366 C7	10.4	334	29.9	338	1.5	242	58.2	372

Data on SP labeling in r341 and in m96 are not available because and these animals did not receive colchicine injections. Therefore, data concerning single- and double-labeled neurons in these animals are not directly comparable with those in the same columns. The percentages refer to each of the three categories, and not to the total sampled neurons from each ganglion

neurons may utilize a pathway other than the glutamine cycle for the synthesis of neurotransmitter, which may be GA or a GA-containing dipeptide.

The majority of small SP+ DRG neurons are also immunoreactive for the anti-GA serum. This finding suggests the possibility that some of the neurons containing SP are glutaminergic. Urban and Randić (1984) observed that repetitive stimulation of a dorsal root elicited, after an initial burst of monosynaptic excitatory potentials, a prolonged slow depolarization of dorsal horn neurons, possibly mediated by SP. The two distinct phases of depolarization may be attributable to the release of an excitatory amino acid and a peptide respectively, and may be functionally important in determining the firing pattern of second-order sensory neurons.

References

BARBARESI P, RUSTIONI A, CUÉNOD M (1985) Retrograde labeling of dorsal root ganglion neurons after injections of tritiated amino acids in the spinal cord of rats and cats. Somatosens Res 3 : 57–74

CANGRO CB, SWEETNAM PM, WRATHALL JR, HASER WB, CURTHOYS NP, NEALE JH (1985) Localization of elevated glutaminase immunoreactivity in small DRG neurons. Brain Res 336 : 158–161

CONTI F, RUSTIONI A, PETRUSZ P (1985) Morphology and laminar distribution of neurons with glutamate-like immunoreactivity in the rat somatosensory cortex. Neurosci Abstr 11 : 755

CUÉNOD M, STREIT P (1983) Neuronal tracing using retrograde migration of labeled transmitter related compounds. In: BJÖRKLUND A, HÖKFELT T (eds) Handbook of chemical neuroanatomy, vol 1. Elsevier, Amsterdam, pp 365–397

DUCE IR, KEEN P (1983) Selective uptake of [3H]glutamine and [3H]glutamate into neurons and satellite cells of dorsal root ganglia in vitro. Neuroscience 8 : 861–866

HENRY JL (1976) Effects of substance P on functionally identified units in cat spinal cord. Brain Res 114 : 439–451

HÖKFELT T, KELLERTH JO, NILSSON G, PERNOW B (1975) Substance P: localization in the central nervous system and in some primary sensory neurons. Science 190 : 889–890

JOHNSON JL, APRISON MH (1970) The distribution of glutamic acid, a transmitter candidate, and other amino acids in the dorsal sensory neurons of the cat. Brain Res 24 : 285–292

HEPLER JR, PETRUSZ P, RUSTIONI A (1985) Antisera to GABA, glutamate and aspartate: characterization by immunoabsorption and immunocytochemistry. J Histochem 34 : 110

SALT TE, HILL RG (1983) Neurotransmitter candidates of somatosensory primary afferent fibers. Neuroscience 10 : 1083–1103

SCHNEIDER SP, PERL ER (1985) Selective excitation of neurons in the mammalian spinal dorsal horn by aspartate and glutamate in vitro: correlation with location and excitatory input. Brain Res 360 : 339–343

STORM MATHISEN J, LEKNES AC, BORE AT, VAALAND JL, EDMINSON P, HAUG FMS, OTTERSEN OP (1983) First visualization of glutamate and GABA in neurones by immunocytochemistry. Nature 301 : 517–520

URBAN L, RANDIĆ M (1984) Slow excitatory transmission in rat dorsal horn: possible mediation by peptides. Brain Res 290 : 336–341

9 A Comparison of the Relative Numbers and Properties of Cutaneous Nociceptive Afferents in Different Mammalian Species

B. Lynn and R. Baranowski

Nearly two decades have passed since the first detailed accounts of the numbers a properties of nociceptive afferents in mammalian skin were published by Prof. E. R. P and his associates (Burgess and Perl 1967; Bessou and Perl 1969). Working on the limb skin of the cat, and subsequently the monkey (Perl 1968; Kumazawa and Perl 1977), two major classes of nociceptor were identified. These were (1) high-threshold mechanoreceptors (HTMs) with Aδ axons and (2) polymodal nociceptors with unmyelinated (C) axons. This classification has served well in a range of mammalian species for hairy skin, although some modifications are needed for glabrous skin, where, for example, substantial numbers of heat-sensitive A-fiber nociceptors may be present (Beck et al. 1974; Georgopoulos 1976).

Our recent work has involved using the same methods to study the nociceptors in hairy skin in three different mammalian species, the rat (Lynn and Carpenter 1982), the rabbit (Lynn 1979; Fitzgerald and Lynn 1977) and, most recently, the ferret (*Mustela putorius furo* L.). We wish to consider here the relative numbers of nociceptors in the various species and the extent to which their properties, such as heat and mechanical thresholds, vary between species. In particular it will be argued that the wide variations between species in the responses of polymodal nociceptors to heating indicate that heat sensitivity may not be an important part of their function. In addition, we will briefly consider the absolute numbers of nociceptors present in the rat and will make an estimate of the innervation density of nociceptors in this species.

Methods

Afferent units have been studied by recording extracellularly from fine filaments dissected from cutaneous nerves, usually the saphenous nerve innervating the medial aspect of the lower leg, but also the sural and the great auricular nerves in the rabbit. In order to obtain a complete sample of all types of fiber present, the search stimulus was a maximal electrical shock applied to the nerve between the recording point and the skin. This arrangement also allowed the conduction velocity of units to be measured. The electrical stimulus was a rectangular pulse of 0.5 ms duration and with an amplitude that was supramaximal for the C compound action potential (usually 1–3 mA). These large pulses could cause A-fiber conduction block, so the repetition frequency was kept less than 1 Hz. When a clear single unit was present with electrical stimulation, the skin was searched with strong mechanical stimuli. If no field was found, an ice-cold probe was passed over the skin and sometimes also a probe at 55°C. Mechanical sensitivity was estimated for slowly adapting units by using a series of calibrated von Frey bristles of diameter 0.1–0.4 mm. Heat sensitivity was measured using either a radiant heat lamp (Fitzgerald and Lynn 1977; Lynn 1979) or a contact probe (Lynn 1981) that heated a circular region about 7 mm in diameter. Both probes were controlled by feedback from thermocouples in contact with the skin surface so that skin temperature was raised at a rate of 1°C/s.

Results

Relative Numbers of Different Types of Unit

The data for nerves innervating the lower leg in rat, ferret and rabbit and the pinna in the rabbit are summarized in Table 1. Not included in this table are units that were excited by the electrical search stimulus but for which no receptive field could be found. Such units comprised 0 %–10 % of all A fibers sampled and 12 %–25 % of C fibers. The larger number of C fibers with no receptive field is probably accounted for by the presence of sympathetic efferent C fibers in the sample. In distal nerves to hairy skin, sympathetic fibers are known to comprise 19 %–33 % of all C fibers (Blumberg and Jänig 1982; McLachlan and Jänig 1983).

The A fiber unit sample is dominated by sensitive mechanoreceptors, mostly rapidly adapting hair follicle units. The markedly less sensitive mechanical nociceptors of the A-HTM type form only 16 %–26 % of the total sample of A fibers. Published figures for other mammalian species are similar, e.g. 20 % in monkey (Perl 1968) and 13 % in cat (Burgess et al. 1968). Conversely, with the C fibers it is the nociceptors that are most numerous. Polymodal nociceptors comprise 52 %–79 % of all C units with cutaneous fields. This is rather higher than the 34 % reported for cat hairy skin by Bessou and Perl (1969) in their pioneering study, but not as high as reported for the monkey (80 %; Kumazawa and Perl 1977).

Table 1. Relative numbers of different classes of afferent unit from hairy skin in three mammalian species

Species	Skin region	A fibers Total number	A fibers % classified as RA	SA	HTM	C fibers Total number	C fibers % classified as POLY	SENS	COLD
Rat	Limb	474	74	5	16	241	79	12½	3
Ferret	Limb	30	60	23	17	27	52	18½	15
Rabbit	Limb	82	66	4	26	68	73	20	3
Rabbit	Pinna	55	75	0	25	40	62½	35	0

RA, rapidly adapting mechanoreceptors, mostly from hair follicles; SA, slowly adapting mechanoreceptors, mostly type I; HTM, high-threshold nociceptors; POLY, polymodal nociceptors, plus small number of heat nociceptors; SENS, sensitive C-mechanoreceptors; COLD, cold-sensitive thermoreceptors

Not included in the table are small numbers of units that do not fit the main categories; many of these are insensitive mechanoreceptors with varied properties

Sources: Rat: Lynn and Carpenter (1982), Lynn (1984) and unpublished data; Ferret: unpublished data; Rabbit: Fitzgerald and Lynn (1977), Lynn (1979), Barasi and Lynn (1986)

Conduction Velocities

A-HTM units in all three species conducted predominantly at slow rates in the delta range (5–25 m/s). However, as in cat and monkey (Burgess and Perl 1967; Perl 1968), a few conducted more rapidly, and values up to 32.5 m/s and 40 m/s have been observed in the rabbit and rat respectively (Fitzgerald and Lynn 1977; Lynn and Carpenter 1982). Not surprisingly in view of the large numbers found, C-polymodal nociceptor fibers conducted over the entire C-fiber conduction velocity range in all the species studied. Rat C fibers were slower than those in the rabbit or ferret. The range of C-fiber conduction velocities was wider in the ferret, at 0.5–1.4 m/s ($n = 31$), than in the rabbit (0.7–1.1 m/s, $n = 39$; Lynn 1979) or rat (0.5–0.9 m/s; Lynn and Carpenter 1982).

Responses to Mechanical Stimulation

Both HTMs and polymodal nociceptors were reliably stimulated by local pressure. Receptive fields comprised either a single point or small zone or a number of separated points; polymodal fields were almost always a single point whilst HTMs were only rarely a single point and could comprise more than 10 points. Responses were slowly adapting from both classes of nociceptor, and sensitivity was usually assessed by using calibrated von Frey bristles. Thresholds for such stimuli are given in Table 2. Polymodal units were slightly more sensitive on average than HTMs, but both types showed a wide range of sensitivity. Within this range, polymodal units from the ferret had the lowest average thresholds, whilst the rat units had the highest.

Table 2. Mechanical and heat thresholds of nociceptors in rat, rabbit and ferret

Species				HTM			C-POLYMODAL		
	Mechanical threshold (g)			Mechanical threshold (g)			Heat threshold (°C)		
	Range	*n*	Mean[a]	Range	*n*	Mean[a]	Range	*n*	Mean[b]
Rat	0.2->10	32	1.73[c]	0.08->5	43	0.74[c,g]	36–59	83	47.0[c]
Rabbit	0.3->10	18	2.18[d,g]	0.025–4	148	0.46[e]	41–65	69	54.1[e,f]
Ferret		–		0.05–2	14	0.27[g]	28–54	13	40.5[g]

[a]Geometric mean
[b]Normal arithmetic mean
[c]Lynn and Carpenter (1982)
[d]Barasi and Lynn (1986)
[e]Fitzgerald (1978)
[f]Lynn (1979)
[g]Unpublished data

Responses to Heat Stimulation

A-HTM units in hairy skin only rarely respond to heating, although they can become sensitized by repeated heat stimulation (Fitzgerald and Lynn 1977). Polymodal nociceptors are required to be heat-sensitive to be so classified, and the heat thresholds for rat, rabbit and ferret polymodal units are given in Table 2. Thresholds in the ferret are lower than in the rat, which in turn has lower thresholds than the rabbit. There is considerable overlap, but it is still found that half the ferret units fire at temperatures that never excite units in the rabbit. Suprathreshold responses also vary between species. Typical plots of firing frequency against skin temperature are shown for a ferret polymodal nociceptor in Fig. 1. Firing frequency increases approximately exponentially during the 1°C/s ramp stimulus, although the firing is rather variable from moment to moment. This pattern is similar to

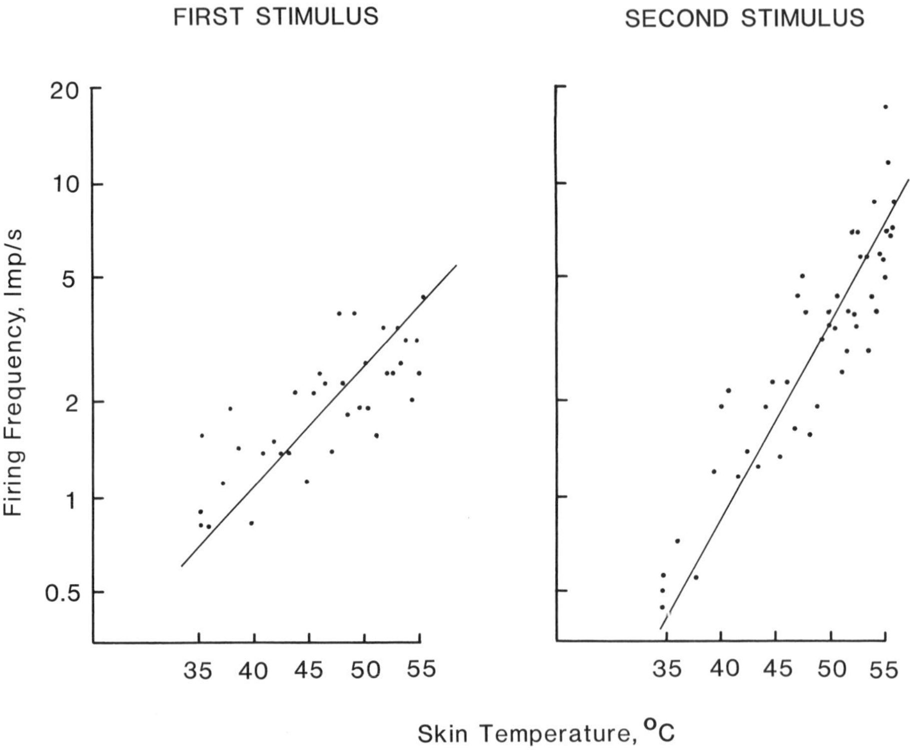

Fig. 1. Heat responses of polymodal nociceptor unit from ferret saphenous nerve. Left plot is from the first heat stimulus, a "ramp" at 1°C/s from a holding temperature of 35.2°C; right plot for second identical ramp from 34.9°C hold 4 min later. Each interspike interval is plotted as instantaneous firing frequency, on a log scale, against the average skin temperature during the interval. The fitted lines are least squares fits for the regression of log frequency against temperature. Note that average firing is little changed but the slope of the firing frequency-temperature relation has increased. Not enough data are available to establish whether this is a regular feature of ferret nociceptors when given repeated heat stimuli

most rabbit units (Lynn 1979) although rabbit units tended to fire more regularly and to show a steeper frequency-temperature relation. It differs from most rat units, which showed erratic or discontinuous firing during heat ramps (Lynn and Carpenter 1982).

Repeated heating to skin temperatures in excess of 50°–55°C was shown to sensitize polymodal nociceptor units in the cat by Bessou and Perl (1969). Similarly, rabbit units were reliably sensitized by strong skin heating (Lynn 1979) with thresholds falling by as much as 17°C and with an average fall for units heated to 54°–61°C of 5.0°C. Rat units show such sensitization only rarely, and since some rat polymodal units desensitize, the population as a whole is on average not enhanced in its firing by repeated strong heating. The small number of ferret units examined so far with repeated heat stimuli to above 55°C have shown little overall increase in firing, although the unit shown in Fig. 1 clearly has a different response pattern on the second heat trial. In the rat, the least sensitive units tend to show the greatest threshold fall on repeated heating, and a similar trend has been reported for the polymodal nociceptors from the rabbit pinna (Shea and Perl 1985). It therefore appears that the ferret units, with their generally low initial thresholds, are behaving like units with low thresholds in other species by not sensitizing.

Actual Numbers of Nociceptors and the Density of Innervation of Hairy Skin

Recent work has given data on the numbers of A and C fibers in the saphenous nerve in the rat (Lynn 1984; and unpublished). A total of 930 A fibers and 3400 C fibers are present at the level where our electrical search stimulus is applied. Since on average 4 % of A fibers and 15 % of C fibers in the rat have no receptive field, there is a functioning afferent population of 893 A and 2890 C fibers, of which 16 % of the A fibers, that is 143 fibers in all, are A-HTMs and 79 % of C fibers, i.e. 2283 fibers, are polymodal nociceptors.

The area of skin innervated by the saphenous nerve is approximately 650 mm^2, but this area is not uniformly innervated. About half the fibers innervate the foot (area 164 mm^2) whilst the other half innervate the larger area of leg and ankle (486 mm^2). Innervation densities have therefore been calculated separately for these two zones. Overall, 42 % of our sample of polymodal units had fields on the leg (Lynn and Carpenter 1982) giving an innervation density of 1.97/mm^2 (see Fig. 2). For HTMs, 60 % innervated the leg, giving 0.18 units/mm^2. However, each unit had on average five distinct points in its receptive fields, so the density of such "receptors" is 0.88/mm^2, as shown in Fig. 2. Similar calculations for the foot give figures of 8.1 polymodal units/mm^2 and 0.35 HTMs/mm^2 (but 1.22 HTM "receptors"/mm^2, since on average each HTM unit on the foot had 3.5 sensitive points in its receptive field).

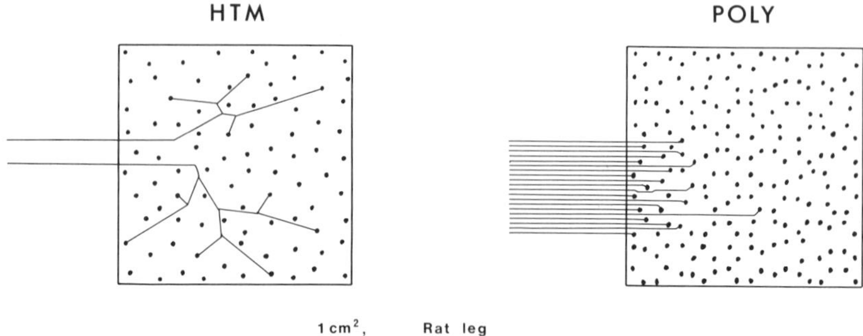

Fig. 2. Density of fields of nociceptors on the limb skin of the rat. Left, high-threshold mechanoreceptors (HTM); right, polymodal nociceptors (Poly). A 1-cm^2 patch of skin is shown. The numbers of fields have been calculated as described in the text. Only 10% of the axons supplying each patch are shown. Data from saphenous nerve for skin of medial aspect of lower leg

Discussion

The provision of information about noxious mechanical stimuli appears to be organized in a rather uniform manner in all the mammalian species studied so far. Both the relatively fast-conducting HTM units and the slowly conducting polymodal nociceptors will signal about such stimuli. Both populations cover a wide range from moderate pressure levels, which are certainly non-painful in normal human skin, to clearly damaging stimuli such as pressure with a needle. The role of the faster-conducting HTMs might appear the most important for triggering rapid defence reactions to threatening mechanical stimuli. However, the greater sensitivity and, especially in the foot, the greater numbers of polymodal units may indicate that this group also plays an important role in mechanical nociception. With slowly increasing mechanical stresses, the greater sensitivity of polymodal units may even lead to these providing the earliest warning to the CNS of impending danger.

Responses to heat present a more variable picture. In hairy skin of non-primates, although the major heat-sensitive group are the polymodal nociceptor units, such units vary quite a lot in their responses between species. It may be that heat responses are not actually very important to most animals in their natural environment. Heat pain stimuli are very convenient for the experimenter, since they are easy to apply in a controlled, repeatable manner. However, in practice they may not be much more "natural" than electric shocks. It seems more likely that the key property of polymodal nociceptors is their ability to respond to irritant chemicals, including several of the mediators known to be released during inflammation (see e.g. Bessou and Perl 1969; Beck and Handwerker 1974; Belcher 1979).

Summary

Mammalian hairy skin is innervated by large numbers of two major classes of nociceptors. Mechanical nociceptors of the HTM type are less numerous than C-polymodal units; estimates of the numbers of "receptors" in rat limb skin are 0.9–1.2/mm^2 for HTMs and 2.0–8.1/mm^2 for polymodal nociceptors. Both types signal about noxious mechanical stimuli in a quantitatively similar way in all species examined. Heat responses are mostly only shown by C-polymodal nociceptors and vary rather a lot from species to species. It is suggested that this may reflect the lesser importance of heat stimuli in the natural environment.

Acknowledgement. This work was supported in part by a project grant from the Medical Research Council.

References

Barasi S, Lynn B (1986) Effects of sympathetic stimulation on mechanoreceptive and nociceptive afferent units from the rabbit pinna. Brain Res 378 : 21–27

Beck PW, Handwerker HO (1974) Bradykinin and serotonin effects on various types of cutaneous nerve fibers. Pfluegers Arch 347 : 209–222

Beck PW, Handwerker HO, Zimmermann M (1974) Nervous outflow from the cat's foot pad during noxious radiant heat stimulation. Brain Res 67 : 373–386

Belcher G (1979) The effects of intra-arterial bradykinin, histamine, acetylcholine and prostaglandin E_1 on nociceptive and non-nociceptive dorsal horn neurones of the cat. Eur J Pharmacol 56 : 385–395

Bessou P, Perl ER (1969) Response of cutaneous sensory units with unmyelinated fibers to noxious stimuli. J Neurophysiol 32 : 1025–1043

Blumberg H, Jänig W (1982) Changes in unmyelinated fibers including sympathetic postganglionic fibers of a skin nerve after peripheral neuroma formation. J Auton Nerv Syst 6 : 173–183

Burgess PR, Perl ER (1967) Myelinated afferent fibers responding specifically to noxious stimulation of the skin. J Physiol (Lond) 190 : 541–562

Burgess PR, Petit D, Warren RM (1968) Receptor types in cat hairy skin supplied by myelinated fibers. J Neurophysiol 31 : 833–848

Fitzgerald M (1978) The sensitization of cutaneous nociceptors. PhD thesis, University of London

Fitzgerald M, Lynn B (1977) The sensitization of high threshold mechanoreceptors with myelinated axons by repeated heating. J Physiol (Lond) 265 : 549–563

Georgopoulos AP (1976) Functional properties of primate afferent units probably related to pain mechanisms in primate glabrous skin. J Neurophysiol 39 : 71–83

Kumazawa T, Perl ER (1977) Primate cutaneous sensory units with unmyelinated (C) afferent fibers. J Neurophysiol 40 : 1325–1338

Lynn B (1979) The heat sensitization of polymodal nociceptors in the rabbit and its independence of the local blood flow. J Physiol (Lond) 287 : 493–507

Lynn B (1981) A microprocessor-controlled stimulator for measuring human heat pain thresholds. J Physiol (Lond) 317 : 13–14P

Lynn B (1984) Effect of neonatal treatment with capsaicin on the numbers and properties of cutaneous afferent units from the hairy skin of the rat. Brain Res 322 : 255–260

Lynn B, Carpenter SE (1982) Primary afferent units from the hairy skin of the rat hind limb. Brain Res 238 : 29–43

McLachlan EM, Jänig W (1983) The cell bodies of origin of sympathetic and sensory axons in some skin and muscle nerves of the cat hindlimb. J Comp Neurol 214 : 115–130

Perl ER (1968) Myelinated afferent fibers innervating the primate skin and their response to noxious stimuli. J Physiol (Lond) 197 : 593–615

Shea VK, Perl ER (1985) Sensory receptors with unmyelinated (C) fibers innervating the skin of the rabbit's ear. J Neurophysiol 54 : 491–501

10 Evidence for and Possible Functional Significance of Multiple Branches of Afferent C Fibres in Peripheral Nerve

S. B. McMahon and P. D. Wall

Electron-microscopic studies on peripheral nerves have shown that unmyelinated axons outnumber myelinated ones by a factor of some 4 : 1 or 5 : 1 in somatic nerves (McLachlan and Jänig 1983) and as much as 10 : 1 in visceral nerves (Kuo et al. 1982). After allowing for the contribution of sympathetic efferents, unmyelinated fibres still constitute the large majority of afferents (McLachlan and Jänig 1983). There has recently been some interest in the possibility that many primary afferents might have two or more branches. Langford and Coggeshall (1979, 1981) have reported that rat dorsal root axons are more numerous than dorsal root ganglion cells by a factor of 2 : 1 for all cells. Similar results have been obtained in the cat (Aldskogius and Risling 1981; Chung and Coggeshall 1984). For peripheral nerves, equivalent counts in sympathectomised rats yielded an axon : cell ratio of 2.3 : 1. The possibility that sympathectomy might induce sprouting of the remaining afferent axons has not been excluded: interestingly, peripheral axotomy can lead to a stable increase in the numbers of unmyelinated axons in some regenerated nerves, whilst there is either no change or a small decrease in the number of DRG cells (Jenq and Coggeshall 1985; Tessler et al. 1985).

These counts suggest multiple axon branches in peripheral nerve and dorsal root. Other supporting evidence for peripheral branching has been put forward by Taylor and Pierau (1982) and Pierau et al. (1982, 1984), who reported that large numbers of lumbosacral DRG cells could be either activated by electrical stimulation of both the peripheral sciatic and pudendal nerves, or double-labelled by tracers applied to these same nerves. Bahr et al. (1981) also found electrophysiological evidence that some afferents in cat splanchnic nerve also have a branch in a lumbar spinal nerve. However, there is a large body of literature which specifically denies the common existence of such spatially widespread branching. Devor et al. (1984) found evidence for branching in only 0.27 % of myelinated fibres and 0.06 % of unmyelinated fibres in various tributaries of rat sciatic nerve. Borges and Moscowitz (1983) found evidence for branches in only 0.23 % of monkey trigeminal axons, and similar results were found by McMahon et al. (1985) in the cat. Laurberg and Sorenson (1985) found less than 1 % of cells in cervical DRG to have widespread peripheral collaterals.

There is one other special case where peripheral branching may be common and that is for ventral root afferents (Clifton et al. 1976). Some of these axons appear to be branches of unmyelinated axons which have receptive fields in the periphery and send axons into dorsal roots (Kim and Chung 1985). It is not clear whether these ventral root branches penetrate the spinal cord: they may peter out or innervate pia (Dalsgaard et al. 1982).

There are a number of other observations which are not consistent with widespread peripheral branching of afferents. There are only occasional reports of afferent fibres in dorsal roots, or dorsal horn cells, exhibiting two distant receptive fields; a few such fibres have been seen innervating the tail (Mense et al. 1980). Transganglionic horseradish peroxidase (HRP) labelling at different peripheral nerves shows that nerves have essentially non-overlapping termination fields in the dorsal horn (Ygge and Grant 1983; Molander and Grant 1985; Sweet and Woolf 1985).

The discrepancy between on the one hand, axon and DRG cell counts, and on the other, a lack of widespread branches, could be explained if all the branches of a given cell were to project through the same peripheral nerve.

To study this possibility we have performed electrophysiological experiments in anaesthetised rats. Single-unit recordings were made from fine dissected filaments of dorsal roots. Strands were dissected until a unitary all-or-none potential could be recorded at C-fibre latency (i. e. impulse conduction velocity less than 1.5 m/s) by supramaximal stimulation of the sural nerve. When isolated, the response of the fibres to graded electrical stimulation with a fine intraneural microelectrode was carefully studied.

For 17 of 44 fibres (39 %) the latency of response showed a small and gradual decrease from an average of 91 ms as the peripheral stimulus was increased to 10 times threshold. The magnitude of the decrease varied from 0.5 to 1.5 ms and this expected response presumably reflects the spread of stimulus to more proximal portions of the axon. In the remaining 27 fibres (61 %), sudden jumps in latency were observed as the stimulus was raised above threshold. Figure 1 shows, on an expanded time base, such a shift in latency for one fibre.

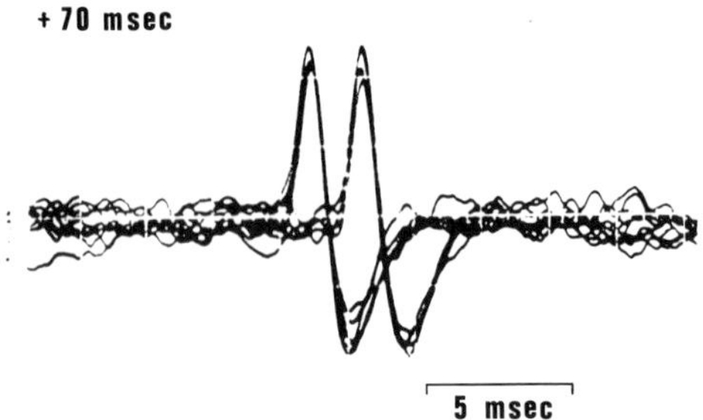

Fig. 1. Responses recorded in a dorsal root filament to stimuli applied with a single stimulating electrode at one locus in the sural nerve. Five stimuli were of 180 μA and 250 μs, and these produced the longer latency responses. Five more stimuli, of 210 μA and 250 μs, were then delivered and the response latency can be seen to have jumped to a new stable latency some 2 ms earlier. The sweeps did not begin until 70 ms after the stimuli were delivered. (From McMahon and Wall 1986, with permission)

Table 1. Magnitude and frequency of occurrence of latency jumps and relative stimulus strengths necessary to elicit them.

Number	Fibres with 1 Latency (n=17)	2 Latencies (n=18)	3 Latencies (n=7)	4 Latencies (n=2)
Conduction velocity (m/s)	0.85 (0.58-0.13)	0.98 (0.68-1.5)	1.01 (0.81-1.24)	0.94
Latency jump (ms)				
First	–	2.2 (0.5–15)	1.8 (0.3–7.2)	0.6
Second	–	–	1.8 (0.4–7.7)	1.9
Third	–	–	–	0.9
Stimulus ratio				
Latency 1–2	–	1.2 (1.2–1.3)	1.4 (1.2–15)	1.5
Latency 2–3	–	–	1.3 (1.1–1.7)	1.1
Latency 3–4	–	–	–	1.2

The figures in the first three columns are means, with ranges in parentheses. The figures in the fourth column are for a single example.

The shift in latency was repeatedly demonstrated for each fibre. In 18 cases only one shift in latency was apparent. It occurred with stimulus amplitudes between 120 % and 130 % of the threshold for the first response. The average shift was 2.2 ms (range 0.5-15 ms). Seven and two fibres showed three and four fixed latencies respectively. The details of magnitude of latency shift and stimuli necessary to elicit them are shown in Table 1.

It is not surprising that such jumps in latency have not previously been reported; they are relatively small (less than 3 % of overall latency on average) and might easily be missed if the response is examined with a only slow sweep. Further, they occur over a relatively small range of stimulus intensities.

We suspected that the observation of two latencies for the action potential recorded in a single axon was produced by the presence in the peripheral nerve of two branches of the axon. It is proposed that under favourable circumstances, the smaller branch was closer to the stimulating electrode and therefore a delayed action potential was recorded. As the stimulus was raised, the larger branch was stimulated and an earlier action potential recorded. With this higher stimulus the orthodromic impulse in the faster fibre would be expected to invade the smaller fibre at the branch point and to collide with the impulse in the smaller fibre, so that only one impulse would be recorded. To test this suggestion further, we measured the conduction velocity of the fast and slow spikes from different stimulus positions, since if two branches were present we would expect a consistent relationship between the two action potential latencies.

Figure 2 shows an example of one fibre tested at six progressively shorter conduction distances from 96 to 71 mm. The velocity of the fast potential was 1.23 m/s over this range. The slower potential could be evoked at four of the six stimulus positions. From the two-branch hypothesis one would not expect to evoke both potentials at each locus, since there is a good chance that the faster fibre will in some cases be closer to the stimulating electrode

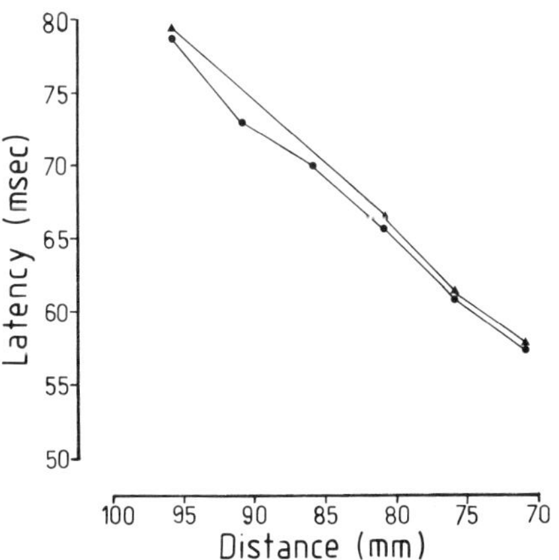

Fig. 2. Graph of the latencies of response of a single C afferent fibre to stimuli applied to different sites in the sural nerve. The circles connect the shortest fixed latency response seen at each location tested when the stimulus was raised from zero to above threshold. The triangles connect the slower latencies found when there were two stable latencies of response with increasing stimulus strengths. For this unit there were never more than two latencies recorded at one stimulus point. Note that the two lines are approximately parallel. (From McMahon and Wall 1986, with permission)

and then only the faster potential will be recorded because it will collide with the slower. In Fig. 2 it can be seen that the slow potential arrived at the recording electrode 1 ms later than the fast potential from the most distal locus and 0.5 ms later than the fast potential from the most proximal locus, giving this impulse a conduction velocity an average of 4.4 % slower than that of the fast impulse. Six other fibres were found to show consistent latency shifts at different stimulus locations.

We tested whether fibres yielding evidence of branching within the sural nerve could also be activated from other branches of the sciatic. In agreement with our earlier studies (Devor et al. 1984), no such widespread branches were seen.

There are a number of possible explanations for these latency shifts and we show some of these in Fig. 3.

The simplest possibility is that the unmyelinated afferents have only one branch, and that because of specialised nodal points on this axon, an increasing stimulus causes spike initiation to jump to more proximal sites (Fig. 3A). Although such nodes exist for myelinated fibres, they apparently do not for unmyelinated ones (Waxman 1984). Moreover, the latency jumps we have seen would imply a stimulus spread of over 2 mm on average for stimulus increases of only 20 %-30 % (Table 1). Our negative findings for 17 fibres, where a tenfold increase in stimulus intensity produced latency shifts of only 0.5-1.5 ms, argue against this, as do other measurements of the likely current necessary to spread such distances (Devor et al. 1984; McMahon and Wall 1985). Finally, if nodes are proposed, changing the stimulation location should result in unpredictable latency jumps at different sites. This was not observed (Fig. 2). We therefore think that the data suggest the presence of multiple

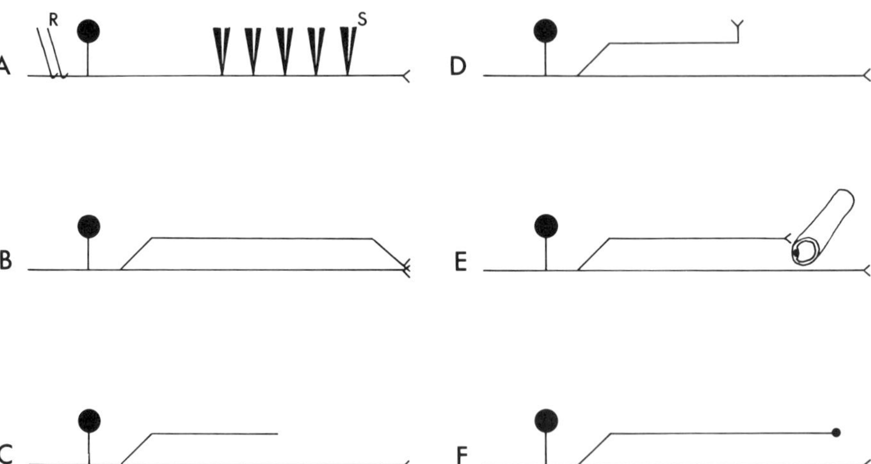

Fig. 3 A–F. Six possible explanations for the observed latency shifts in potentials recorded from dorsal root filaments (R). **A** Discontinuities of threshold along the course of a single axon either normally existing or produced by the presence of stimulating microelectrodes (S). **B** The presence of branches peripheral to the dorsal root ganglion which terminate in the same area of tissue. **C** The presence of branches one of which ends in a non-functioning terminal. **D** Branches terminating in widely separated areas. **E** Branches one of which ends in a normal sensory ending and the other on a blood vessel to produce the axon reflex. **F** Branches one of which ends in a normal sensory ending and the other specialised in the absorption of chemicals which are transported centrally

branches in over 60 % of sural C afferents. Of course, our techniques will underestimate the degree of branching, since when the stimulating electrode lies closer to the faster conducting branch, branch point invasion and collision will prevent the detection of slower branches.

Figure 3B suggests that different branches within a nerve converge on the same area of skin, and this is proposed to account for the lack of dual receptive fields in dorsal root unmyelinated axons. It is also consistent with the report by Kenins (1984) who claimed that electrical stimulation of fine dissected nerve filaments produces neurogenic extravasation only at one small site in the periphery.

Another possible arrangement is shown in Fig. 3C, where some branches remain undeveloped within the nerve and do not form functional connections with the periphery. Such branches may be the remnants of the original developmental process where multiple branches are present. Since the ventral root branches of unmyelinated afferents do not appear to produce post-synaptic actions on spinal cord cells, they too may be examples of this type of arrangement.

Widely separated peripheral branches (Fig. 3D) were not observed in this study. Figure 3E shows an arrangement of nerves suggested by Lewis (1942) to explain the axon reflex. Activity in some fibres following noxious stimulation was proposed to invade other branches ending on blood vessels and there produce an increase in blood flow, increased vascular permeability and oedema. Unmyelinated afferents are necessary for such an axon reflex (Jancso et al. 1967; Lembeck and Gamse 1982). However, the branches we have observed here are unlikely to form the afferent and efferent limbs of this reflex, since it is known that neurogenic oedema can be elicited for some time after peripheral nerve block or section, at a site distal to the branching seen here (Chahl 1976; Jansco and Kiraly 1983; McMahon and Wall 1986).

Figure 3F incorporates another important function of afferent nerve fibres – the axonal transport of substances. In this figure we speculate that some branches of unmyelinated afferents are particularly concerned with the transport of chemicals arising from the peripheral tissue, whilst others are concerned with reporting the immediate state of the tissue by transmitting action potentials. It is possible, of course, that a given axon performs both functions. The importance of retrograde axon transport in unmyelinated afferents is shown by several observations. Applying axon transport blockers to a nerve causes a change in expression of certain peptides by the cell bodies of treated unmyelinated afferents (Fitzgerald et al. 1984). Trophic tissue factors such as NGF, when applied to peripheral tissue, can increase the production of substance P by nerves innervating that tissue (Goedert et al. 1981). Peptide levels are also reported to be increased when the state of tissue is changed, as in experimentally induced arthritis (Lembeck et al. 1981).

C fibres with similar electrophysiological properties show very different chemistries, depending on the tissue that they innervate (McMahon et al. 1984). We have taken advantage of this to test the effects of peripheral environment on primary afferent nerve function (McMahon and Gibson 1986). In rats, many cutaneous afferents in the sural nerve contain the peptide substance P and the enzyme fluoride-resistant acid phosphatase (FRAP), but muscle afferents in the gastrocnemius nerves do not (McMahon et al. 1984). In adult rats these nerves were cut and cross-anastomosed. Electrophysiological experiments revealed that most nerves had regrown along the inappropriate path and formed functional endings in inappropriate tissue. Two thirds of the gastrocnemius nerves which grew along the sural

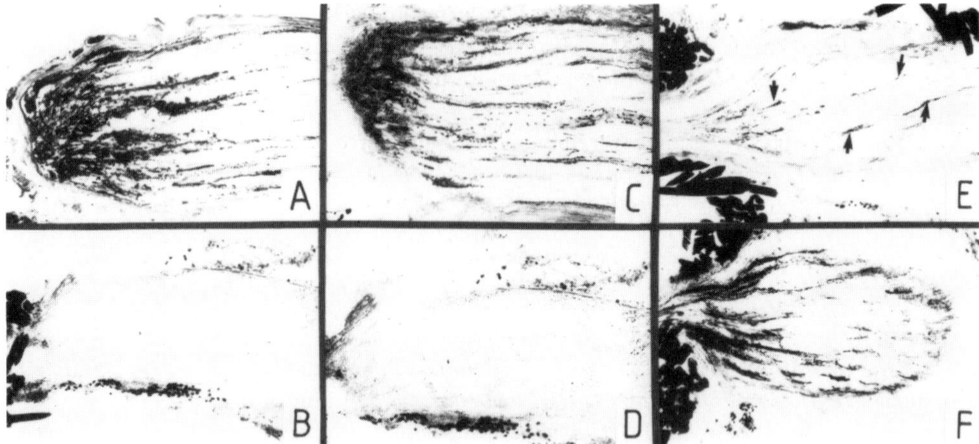

Fig. 4 A, B. Normal sural **(A)** and gastrocnemius **(B)** nerves of rat, immunostained for substance P immunoreactivity, 24 h after ligation (note black threads visible in **B**) . Heavy immunoreactivity is present in **A,** but no fibres are visible in the gastrocnemius. **C, D** Substance P-immunoreactive fibres in the sural nerve **(C)** and gastrocnemius nerve **(D)** following appropriate regeneration of the nerves to innervate their original targets. Much substance P-immunoreactivity is present in the sural nerve but not in the gastrocnemius nerve. **E, F** Sural and gastrocnemius nerves reinnervating inappropriate tissue, i.e. sural directed to muscle **(E)** and gastrocnemius to skin **(F)** . Note marked decrease in immunoreactive staining in **E** compared with **A** and **C** and marked increase in **F** compared with **B** and **D**. All photographs show nerves proximal to the ligature. Magnification x 110. (Courtesy Dr. Sally Gibson)

nerve tract to skin showed many fibres positively stained for substance P-like immunoreactivity and FRAP, in contrast to nerves regrowing appropriately to innervate muscle (Fig. 4). Qualitative assessment showed that peptide levels in sural nerves inappropriately reinnervating muscle were lower than in intact or appropriately reinnervating nerves (McMahon and Gibson 1986).

These results suggest that tissue-specific trophic factors are sampled by unmyelinated afferent nerve fibres and that these can markedly affect the properties of the afferent fibres.

Of the interpretations shown in Fig. 3, we have direct evidence against only 3D. The other options are all possible with, as discussed, varying degrees of likelihood on the basis of indirect evidence. Additionally, they are not all mutually exclusive.

References

Aldskogius H, Risling M (1981) Effect of sciatic neurectomy on neuronal number and size distribution in the L7 ganglion of kittens. Exp Neurol 74: 597–604

Bahr R, Blumberg H, Jänig W (1981) Do dichotomizing afferent fibres exist which supply visceral organs as well as somatic structures? A contribution to the problem of referred pain. Neurosci Lett 24: 25–28

BORGES M, MOSCOWITZ H (1983) Do intracranial and extracranial trigeminal afferents represent divergent axon collaterals. Neurosci Lett 35: 265–270

CHAHL LA (1976) Interactions of bradykinin, prostaglandin E_1, 5-hydroxytryptamine, histamine and adenosine-5-triphosphate on the dye leakage response in rat skin. J Pharm Pharmacol 28: 753–757

CHUNG R, COGGESHALL RE (1984) The ratio of DRG cells to dorsal root axons in sacral segments of the rat. J Comp Neurol 225: 24–30

CLIFTON GL, COGGESHALL RE, VANCE WH, WILLIS WD (1976) Receptive fields of unmyelinated ventral root afferent fibres in the cat. J Physiol (Lond) 256: 573–600

DALSGAARD GJ, RISLING M, CUELLO C (1982) Immunohistochemical localisation of substance P in lumbosacral pia matter and ventral roots of the cat. Brain Res 246: 168–171

DEVOR M, WALL PD, MCMAHON SB (1984) Dichotomizing somatic nerve fibres exist in rats but they are rare. Neurosci Lett 49: 187–192

FITZGERALD M, WOOLF CJ, GIBSON SJ, MALLABURN PS (1984) Alterations in the structure, function and chemistry of C fibres following local application of vinblastine to the sciatic nerve of the rat. J Neurosci 4: 430–441

GOEDERT M, STOECKEL R, OTTEN V (1981) Biological importance of the retrograde axonal transport of nerve growth factor in sensory neurons. Proc Natl Acad Sci USA 78: 5895–5898

JANSCO G, KIRALY E (1983) Cutaneous nerve regeneration in the rat: reinnervation of the denervated skin by regenerative but not collateral sprouting. Neurosci Lett 36: 133–137

JANCSO G, JANCSO-GABOR A, SZOLCSANYI J (1967) Direct evidence for neurogenic inflammation and its prevention by denervation and by pretreatment with capsaicin. Br J Pharmacol Chemother 31: 138–151

JENQ C, COGGESHALL RE (1985) Long-term patterns of axonal regeneration in the sciatic nerve and its tributaries. Brain Res 345: 34–44

KENINS P (1984) Electrophysiological and histological studies of vascular permeability after antidromic sensory nerve stimulation. In: Chahl LA, Szolcsanyi J, Lembeck F (eds) Antidromic vasodilation and neurogenic inflammation. Academaia Kiado, Budapest pp 175–188

KUO DC, YANG GCH, YAMASAKI DS, KRAUTHAMER GM (1982) A wide field electron microscopic analysis of the fibre constituents of the major splanchnic nerve in the cat. J Comp Neurol 210: 49–58

KIM J, CHUNG JM (1985) Electrophysiological evidence for the presence of fibres in continuity between dorsal and ventral roots in the cat. Brain Res 338: 355–359

LANGFORD LA, COGGESHALL RE (1979) Branching of sensory axons in the dorsal root and evidence for the absence of dorsal root efferent fibres. J Comp Neurol 184: 193–204

LANGFORD LA, COGGESHALL RE (1981) Branching of sensory axons in the peripheral nerve of rat. J Comp Neurol 203: 745–750

LAURBERG S, SORENSEN KE (1985) Cervical dorsal root ganglion cells with collaterals to both shoulder skin and the diaphragm. A fluorescent double labelling study in the rat. A model for referred pain? Brain Res 331: 160–163

LEMBECK F, GAMSE R (1982) Substance P in peripheral sensory processes. Ciba Found Symp 91

LEMBECK F, DONNERER J, COLPAERT FC (1981) Increase in substance P in primary afferent nerves during chronic pain. Neuropeptides 1: 175–180

Lewis T (1942) Pain. Macmillan, London

McLachlan EM, Jänig W (1983) The cell bodies of origin of sympathetic and sensory axons in some skin and muscle nerves of the cat hindlimb. J Comp Neurol 214: 115–130

McMahon MS, Nopregaard TV, Deyerl BD, Borges LF, Moscowitz MA (1985) Trigeminal afferents to collateral arteries and forehead are not divergent axon collaterals in cat. Neurosci Lett 60: 63–68

McMahon SB, Gibson S (1987) Peptide expression is altered when afferent nerves reinnervate inappropriate tissue. Neurosci Lett 73 : 9–15

McMahon SB, Wall PD (1985) The distribution and central termination of single cutaneous and muscle unmyelinated fibres in rat spinal cord. Brain Res 359: 39–48

McMahon SB, Wall PD (1986) Physiological evidence for branching of peripheral unmyelinated sensory afferents. J Comp Neurol. In press

McMahon SB, Sykova E, Wall PD, Woolf CJ, Gibson SJ (1984) Neurogenic extravasation and substance P levels are low in muscle as compared to skin in the rat hindlimb. Neurosci Lett 52: 235–240

Mense S, Light A, Perl E (1980) Spinal terminations of subcutaneous high threshold mechanoreceptors. In: Brown AG, Rethelyi M (eds) Spinal cord sensation. Scottish Academic Press, Edinburgh, pp 79–86

Molander C, Grant G (1985) Cutaneous projections from the rat hindlimb foot to the substantia gelatinosa of the spinal cord studied by transganglionic transport of WGA-HRP conjugate. J Comp Neurol 237: 476–484

Pierau F-K, Abel W, Friedrich B (1982) Dichotomizing peripheral fibres revealed by intracellular recording from rat sensory neurones. Neurosci Lett 31: 123–128

Pierau F-K, Fellner G, Taylor DCM (1984) Somatovisceral convergence in cat dorsal root ganglia neurones demonstrated by double labelling with fluorescent traces. Brain Res 321: 63–70

Sweet J, Woolf CJ (1985) The somatotopic organisation of primary afferent terminals in the superficial laminae of the dorsal horn of the rat spinal cord. J Comp Neurol 231: 66–77

Taylor DCM, Pierau F-K (1982) Double fluorescent labelling supports electrophysiological evidence for dichotomizing peripheral sensory nerve fibres in rats. Neurosci Lett 33: 1–6

Tessler A, Himes BT, Krieger NR, Murry M, Goldberger M (1985) Sciatic nerve transection produces death of DRG cells and reversible loss of SP in spinal cord. Brain Res 332. 209–218

Waxman S (1984) Nodelike membrane at extranodal sites: comparative morphology and physiology. In: The node of Ranvier. Academic, New York, pp 311–351

Ygge J, Grant G (1983) The organisation of the thoracic spinal nerve projection in the rat dorsal horn demonstrated with transganglionic transport of horseradish peroxidase. J Comp Neurol 216: 1–9

11 Chemosensitivity of Nerve Sprouts in Experimental Neuroma of Cutaneous Nerves of the Cat

M. Zimmermann and G.-M. Koschorke

Introduction

Neuromas produced experimentally in peripheral nerves of animals have been considered to mimic conditions of clinical pain syndromes which may occur in patients after nerve trauma (Sunderland 1978; Siegfried and Zimmermann 1981). Several laboratories have contributed to the analysis of the conditions of impulse generation in neuromas, using direct electrophysiological recording from the fibers of the neuroma nerve (Korenman and Devor 1981; Scadding 1981; Blumberg and Jänig 1984; Burchiel 1984), or, more indirectly, the behavioral pattern of self-mutilation as an indicator of impulse activity (Wall et al. 1979 a, b; Levitt 1985). Thus, it has been found in mice, rats, cats, and monkeys that the sprouts of regenerating fibers in the neuroma show discharges in response to mechanical stimulation (Blumberg and Jänig 1984), to intravenous or local administration of adrenaline (Korenman and Devor 1981), and to activation of the sympathetic trunk (Devor and Jänig 1981). Ongoing activity was also observed in the absence of obvious intentional stimulation (Govrin-Lippmann and Devor 1978; Scadding 1981; Blumberg and Jänig 1984; Meyer et al. 1985). Our interest was to study the modulation of excitability of neuroma sprouts by chemical substances other than adrenaline and noradrenaline. Here, we report on the excitatory effects of bradykinin and histamine. These substances have long been known to produce pain and/or itch (Keele and Armstrong 1964), to excite sensory receptors in skin, muscle, and viscera, and to be endogenous factors in inflammatory diseases (Armstrong 1970).

Methods

The sural nerve was transected and ligated unilaterally in cats, as far distally as possible on the leg. Surgery was performed under sterile conditions, the animals being anesthetized with pentobarbital sodium (35 or 40 mg/kg intraperitoneally). The animals recovered without complications. No signs of pain or discomfort could be observed: in particular, grooming, scratching, or self-mutilation (autotomy) of the denervated territory, which have been observed in rats following transection of the sciatic nerve (Wall et al., 1979 b; Levitt, 1985), did not occur. This absence of autotomy may have two reasons. First, there are no records of autotomy in cats (Levitt 1985), although no systematic study has been performed. Second, from work in rats it is known that a neuroma of a large nerve (e.g., the sciatic nerve) results in autotomy, whereas a small nerve neuroma (e.g., the saphenous nerve) does not (Wall et al. 1979 b).

Several weeks after the nerve sections animals were again anesthetized (pentobarbital sodium, 35 or 40 mg/kg intraperitoneally, supplemental doses given intravenously if required). The sural nerve was exposed in a pool of mineral oil, and prepared for electrophysiological recording at a site close to its origin from the sciatic nerve. The perineurial sheath around the neuroma was opened or removed and the neuroma was put into a small perspex chamber for continuous superfusion with physiological solution or solutions containing bradykinin, histamine, adrenaline, noradrenaline, or substance P. After superfusions with bradykinin or histamine no other chemical stimuli were given within at least 15 min. A filament was separated from the desheathed proximal part of the nerve for recording of unit action potentials in A and C fibers, which could be identified by electrical nerve stimulation close to the neuroma. In order to have sufficient yield from these time-consuming experiments, filaments were selected containing about 10 C fibers (Fig. 1). Multifiber discharges were counted at 5-s intervals and plotted as histograms.

Results

As the perineurial sheath was still closed by the ligature at the time of neurophysiological analysis we can assume that the sprouts of regenerating fibers had accumulated within the neuroma. After 3 weeks the neuroma had a length of about 3 mm and a largest diameter of 50 % greater than the nerve. Single fibers could be discerned by recording unit action potentials from small nerve filaments in Aβ, Aδ, and C fibers.

In most filaments ongoing activity was seen, usually arising in one or two single C fibers, at discharge rates well below 1 imp/s. No ongoing activity was seen in A fibers. Mechanical probing with Frey hairs before the neuroma was put into the perfusion chamber showed

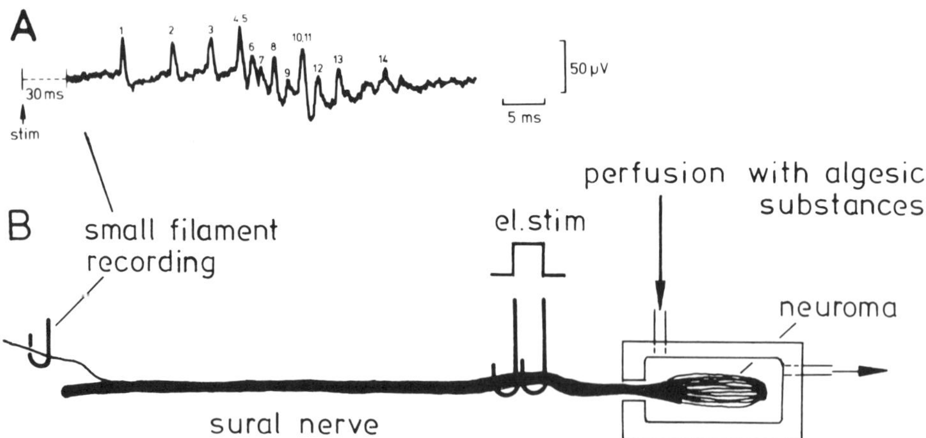

Fig. 1 A, B. Neurophysiological recording of fibers from an experimental neuroma. **A** Oscilloscope display of electrical recording from a small filament dissected out of the sural nerve of a cat after supramaximal electrical stimulation at a more distal site. Unit action potentials can be discriminated; C fibers labeled 1 to 14 are shown. The conduction distance was 40 mm. **B** Experimental arrangement in vivo of the sural nerve which had been transected and ligated some weeks before to produce a neuroma. The neuroma was put into a chamber for superfusion with various solutions. Superfusion at a rate of 0.5 ml/min was maintained by a roller pump

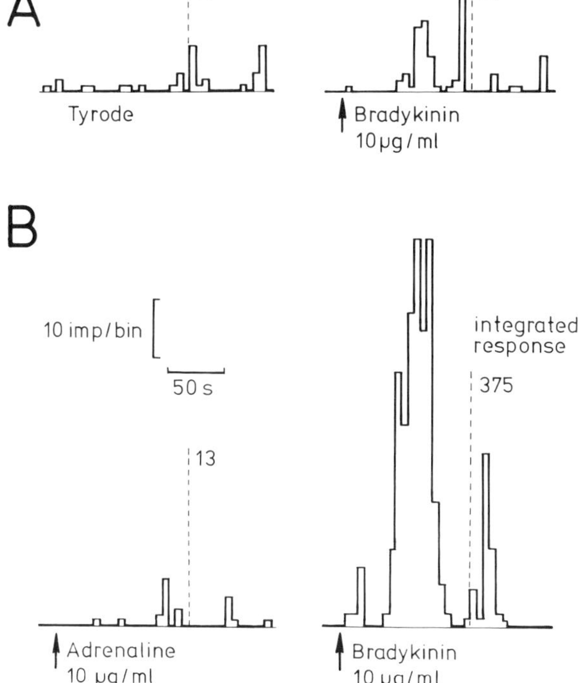

Fig. 2 A, B. Discharges of neuroma fibers evoked and sensitized by chemical substances. **A** Histogram of C-fiber discharges recorded from a multiunit filament during superfusion with Tyrode solution (left) or with solution containing bradykinin at a concentration of 10 μg/ml (right). The numbers at the broken vertical lines indicate the integrated responses during 100–105 s from start of superfusion (arrow). **B** Discharges during superfusion of the neuroma with a solution containing adrenaline, 10 μg/ml (left) or bradykinin, 10 μg/ml, (right). Bradykinin superfusion was started immediately at the end of a 5-min superfusion with adrenaline. Calibrations in **B** hold also for records in **A**

that responses could be elicited in A and C fibers by mild mechanical stimuli. We did not quantify these responses, as they have been extensively studied by others (Wall and Devor 1978; Scadding 1981; Blumberg and Jänig 1984).

Prolonged discharges were elicited in C fibers when the neuroma was irrigated with bradykinin (Fig. 2) or histamine. Usually, the total duration of the evoked discharges was around 60 s. In some of the filaments, repeated periods of discharges appeared during a continuous irrigation with bradykinin, separated by intervals during which the discharge rate could not be distinguished from that recorded before the superfusion with the chemical substance. After exposure to bradykinin or histamine the responding fibers showed prolonged desensitization or tachyphylaxis to a subsequent administration of the same substance, which could last for more than 15 min.

It was a prominent feature of the discharges elicited from the neuroma that they began after a latency between 15 and 125 s from the start of superfusion with bradykinin or histamine. The maximum discharge rate or the total number of impulses elicited during super-

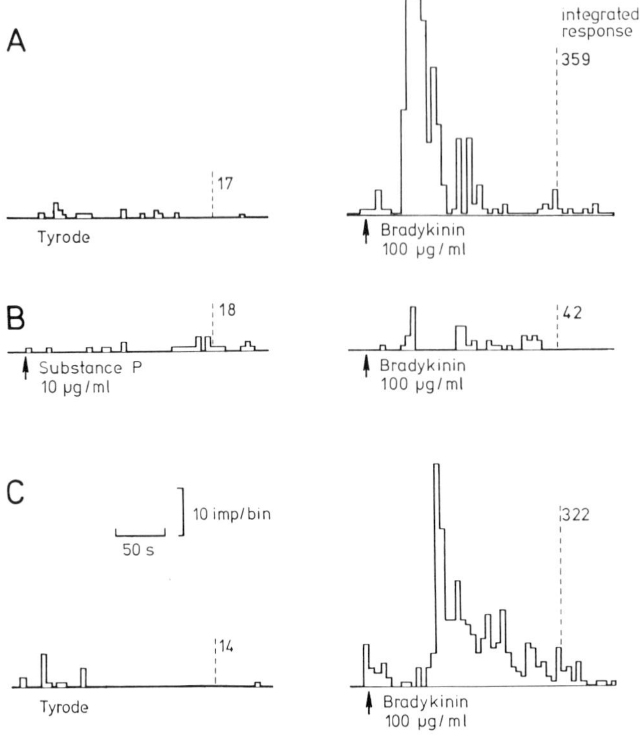

Fig. 3 A, B. Suppression of the bradykinin response in neuroma fibers by substance P. **A** Histograms of C-fiber discharges recorded from a multiunit filament during superfusion of the neuroma with Tyrode solution (left) or a solution containing bradykinin (right) at a concentration of 100 µg/ml. **B** Histograms of the same filament as in **A** during superfusion with a solution containing substance P at 10 µg/ml (left) or bradykinin at 100 µg/ml (right) given after the end of the superfusion with substance P. **C** Histograms of the same filament as in **A** and **B** during superfusion with Tyrode solution (left) or a solution containing bradykinin at 100 µg/ml (right), administered 30 min after the end of the superfusion with substance P shown in **B**. Calibrations in **C** hold for all records. The numbers at the vertical broken lines indicate the integrated responses during periods of 190 s from the starts of superfusions (arrows)

fusion increased dose-dependently. Thresholds of discharges were between 1 and 10 µg/ml superfusion fluid, i.e. between 1 and 10 µM.

The fibers responding to irrigation of the neuroma with bradykinin or histamine were almost exclusively C fibers. Usually, more than one C fiber in a filament responded to the substances. The fibers responding could be identified by displaying the action potentials on a digital storage oscilloscope; various fibers could be discerned by the different shapes of their action potentials. Thus, we found that 26% of all the C fibers contained in the recorded filaments responded to bradykinin, and 16% to histamine. No responses occurred in Aβ fibers to any of the chemical substances used for superfusion. Of 50 Aδ fibers only two responded to bradykinin.

An outstanding feature of the chemosensitivity of fiber sprouts in the neuroma was that responses to bradykinin were greatly facilitated by a preceding superfusion with a solution containing adrenaline or noradrenaline at concentrations of 10 or 100 μg/ml. However, when given alone these catecholamines produced responses only in rare cases, which differs markedly from the findings of other investigators regarding responses to adrenaline and noradrenaline in rat neuroma (Korenman and Devor 1981). An example of the potentiating effect of adrenaline is shown in Fig. 2B. We have seen this enhancement of discharges by one or the other of the catecholamines in the majority of filaments tested in this way. The facilitated responses were greater by up to 10 times the original response; average facilitation of all filaments tested was up to about 5 times the control responses. We have observed that new fibers were recruited in some filaments after the catecholamine superfusion, whereas in others the facilitation was not associated with an increase in the numbers of fibers active. Thus, catecholamine can increase the responsiveness of sprouts to bradykinin, and may also recruit fibers not responding beforehand.

We have also tested the effect of superfusion with substance P preceding bradykinin. Responses to bradykinin were suppressed by substance P at concentrations of 1–100 μg/ml (Fig. 3). Discharges evoked in C fibers by heating the neuroma to 50 °C by irrigation with hot solutions were also suppressed by preceding superfusion with substance P.

Discussion

Our results show that sprouts of regenerating C fibers in cutaneous nerves respond to bradykinin and histamine. The threshold concentrations can be compared with the concentrations of kinins in human plasma, which may rise to 8 μg/ml in pathological conditions (Armstrong 1970). It is likely that the actions of these substances are mediated by specific biochemical receptors for bradykinin and histamine, as fibers in normal or acutely damaged nerve do not respond (Klumpp and Zimmermann, in Zimmermann and Sanders 1982; and unpublished observation).

Bradykinin and histamine are excitants of sensory receptors in skin, muscle, joints, and viscera (Beck and Handwerker 1974; Mense 1977; Mense and Schmidt 1977; Floyd et al. 1977; Kumazawa and Mizumura 1980; Kanaka et al. 1985; Kumazawa et al., this volume), and these excitatory actions have been associated with pain produced by these chemical substances in human subjects (Keele and Armstrong 1964). Therefore, it is conceivable that our results are related to pain originating from a neuroma in patients when algesic substances are present.

We observed significant modifications of responses to bradykinin when the neuroma was superfused beforehand with adrenaline, noradrenaline, or substance P. Remarkable enhancements of responsiveness were induced by superfusion with adrenaline or noradrenaline, although the regenerating sprouts usually did not show responses to these catecholamines alone, except in a few cases. Thus, an interaction between a catecholamine and bradykinin occurs at the sprouts. The underlying mechanisms of this interaction could involve a specific biochemical process at a complex receptor site with binding capabilities for both catecholamines and bradykinin.

Whatever the mechanism is behind the facilitation observed, the phenomenon is reminiscent of the interaction between prostaglandin E 2 or 5-hydroxytryptamine and bradykinin observed at nociceptors of skeletal muscle (Mense 1981). We hypothesize here that facilitatory interactions of two or more neuroactive substances may be a mechanism by which nociceptive nerve endings are sensitized during disease processes involving the release of endogenous substances, such as is known for inflammatory processes.

The phenomena reported here might form part of the pathophysiological functions by which pain due to nerve lesions is enhanced in states of sympathetic activation (Nathan 1983): as regenerating sympathetic efferent (postganglionic) fibers are certainly contained in the neuroma, the catecholamines released during sympathetic activation could have the same facilitatory effect as we have observed upon irrigation of the neuroma with exogenous adrenaline or noradrenaline. Interestingly, excitatory effects of sympathetic trunk stimulation have been observed in experimental neuroma of the rat (Devor and Jänig 1981).

Suppression by substance P of discharges evoked from the neuroma by bradykinin or noxious heating is an unexpected effect, as substance P was considered a pain-producing substance previously, before synthetic substance P was available (Keele and Armstrong 1964). More recently, substance P released from sensory nerve endings in the skin and viscera was found to be the mediator of neurogenic inflammation and related phenomena (Chahl et al. 1984). Functionally, neurogenic inflammation can be considered a regulatory response to counteract the trauma eliciting it. As we know that substance P is released from neuroma sprouts (Koschorke et al. 1985), suppression of afferent activity in neuroma sprouts might have a similar regulatory function. Further studies will hopefully contribute to a better understanding of the functional significance of the phenomena we have reported here.

Acknowledgements. The authors are grateful to Hannelore Ehlers for typing the manuscript and Almuth Manisali for the graphics. This work is being supported by the Deutsche Forschungsgemeinschaft (Grant Zi 110).

References

Armstrong D (1970) Pain. In: Eichler O, Farah A, Herken H, Welch AD (eds) Handbook of experimental pharmacology, vol 25. Springer Berlin, pp 434–473

Beck PW, Handwerker HO (1974) Bradykinin and serotonin effects on various types of cutaneous nerve fibers. Pflugers Arch 347 : 209–222

Blumberg H, Jänig W (1984) Discharge pattern of afferent fibers from a neuroma. Pain 20 : 335–353

Burchiel KJ (1984) Spontaneous impulse generation in normal and denervated dorsal root ganglia: sensitivity to alphaadrenergic stimulation and hypoxia. Exp Neurol 85 : 257–272

Chahl LA, Szolcsanyi J, Lembeck F (eds) (1984) Antidromic vasodilatation and neurogenic inflammation. Akademiai Kiado, Budapest

Devor M, Jänig W (1981) Activation of myelinated afferents ending in a neuroma by stimulation of the sympathetic supply in the rat. Neurosci Lett 24 : 43–47

Floyd K, Hick VE, Koley J, Morrison JFB (1977) The effects of bradykinin on afferent units in intra-abdominal sympathetic nerve trunks. QJ Exp Physiol 62 : 19–25

Govrin-Lippmann R, Devor M (1978) Ongoing activity in severed nerves: source and variation with time. Brain Res 159 : 406–410

Kanaka R, Schaible H-G, Schmidt RF (1985) Activation of fine articular afferent units by bradykinin. Brain Res 327 : 81–90

Keele CA, Armstrong D (1964) Substances producing pain and itch. Arnold, London

Korenmann EMD, Devor M (1981) Ectopic adrenergic sensitivity in damaged peripheral nerve axon in the rat. Exp Neurol 72 : 63–81

Koschorke GM, Helme RD, Zimmermann M (1985) Substance P suppresses the response to bradykinin and to heat of nonmyelinated fibers in experimental neuroma of the cat's sural nerve. Soc Neurosci Abstr 11 : 118

Kumazawa T, Mizumura K (1980) Chemical responses of polymodal receptors of the scrotal contents in dogs. J Physiol (Lond) 299 : 219–231

Levitt M (1985) Dysesthesias and self-mutilation in humans and subhumans: a review of clinical and experimental studies. Brain Res 10 : 247–290

Mense S (1977) Nervous outflow from skeletal muscle following chemical noxious stimulation. J Physiol (Lond) 267 : 75–88

Mense S (1981) Sensitization of group IV muscle receptors to bradykinin by 5-hydroxytryptamine and prostaglandin E2. Brain Res 225 : 95–105

Mense S, Schmidt RF (1977) Muscle pain: which receptors are responsible for the transmission of noxious stimuli? In: Clifford Rose F (ed) Physiological aspects of clinical neurology. Blackwell, Oxford, pp 265–278

Meyer RA, Raja SN, Campbell JN, Mackinnon SE, Dellon AL (1985) Neural activity originating from a neuroma in the baboon. Brain Res 325 : 255–260

Nathan PW (1983) Pain and the sympathetic nervous system. In: Yokota T, Dubner R (eds) Current topics in pain research and therapy. Excerpta Medica, Amsterdam, pp241–247

Scadding JW (1981) The development of ongoing activity, mechanosensitivity and adrenaline sensitivity in severed peripheral nerve axons. Exp Neurol 73 : 345–364

Siegfried J, Zimmermann M (1981) Phantom and stump pain. Springer, Berlin

Sunderland S (1978) Nerves and nerve injuries. Churchill Livingstone, London

Wall PD, Devor M (1978) Physiology of sensation after peripheral nerve injury, regeneration and neuroma formation. In: Waxman SJ (ed) Physiology and pathobiology of axons. Raven, New York, pp 377–388

Wall PD, Scadding JW, Tomkiewicz MM (1979 a) The production and prevention of experimental anesthesia dolorosa. Pain 6 : 175–182

Wall PD, Devor M, Inbal R, Scadding JW, Schonfeld D, Seltzer Z, Tomkiewicz MM (1979 b) Autotomy following peripheral nerve lesions: experimental anesthesia dolorosa. Pain 7 : 103–113

Zimmermann M, Sanders K (1982) Responses of nerve axons and receptor endings to heat, ischemia and algesic substances. In: Culp WJ, Ochoa J (eds) Abnormal nerves and muscles as impulse generators. Oxford University Press, New York, pp 513–532

12 Comparison Between Human Subjective Ratings and Response Properties of Cat Intradental Fine Afferents to Cold Stimulation of Teeth

E. Jyväsjärvi and K.-D. Kniffki

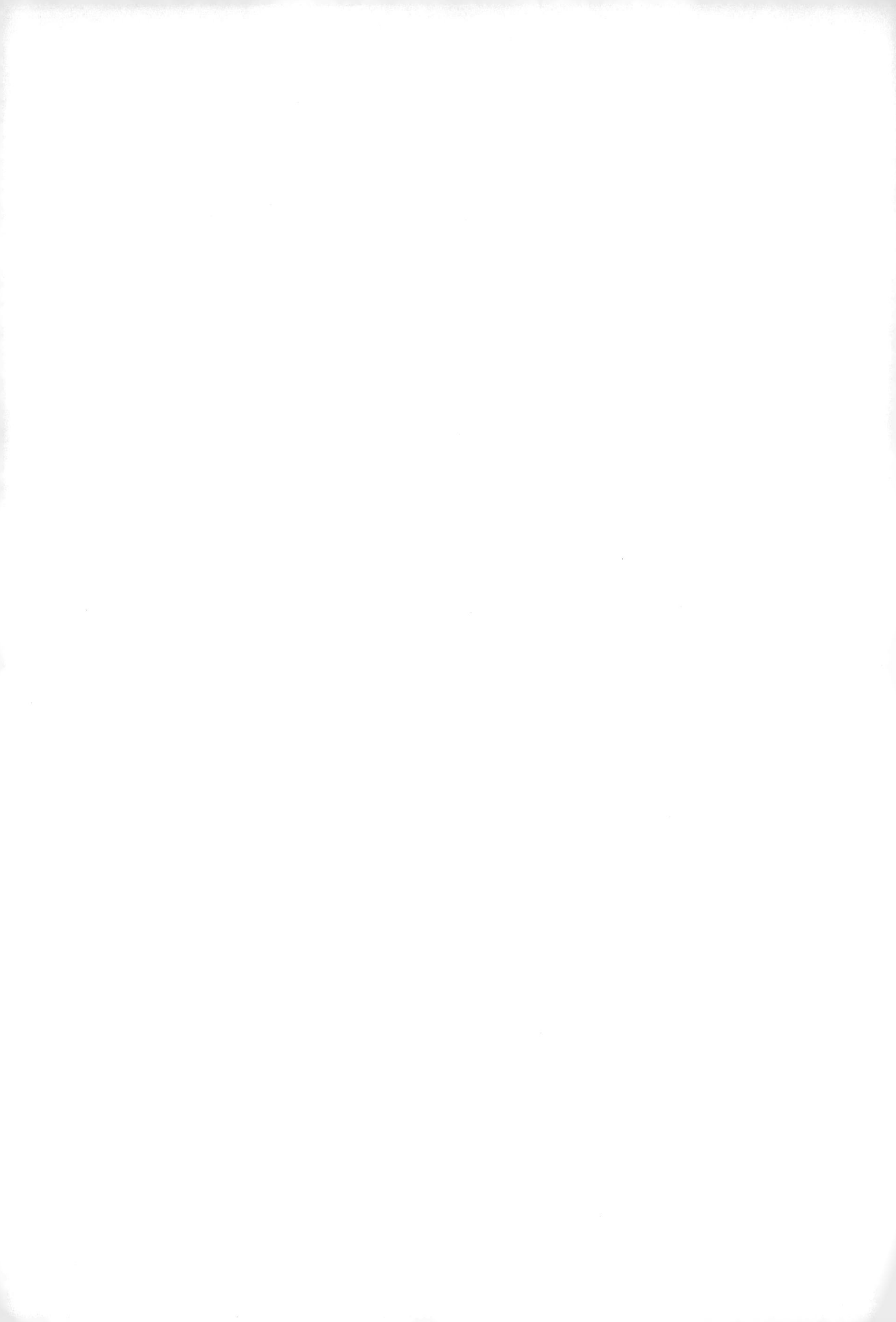

Introduction

It has been observed that if a tooth is subjected to cold, a painful sensation will result, whose quality obviously depends on the intensity of the stimulus (Hensel and Mann 1956) but is usually described as sharp and stabbing (Naylor 1964; Trowbridge et al. 1980). Ahlquist et al. (1984) have found that the pain evoked by cold stimulation of the tooth in human subjects correlates with the electrical activity recorded from the dentine of the same tooth. Such a dentine recording technique is said to pick up the neuronal discharges of Aδ fibres (Haegerstam 1976).

In animal experiments, recordings of the activity of intradental afferent fibres evoked by cold stimulation of the tooth are rare (Wagers and Smith 1960; Funakoshi and Zotterman 1963; Yamada et al. 1968; Matthews 1977; Kollmann and Matthews 1982; Närhi et al. 1982) and no clear description of the response behaviour of intradental afferent Aδ and C fibres to cold stimulation of the tooth has been given. Also, the contribution of these two different fibre types to the perceived dental pain is unknown.

The aim of the present study was to record the neuronal discharges of single intradental afferent Aδ and C fibres to cold stimulation of the tooth in cats and compare the responses with the perceived sensation in humans using similar stimulating conditions.

Methods

Animal Experiments

The experiments were carried out on 29 adult cats initially anaesthetized with an intraperitoneal injection of pentobarbitone sodium. The right femoral artery and vein were cannulated for measurement of blood pressure and administration of injections. The trachea was cannulated to allow undisturbed ventilation. Anaesthesia was subsequently maintained by intravenous injections of the same anaesthetic. Arterial blood pressure and body core temperature were monitored and kept within normal physiological limits.

The mandible was fixed to the maxilla in an open position using self-curing dental acrylic between the upper and lower posterior teeth. The lower margin of the left mandible was removed posterior to the mental foramen and the inferior alveolar nerve lying in the bony canal was exposed, freed from the connective tissue and cut as far proximally as possible. A pool was formed out of the skin flaps and filled with paraffin oil at 37 °C.

The crown of the left lower canine tooth was cleaned, dried and isolated from the surrounding tissue using a Teflon plate cemented around the neck of the tooth (Fig. 1A). A polyethylene tube was fitted over the tip of the crown and fixed with dental acrylic so that

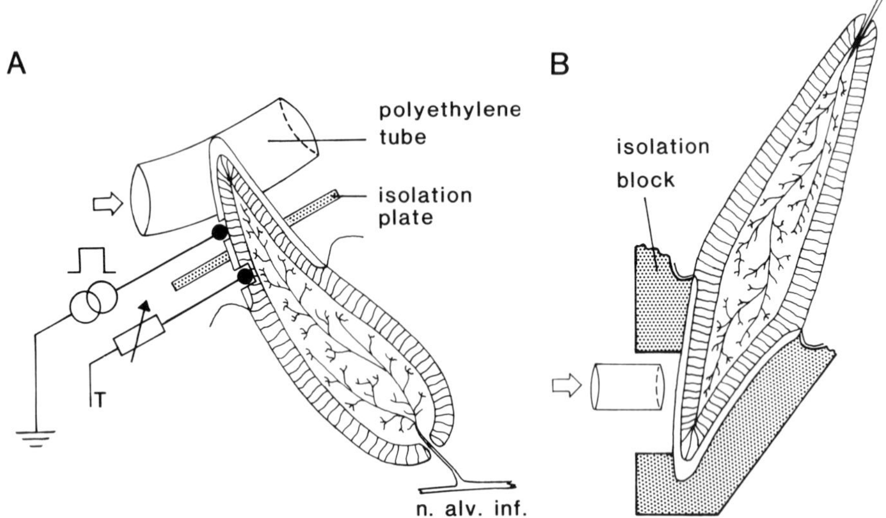

Fig. 1 A, B. Schematic illustration of the experimental arrangements for animal **(A)** and human **(B)** studies. **A** The lower canine tooth of the cat. By monopolar electrical stimulation of the tooth using a constant current stimulator, single intradental nerve fibres were identified from fine afferent filaments split from the inferior alveolar nerve (n. alv. inf.). For cold stimulation, an area of the tooth was isolated from the surrounding tissue and dichlorodifluoromethane (Frigen-12, Provotest) as a cold spray was guided (arrows) through a polyethylene tube to the stimulation area. In animal experiments the temperature of the tooth near the pulp was recorded with a thermistor (T)

approximately 15% of the surface area of the crown was within the tube. To measure the temperature near the pulp, a thermistor probe was sealed into a deep cavity drilled proximal to the plate (Fig. 1A). Another cavity, just penetrating the enamel layer, was drilled between the tube and the plate. A platinum wire electrode was inserted into the cavity for electrical stimulation of the tooth; the indifferent electrode was attached to the ipsilateral lower lip. The impedance of this circuit varied between 30 and 120 kΩ, while that along the dried enamel surface and over the plate exceeded 10 MΩ.

Neuronal activity was recorded extracellularly from fine filaments split from the cut end of the nerve using platinum wire electrodes; it was amplified, filtered, displayed on an oscilloscope, audiomonitored and stored on magnetic tape.

Functional single units were identified by cathodal square wave current pulses applied to the tooth using a constant current stimulator. The responding fibres were classified as Aδ fibres if their conduction velocity was between 2.5 and 30.0 m/s, and as C fibres if it was below 2.5 m/s. After identification, the response behaviour of the fibres to rapid cooling of the tooth was studied by applying volatile dichlorodifluoromethane fluid (Frigen-12, Provotest) as a cold spray through the tube. Stimulus duration, tooth temperature, and response latency and duration were recorded. In 11 experiments, after several cold stimuli the pulp was exposed and the receptive fields to mechanical stimulation were determined for Aδ and C fibres.

Human Experiments

Seven volunteers (four female and three male) participated in the experiments. Altogether 10 intact upper central incisors and one devitalized lateral one with a root filling were isolated from the surrounding oral tissue by a block made of dental impression material (Fig. 1B). A hole was cut into the block, exposing about 15% of the surface of the tooth crown to be tested.

The subjects were trained to estimate the magnitude of the perceived pain sensation evoked by cold stimulation of the tooth by using a 50-point categorical division procedure according to Göbel and Westphal (1984): 0, no pain; 1–10, very weak pain; 11–20, weak pain; 21–30, moderate pain; 31–40, strong pain; 41–50, very strong pain; above 50, intolerable pain. Recordings of the ratings were obtained with a hand-driven potentiometer, whose output voltage was displayed on an oscilloscope and stored on magnetic tape. The cold stimulus to the human tooth was the same as that used in the animal experiments. The root-filled tooth served as a control for stimulus spread. The test teeth were stimulated four to five times at intervals of several minutes. Stimulus duration and response latency and duration were recorded. The quality of the sensation was ascertained after every stimulation.

Results

Animal Experiments

A total of 86 single intradental nerve fibres were isolated. Of these 43 were classified as Aδ fibres with a mean conduction velocity (c.v.) of 13.9 ± S.D. 6.4 m/s (range: 3.6–26.0 m/s) and 43 as C fibres with an average c.v. of 1.3 ± 0.5 m/s (range: 0.5–2.2 m/s). The mean electrical threshold using 1-ms cathodal current pulses was 62.3 ± 41.1 μA (range: 10–180 μA) for Aδ fibres and 104.4 ± 53.7 μA (range: 25–200 μA) for C fibres. None of the intradental fibres showed an ongoing discharge unless being stimulated.

Of the 43 Aδ fibres, 36 responded to the cold stimulus used. A typical example of a response of an Aδ fibre to cold stimulation of the tooth is given in Fig. 2A. The fibre started to fire at a high rate as the tooth temperature (lower trace) rapidly decreased. The discharge rate fell as the rate of change of temperature became smaller and the firing stopped completely as the temperature reached a steady level. No firing occurred as the temperature of the tooth returned to the initial value.

This response behaviour was rather uniform for all cold-sensitive Aδ fibres. The mean stimulus duration to evoke a response was 2.0 ± 1.1 s (range: 0.3–4.5 s) and the average response latency was 1.7 ± 1.1 s (range: 0.1–3.9 s). At that time the mean temperature decrease was 4.9 ± 3.6 °C (range: 0.1–12.6 °C) starting from a mean initial value of

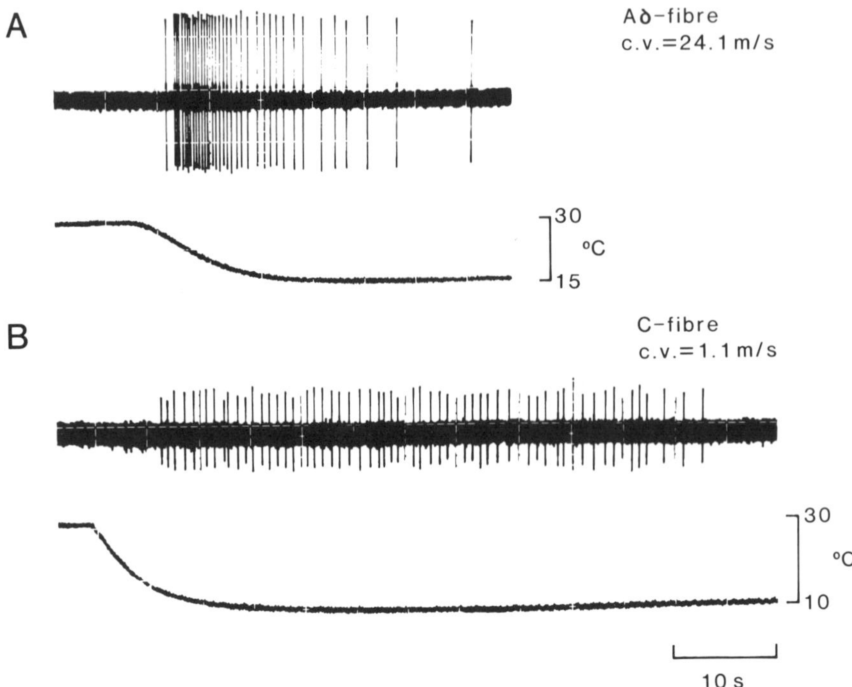

Fig. 2 A, B. Responses of an intradental Aδ fibre **(A)** and a C fibre **(B)** to cold stimulation of the tooth in the cat. The calculated conduction velocity (c.v.) is indicated at the upper right corner of both recordings. The lower traces represent the recorded temperature near the pulp

29.2 ± 1.7 °C (range: 26.1-33.7 °C). The mean duration of the responses was 21.0 ± 9.2 s (range: 3-42 s). A good correlation (r = 0.89) was found between the initially high discharge rate of the Aδ fibres and the maximum temperature change.

Of the 43 intradental C fibres, 38 were sensitive to cold stimulation of the tooth. However, their response behaviour was completely different from that of the Aδ fibres. Figure 2B shows an example of the discharge pattern of C fibres. The recorded fibre started to fire regularly without any dynamic response component after a long latency when the rate of change of tooth temperature was already very small. It continued to discharge as the temperature reached a steady level. The firing stopped soon after the temperature started to rise and did not reappear as the temperature returned to the initial level.

The mean stimulus duration to evoke a response was 6.3 ± 1.7 s (range: 3.3–10.0 s) and the average latency was 7.3 ± 2.5 s (range: 3.9–13.0 s). At that time the mean tooth temperature had decreased to 10.1 ± 3.2 °C (range: 18.4-7.2 °C). On average the response lasted 52.0 ± 15.5 s (range: 25-93 s). The firing rate of the C fibres was independent of the rate of change of tooth temperature, but had a weak correlation (r = 0.6) to the end temperature achieved, i.e. at lower temperatures the firing rate was higher.

After repeatedly eliciting responses to cold stimuli, the receptive fields of four Aδ and seven C fibres were determined by mechanical stimulation of the exposed pulp tissue. Those of Aδ fibres were located superficially at the pulp-dentine border, whereas those of C fibres were much deeper in the pulp tissue and tended to have higher activation thresholds.

Human experiments

The subjects described the sensation evoked by cold stimulation of their teeth as a sharp, shooting pain, which could strictly be localized in the tooth being tested. Stimulation of the devitalized tooth did not evoke any sensation. Sensations other than pain were not perceived. Figure 3 shows three superimposed recordings of the ratings of the perceived pain sensation to cold stimulation of a tooth in one particular human subject. After a short latency, the intensity of the perceived pain rapidly increased within a few seconds to a maximum and then gradually decreased to zero. Sometimes, in the declining phase of the rating curves, a shoulder was seen, where the rate of decrease in the pain intensity was reduced for a few seconds.

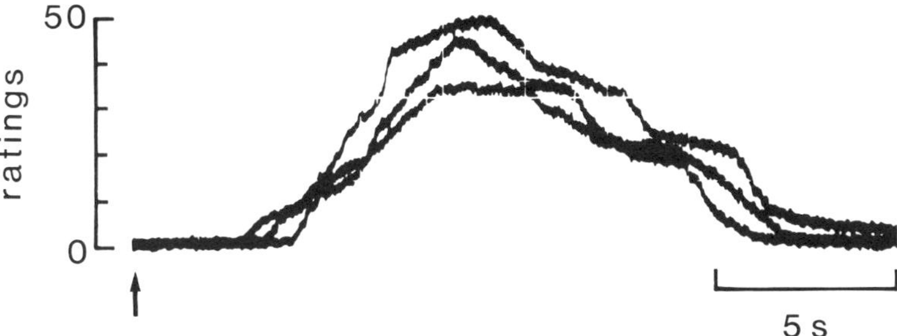

Fig. 3. Ratings of the perceived pain sensation to cold stimulation of a tooth in a human subject. The recordings were obtained by displaying the output voltage of the hand-driven potentiometer on an oscilloscope screen. The arrow indicates the onset of stimulation, which was continued until the subject indicated a response. Rating scale: 0, no sensation; 50, maximum tolerable pain (see text for details). Three ratings are superimposed

The mean stimulus duration to evoke a pain sensation was 3.2 ± 1.6 s (range: 1.0–8.0 s) and the average response latency was 1.5 ± 1.0 s (range: 0.2–6.0 s). The mean duration of the perceived pain was 13.3 ± 4.6 s (range: 6–25 s). The shoulder phase was present in 16 of the 43 trials.

Figure 4 summarizes the results, showing the mean ratings of the perceived pain sensations in human subjects (A) and the mean responses of cat intradental Aδ fibres (B) and C fibres (C) to cold stimulation of the tooth.

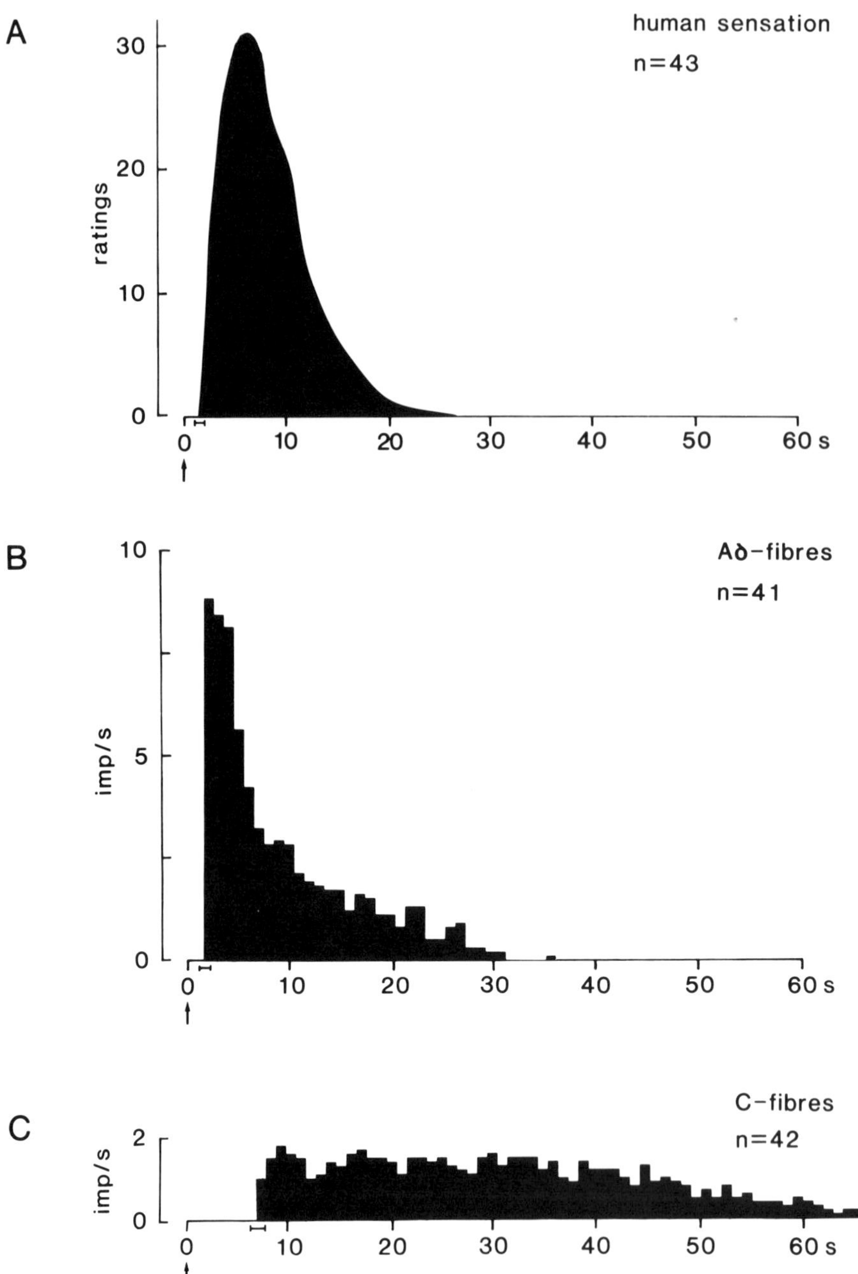

Fig. 4 A–C. Comparison of human pain ratings with the discharges evoked in cat intradental Aδ and C fibres by cold stimulation of the tooth. **A** The mean values of the ratings of 43 trials in ten teeth of seven human subjects. **B** The mean post-stimulus time histogram (bin width 1 s) of the evoked discharges (impulses per second) of 41 trials for 36 Aδ fibres. **C** A similar histogram of the responses of 42 trials for 38 C fibres. Onset of stimulation is marked by the arrows. The short bar under the abscissa indicates ± S.E. of the mean response latency after stimulus onset

Discussion

In the present study the neuronal discharges of intradental fine afferent fibres of the cat and the dental pain sensations in humans in response to cold stimulation of teeth were compared. In spite of the species differences, the similarities in morphological structure of human incisors and cat canines (Byers et al. 1982) justifies this comparison.

The cold stimulus applied to the lower canine tooth of the cat activated most of the identified intradental fibres. This is in contrast to previous reports in which the number of cold-sensitive fibres was reported to be small (Wagers and Smith 1960; Funakoshi and Zotterman 1963; Yamada et al. 1968; Matthews 1977; Kollmann and Matthews 1982; Närhi et al. 1982; Närhi 1985). This difference might be due to the different methods of stimulation used. The cold spray used in the present study is much more effective than ethylchloride, which was used in most of the previous studies.

None of the recorded Aδ fibres showed an ongoing discharge without intentional stimulation. They responded well to cold stimuli while the temperature of the tooth was being reduced, but did not respond when the temperature of the tooth was kept at a constant reduced level. This is in contrast to the properties of cutaneous cold receptors (cf. Hensel 1976) and makes it unlikely that the recorded Aδ fibres innervate thermoreceptors. Some of the recorded Aδ fibres were tested additionally by mechanical stimulation of the exposed pulp tissue at the pulp-dentine border. Their low thresholds to mechanical stimulation suggest that the cold stimulus could have indirectly activated the receptive structures of the Aδ fibres. Brännström and Johnson (1970) have shown that thermal stimuli cause fluid movements in dentinal tubules in vitro and propose that these movements could excite the mechanosensitive receptors of the peripheral pulp.

Most of the recorded C fibres were also sensitive to cold stimulation of the tooth and, like the Aδ fibres, did not show ongoing discharge without intentional stimulation. The C fibres responded to static low temperatures with a regular discharge. Their discharge rate correlated weakly with the static tooth temperature achieved. These response properties are similar to the ones described for cutaneous high-threshold cold receptors (LaMotte and Thalhammer 1982). The high-threshold cold receptors in the skin are insensitive to mechanical stimulation. For some of the cold-responsive dental C fibres, the receptive field for mechanical stimulation was found to be located deep in the pulp and their activation thresholds were higher than for Aδ fibres. The profound difference between C fibres and Aδ fibres in their responsiveness to cold stimulation of the tooth they are innervating may partly be due to the deeper location of the receptive elements of the former.

In human experiments, in almost all cases a cold stimulus similar to the one used in the animal experiments evoked only a sharp, shooting pain sensation. This is in agreement with the studies by Naylor (1964), Trowbridge et al. (1980) and Ahlquist et al. (1984), but contradicts the findings of Grüsser et al. (1982). These latter authors report cold perception also in human teeth. In the present experiments, due to the rapid cooling of the tooth the evoked pain perception might have masked cold perception. If this intradental cold perception is present at all, then, based on their response behaviour, it is likely that the cold-sensitive C fibres could be involved, if the tooth is cooled very slowly in order not to excite the intradental Aδ fibres.

Comparing the required stimulus intensity, the response latency, the response duration and the time course of the ratings of human subjects with the response characteristics of cat intradental Aδ and C fibres to cold stimulation of the tooth, it is tempting to suggest that the sharp, pricking dental pain sensation is predominantly due to activity in intradental Aδ fibres.

Summary

In the present study the neuronal responses of cat intradental fine afferent fibres to cold stimulation of the tooth were compared to cold-evoked dental pain in human subjects.

The results indicated that most of the intradental Aδ and C fibres are sensitive to the cold stimulus used. The recorded Aδ fibres responded with a short latency and their initial dynamic firing rate correlated with the maximum rate of change of temperature. In contrast, the C fibres were activated after a longer latency and their regular firing rate had a weak correlation with the static end temperature.

A comparison of the time course of the subjective ratings of the cold-evoked dental pain in humans with the response properties of cat intradental afferent Aδ and C fibres suggests that the activation of Aδ fibres is responsible for the sharp pain sensation evoked by rapid cooling of a tooth in man.

Acknowledgements. The authors wish to thank Mrs. C. Erhard, Mrs. P. Haumann, and Mrs. M. Schulze for technical assistance. This study was supported by the Wilhelm Sander-Stiftung (grant 83.018.1/2).

References

Ahlquist ML, Edwall LGA, Franzén OG, Haegerstam GAT (1984) Perception of pulpal pain as a function of intradental nerve activity. Pain 19 : 353–368

Brännström M, Johnson G (1970) Movements of the dentine and pulp liquids on application of thermal stimuli. An in vitro study. Acta Odontol Scand 28 : 59–70

Byers MR, Neuhaus SJ, Gierik JD (1982) Dental sensory receptor structure in human teeth. Pain 13 : 221–235

Funakoshi M, Zotterman Y (1963) A study in the excitation of dental pulp nerve fibres. In: Anderson DJ (ed) Sensory mechanisms of dentine. Pergamon, Oxford, pp 60–70

Göbel H, Westphal W (1984) Pain ratings and handedness. Pflügers Arch 404 : R38

Grüsser OJ, Kollmann W, Mijatović E (1982) Evidence for cold perception from human teeth. In: Matthews B, Hill RG (eds) Anatomical, physiological and pharmacological aspects of trigeminal pain. Excerpta Medica, Amsterdam, pp 77–95

Haegerstam G (1976) The origin of impulses recorded from dentinal cavities in the tooth of the cat. Acta Physiol Scand 97 : 121–128

Hensel H (1976) Correlations of neural activity and thermal sensation in man. In: Zotterman Y (ed) Sensory functions of the skin in primates. Pergamon, Oxford, pp 331–352

Hensel H, Mann G (1956) Temperaturschmerz und Wärmeleitung im menschlichen Zahn. Stoma 9 : 76–85

Kollmann W, Matthews B (1982) Responses of intradental nerves to thermal stimulation of teeth in the cat. In: Matthews B, Hill RG (eds) Anatomical, physiological and pharmacological aspects of trigeminal pain. Excerpta Medica, Amsterdam, pp 51–65

LaMotte RH, Thalhammer JG (1982) Response properties of high-threshold cutaneous cold receptors in the primate. Brain Res 244 : 279–287

Matthews B (1977) Responses of intradental nerves to electrical and thermal stimulation of teeth in dogs. J Physiol (Lond) 264 : 641–664

Närhi MVO (1985) The characteristics of intradental sensory units and their responses to stimulation. J Dent Res 64 : 564–571

Närhi MVO, Hirvonen TJ, Hakumäki MOK (1982) Activation of intradental nerves in the dog to some stimuli applied to the dentine. Arch Oral Biol 27 : 1053–1058

Naylor MN (1964) Studies on sensation to cold stimulation in human teeth. Br Dent J 117 : 482–486

Trowbridge HO, Franks M, Korostoff E, Emling R (1980) Sensory response to thermal stimulation in human teeth. J Endodontics 6 : 405–412

Wagers PW, Smith CM (1960) Responses in dental nerves of dogs to tooth stimulation and the effect of systemically administered procaine, lidocaine and morphine. J Pharmacol Exp Ther 130 : 84–105

Yamada M, Suzuta K, Higuchi H (1968) Sensitivity of the tooth to thermal stimulation. Jpn J Physiol 18 : 310–325

13 Uterine Afferent Fibers in the Rat

K. J. Berkley, A. Robbins, and Y. Sato

As discussed by Kumazawa (1986), little information exists regarding the sensory supply of the uterus. The few studies published so far have demonstrated that uterine afferent fibers exist in the hypogastric nerve of the rabbit and cat and that they are predominantly unmyelinated and responsive to mechanical stimulation of the uterus and broad ligament (Bower 1959, 1966; Abrahams and Teare 1969; Floyd et al. 1976). Although units responsive to cervical probing have been observed in the pelvic nerve of the rat (Komisaruk et al. 1972), other studies have questioned the existence of uterine afferents in this nerve (e. g. Bower 1966). Accordingly, the purpose of the present study was to determine by anatomical means whether uterine afferents exist in both of these nerves in the rat and, if so, to examine some of their mechanoreceptive and chemoreceptive response properties. The work was done on 48 Wistar strain rats, 3–12 months old.

Methods and Results

Anatomical Study of Route to Spinal Cord.

Pelvic nerve afferent fibers in the rat enter the spinal cord through the L5-S1 dorsal roots (Nadelhaft and Booth 1984), whereas hypogastric nerve afferent fibers enter through the T10-L4 roots (Neuhuber 1982). Because of this separation, examination of the segments through which uterine afferents enter the spinal cord should provide evidence as to whether they travel in one or both nerves. Accordingly, the wall of the body of the uterus of four rats was multiply injected bilaterally with a total of 10 μl of a 50 % solution of Sigma type VI horseradish peroxidase (HRP). Leakage of HRP to nearby organs was minimized by immediately wiping up excess solution during the injection process and covering the injection tracks with small pieces of dissected fat. (The injection site was located as illustrated in Fig. 1.) Following 45- to 72-h survival, dorsal root ganglia T13-S4 on both sides were examined for the presence of HRP-labeled ganglion cells, using tetramethyl benzidine as a chromogen.

Figure 1 illustrates the results. Although relatively few in number (4 – 36 per ganglion), labeled ganglion cells were consistently observed in the L1-S1 ganglia. They ranged in diameter from 25 μm to 60 μm and were bimodally distributed, one group centered around L2, the other around L6. These results indicate that uterine afferent fibers travel to the spinal cord in the rat via the pelvic as well as the hypogastric nerve.

The projections of uterine afferent fibers were also studied in three other rats whose uteri were abnormal because their light-dark cycle had inadvertently been disrupted. A **total** of only three labeled ganglion cells were observed in these rats.

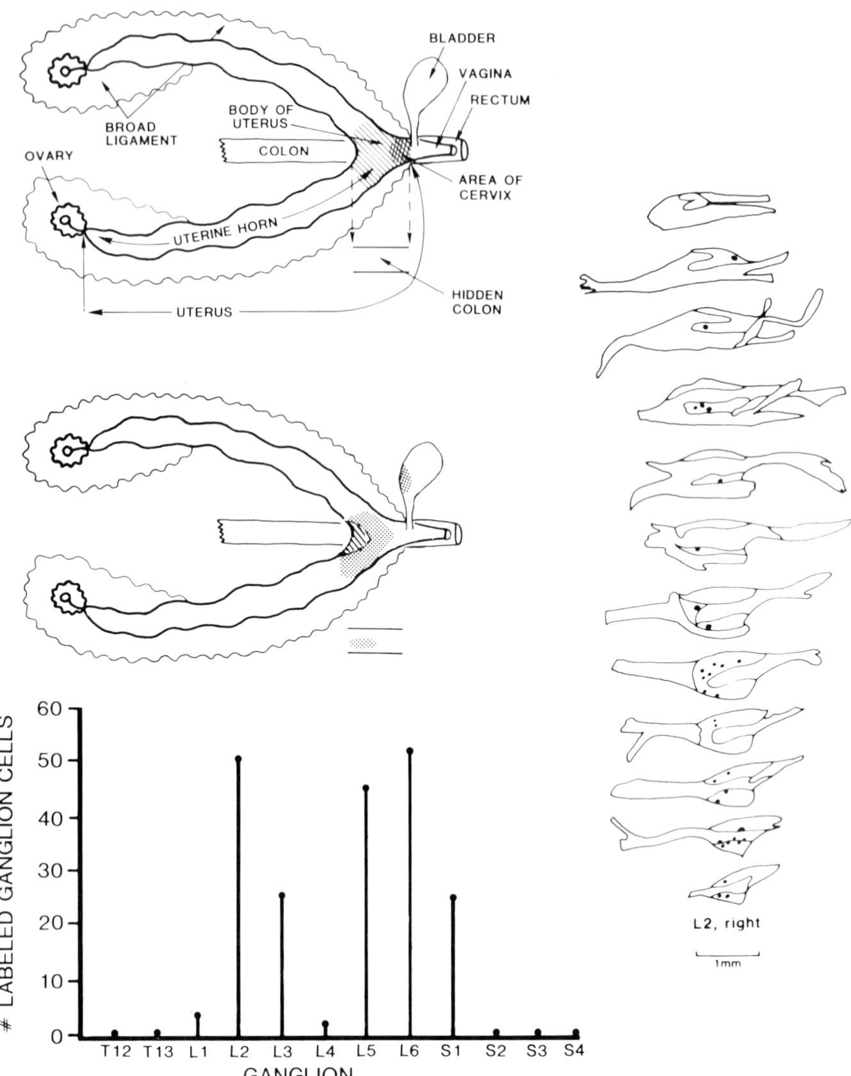

Fig. 1. Labeling of dorsal root ganglion cells following injections of HRP into the wall of the body of the uterus. The labeled diagram at the top, provided for orientation, presents a view of the ventral surface of the uterus and adjacent pelvic viscera, with the bladder retracted to expose the body of the uterus. The middle diagram depicts the HRP injection site in one rat. The shaded part indicates the injection site on the ventral surface; the hatched area, the dorsal surface. Note that although the injection site in this rat extended slightly into adjacent parts of the bladder and colon, the results were virtually identical to those from two other rats whose injections had not invaded adjacent viscera. (The injection site was characterized by localizing the dark-brown reaction product produced by soaking the dissected pelvic viscera in a solution of diaminobenzidine immediately following perfusion.) The column on the right illustrates the labeled ganglion cells (dots) observed in serial 50-µm-thick sections taken through the right L2 ganglion of the rat whose injection site is illustrated. The histogram at the bottom presents the total number of labeled ganglion cells observed in each ganglion from both sides of all four of the rats studied (i. e., **n** = 8 for each ganglion). Note the bimodal distribution of ganglion cell labeling, a finding which was consistent for each rat

Responses to Mechanical Stimulation of the Uterus of Fibers in the Hypogastric nerve

Responses were studied in vivo from 12 single units and 11 multiunits in nerve strands teased from the distal end of the cut nerve in 17 virgin rats maintained on a 12 : 12 light-dark cycle and anesthestized IP with sodium pentobarbital or its mixture with chloral hydrate.

The receptive fields of all units were confined to small portions of the uterus and/or broad ligament, never extending to other pelvic viscera. Most fields contained the cervix part of the body of the uterus (crosshatched area on Fig. 1, top left). Effective stimuli were external probing, stretching, and, in the few cases tested, intraluminal distension. The stimuli were delivered at pressure levels that, although innocuous when tested on human skin, usually produced visible, temporary ischemia at the uterine stimulation site (Fig. 2B, top unit). However, gentle rubbing sometimes produced a response (Fig. 2A, area 2).

Responses varied in two ways as a function of the status of the uterus. First, areas that had been surgically prepared for stimulation were particularly sensitive (Fig. 2A, area 1; Fig. 2B, bottom unit). Second, of the 17 rats used, seven were in estrus at the time of recording (as determined by vaginal smear) and six were in other stages. (The other four rats were in unknown stages.) The hypogastric nerve appeared more "sensitive" in the rats in estrus than in the rats in other stages. This difference was evidenced by comparing the number of single units and multiunits responsive to uterine stimulation that were obtained in the two groups (13 for rats in estrus, six for others), the ratio of single unit to multiunit records (9 : 4 for estrus, 1 : 5 for other stages), and percentages of receptive fields that were smaller than 1 cm^2 (69 % of the 13 units from the seven rats in estrus, 33 % of the six units from the other six rats).

Responses to Algesic and Other Chemical Stimuli in the Hypogastric and Pelvic Nerves

Responses were obtained from 11 single and nine multiunits in nerve strands teased from the distal end of the cut hypogastric nerve in 15 rats. In nine other rats, mass and single unit activity was recorded from the distal cut end of the pelvic nerve. In six of these nine experiments, simultaneous recordings were made from the hypogastric nerve for direct comparison of the two nerve responses.

Responses in all 24 rats were studied in an in vitro preparation of the isolated uterus. This preparation was obtained by dissecting the uterus and its arterial supply free from the rat, placing the uterus in warm paraffin oil, and perfusing it through the uterine artery with oxygenated Lock's solution. The stimuli were delivered by introducing a 0.3 ml aliquot of the chemical into the uterine artery followed by a 0.3 ml wash with Lock's solution. The algesic chemicals used were bradykinin triacetate (BRAD: 0.3, 3.0, and 30 μg dissolved in Lock's solution), 5-hydroxytryptamine creatine sulphate (5-HT: 1.35, 13.5, and 135 μg dissolved in Lock's solution), and potassium chloride (KCl: 0.072, 0.72, and 7.2 mg dissolved in distilled water). In addition, to test whether the units were responsive to some aspect of ischemia

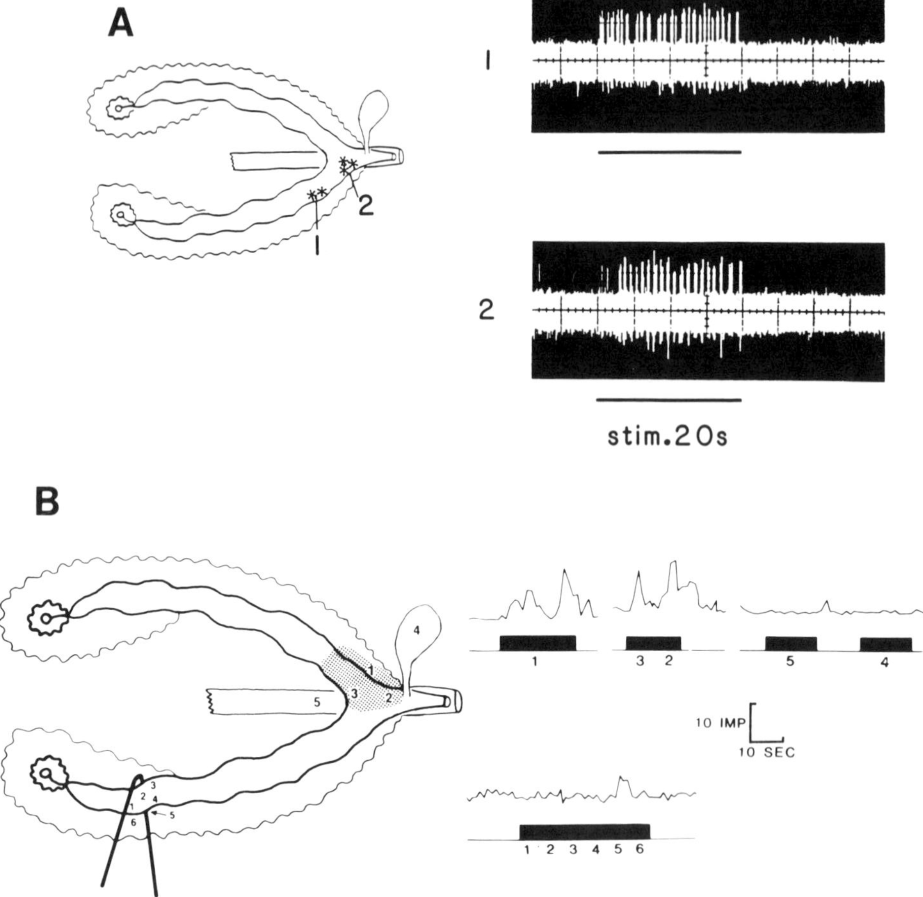

Fig. 2 A. Response of a single unit in the hypogastric nerve to gentle rubbing of the uterine surface. Note discontinuous receptive field (asterisks). In this case, a balloon inside uterine horn is located under area 1. (The conduction velocity of this unit was 1.0 m/s.) The range of conduction velocities of hypogastric units, tested in 4 cases, was 0.5–1.0 m/s.). **B** Response histograms of two other single units in the hypogastric nerve. The receptive field of one unit to moderately intense probing (see text) of the body of the uterus and adjacent ligament with a blunt-tipped glass rod (diameter about 5 mm) is shown by the shaded area. The responses of this unit to probing each of the numbered regions are shown at the top right. The responses of a unit from another rat to probing or steady pressure delivered to each of the numbered areas on the uterine horn (bottom of diagram) with a fine-tipped nylon probe (diameter about 0.5 mm) is shown at the bottom right. The black line depicts a piece of thread that had been placed through the broad ligament around the uterine horn at the beginning of the experiment (to permit suspension of the horn during stimulation). Units with receptive fields this far rostrally on the uterine horn were rarely found except in association with such surgical irritations. Note that the unit was discretely responsive to probing at point #5 (i. e., the point directly adjacent to where the thread passed through the broad ligament)

(e. g., anoxia, CO_2), sodium cyanide (NaCN: 6.0, 60, and 600 μg) and saline mixed with CO_2 (CO_2: 10% - 100%) were used.

The algesic substances produced an increase in activity in both the hypogastric and pelvic nerves. A typical response to BRAD is shown in the multiunit activity of the hypogastric nerve in Fig. 3A and single unit activity in the pelvic nerve in Fig. 3B. Although each unit was usually responsive to more than one algesic chemical, the character of the responses in mass activity to each chemical was unique (latency, duration, frequency, etc.). A comparison of the simultaneously recorded mass activity responses of both nerves to 5-HT, BRAD, and KCl showed them to be similar in this respect (Fig. 3C). However, the 5-HT response for the pelvic nerve always consisted of an initial phase of large amplitude and short duration, which was never observed in the hypogastric nerve response to 5-HT. When tested, these responses were independent of uterine contractions (as measured by uterine EMG recording) and dose-dependent.

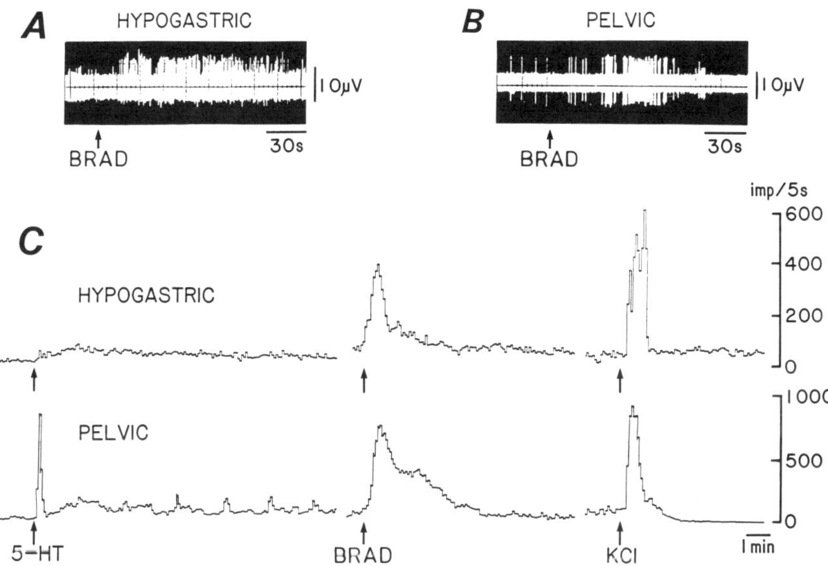

Fig. 3. Responses of the hypogastric and pelvic nerves to chemical stimulation of the uterus in an in vitro preparation (see text). **A** Response of multiunit activity in the hypogastric nerve to an injection of bradykinin triacetate (BRAD) immediately followed by a saline rinse. **B** Single unit activity in the pelvic nerve to a BRAD injection. **C** Histograms of simultaneously recorded mass activity in the hypogastric and pelvic nerves in one rat. Doses used were: 5-HT, 135 μg; BRAD, 30.0 μg: KCl, 7.2 mg

Units were also responsive to NaCN or CO_2, although more inconsistently and less vigorously than to the algesic chemicals. In the hypogastric nerve, the higher doses of NaCN (60–600 μg) were usually necessary to elicit clear responses. In the pelvic nerve, responses were clearer at the lowest (6.0 μg) doses. Effects of stage of estrous were not examined.

Discussion

Anatomical Results

It is evident from gross anatomical dissection that the uterus of the rat is innervated by both sympathetic (hypogastric) and parasympathetic (pelvic) nerves (Baljet and Drukker 1980; Reiner et al. 1981). The results from the present experiment indicate that both of these nerves contain uterine afferent fibers. Such dual afferent innervation from sympathetic and parasympathetic nerves appears to be the case for other visceral organs as well (Mei 1983; Aldskogius et al. 1986). It remains to be determined where these uterine afferent fibers terminate in the central nervous system.

Response Properties

The electrophysiological results indicate that, like afferent fibers from many other visceral structures (e. g., Newman 1974), afferent fibers in the hypogastric nerve arising from the uterus can convey both mechanical and chemical information to the spinal cord. Although the hypogastric afferents sometimes responded to innocuous stimuli, the mechanical stimuli necessary to activate many of them were noxious, in the sense that they threatened tissue damage by the production of ischemia. Effective chemical stimuli were similarly potentially "noxious," in that BRAD, 5-HT, and KCl produce pain in humans or pseudoaffective reactions in animals (Handwerker 1980; Keele and Armstrong 1964; Lim et al. 1962) and the responses to high doses of NaCN and CO_2 are consistent with a responsiveness to severe ischemia (such as may occur with strong uterine contractions).

Thus, uterine afferent fibers traveling in the hypogastric nerve may be responsible for conveying nociceptive information to the spinal cord, as has been suggested as a general feature for afferent fibers traveling in the sympathetic nerves serving the thoracic and some pelvic viscera, including the uterus (Ruch 1960). It should be pointed out, however, that since the effective "algesic" substances used in the present study are known to excite both nociceptive and non-nociceptive afferent units, such conclusions remain speculative and other physiological or functional roles cannot be ruled out.

Since pelvic nerve fibers responded to stimulation of the uterus with algesic and other chemicals in a manner similar to hypogastric nerve fibers, it is possible that fibers in the pelvic nerve also contribute to nociception in the rat, a conclusion consistent with recent evidence from other visceral structures (Malliani et al. 1984). Nevertheless, it will be of interest to determine whether, as suggested by Ruch (1960), the pelvic nerve afferents (i.e., afferents traveling in the parasympathetic nerve) are more likely to convey information relevant to homeostatic aspects of uterine function than nociceptive information. The possibility of a partial division of sensory function in the two nerves is supported by the fact that the pelvic nerves are crucial for such physiological events as pseudopregnancy induction (Kollar 1953; Carlson and de Feo 1965) and that the pelvic, but **not** the abdominal sympathetic nerves, are required for normal pregnancy and parturition (Carlson and de Feo 1965).

Effects of Status of Uterine Tissue

Results from the mechanoreceptive studies suggest that the responses of uterine hypogastric afferent fibers may vary as a function of estrous stage or other aspects of the condition of the uterus (such as its irritation). The results from the anatomical experiments suggest that the axonal transport properties may also vary as a function of uterine condition. Such changes in response or transport properties are not completely surprising as they have been observed in other systems such as, for example, the arthritic knee joint (Guilbaud et al. 1985; Grigg et al. 1986), the pudendal nerve of the estrogen-treated rat (Komisurak et al. 1972; Kow and Pfaff 1973), during aging (Sato et al. 1985) and in the deafferented dorsal column or lateral geniculate nuclei (Singer et al. 1977; Berkley and Vierck 1986). Further studies are needed to confirm, document, and characterize these variations for uterine afferent fibers as well as to determine their mechanism of action.

Acknowledgements. This work was supported by grant RO1 NS 11892 from the National Institutes of Health, U.S.A. and by Grants-in-Aid for Research 57480129 and 5887007 from the Ministry of Education, Science and Culture, Japan. We thank Richard Budell, Stan Warmath, Linda Rinaman, Sybil Core, and Harumi Hotta for technical assistance and Elizabeth Wood and Cindy Dodson for help with the illustrations.

References

Abrahams VC, Teare JL (1969) Peripheral pathways and properties of uterine afferents in the cat. Can J Physiol Pharmacol 47 : 576–577

Aldskogius H, Elfvin L-G, Forsman CA (1986) Primary sensory afferents in the inferior mesenteric ganglion and related nerves of the guinea pig. J Auton Nerv Syst 15 : 179–190

Baljet B, Drukker J (1980) The extrinsic innervation of the pelvic organs in the female rat. Acta Anat (Basel) 107 : 241–267

Berkley KJ, Vierck CJ III (1986) Transient changes in retrograde labeling of diencephalic-projecting neurones in the monkey dorsal column nuclei following dorsal column lesions. Soc Neurosci Abstr 12, p 1049

Bower EA (1959) Action potentials from uterine sensory nerves. J Physiol (Lond) 48 : 2P–3P

Bower EA (1966) The characteristics of spontaneous and evoked action potentials recorded from the rabbit's uterine nerves. J Physiol (Lond) 183 : 730–747

Carlson, RR, de Feo VJ (1965) Role of the pelvic nerve vs. the abdominal sympathetic nerves in the reproductive function of the female rat. Endocrinology 77 : 1014–1022

Floyd K, Hick VE, Morrison JFB (1976) Mechanosensitive afferent units in the hypogastric nerve of the cat. J Physiol (Lond) 259 : 457–771

Grigg P, Schaible H-G, Schmidt RF (1986) Mechanical sensitivity of group III and IV afferents from posterior articular nerve in normal and inflamed cat knee. J Neurophysiol 55 : 635–643

Guilbaud G, Iggo A, Tégner R (1985) Sensory receptors in ankle joint capsules of normal and arthritic rats. Exp Brain Res 58 : 29–40

Handwerker HO (1980) Pain producing substances. In: Kosterlitz HW, Terenius HW (eds) Pain and society. Verlag Chemie, Weinheim, pp 325–338

Keele CA, Armstrong D (1964) Substances producing pain and itch. Arnold, London

Kollar EJ (1953) Reproduction in the female rat after pelvic neurectomy. Anat Rec 115 : 641–658

Komisaruk BR, Adler N, Hutchinson J (1972) Genital sensory field: enlargement by estrogen treatment in female rats. Science 178 : 1295–1298

Kow LM, Pfaff DW (1973) Effects of estrogen treatment on the size of receptive field and response threshold of pudendal nerve in the female rat. Neuroendocrinology 13 : 299–313

Kumazawa T (1986) Sensory innervation of reproductive organs. Prog Brain Res (in press), pp 115–132

Lim RKS, Liu CN, Guzman F, Braun C (1962) Visceral receptors concerned in visceral pain and pseudaffective responses to intra-arterial injection of bradykinin and other algesic agents. J Comp Neurol 118 : 269–293

Malliani A, Pagani M, Lombardi F (1984) Visceral versus somatic mechanisms. In: Wall PD, Melzack R (eds) Textbook of pain. Livingston, Edinburgh, pp 100–109

Mei N (1983) Sensory structures in the viscera. In: Autrum H, Ottoson D, Perl ER, Schmidt RF, Shimazu H, Willis WD Jr. (eds) Progress in sensory physiology, vol 4. Springer Berlin Heidelberg New York, pp 1–42

Nadelhaft I, Booth AM (1984) The location and morphology of preganglionic neurons and the distribution of visceral afferents from the rat pelvic nerve: a horseradish peroxidase study. J Comp Neurol 226 : 238–245

Neuhuber W (1982) The central projections of visceral primary afferent neurons of the inferior mesenteric plexus and hypogastric nerve and the location of the related sensory and preganglionic sympathetic cell bodies in the rat. Anat Embryol (Berl) 164 : 413–425

Newman PP (1974) Visceral afferent functions of the nervous system. Arnold, London

Reiner P, Woolsey J, Adler N, Morrison A (1981) A gross anatomical study of the peripheral nerves associated with reproductive function in the female albino rat. In: Adler N (ed) Neuroendocrinology of reproduction. Plenum, New York, pp 545–549

Ruch T (1960) Pathophysiology of pain. In: Ruch T, Fulton JF (eds) Medical physiology and biophysics, 18th edn. Saunders, Philadelphia, pp 350–368

Sato A, Sato Y, Suzuki H (1985) Aging effects on conduction velocities of myelinated fibers of peripheral nerves. Neurosci Lett 53 : 15–20

Singer W, Hollander H, Vanegas H (1977) Decreased peroxidase labeling of lateral geniculate neurons following deafferentation. Brain Res 120 : 133–137

14 Receptor Properties of Unmyelinated Afferent Fibres Innervating the Rat Small Intestine: An In Vitro Study

K.A. Sharkey and F. Cervero

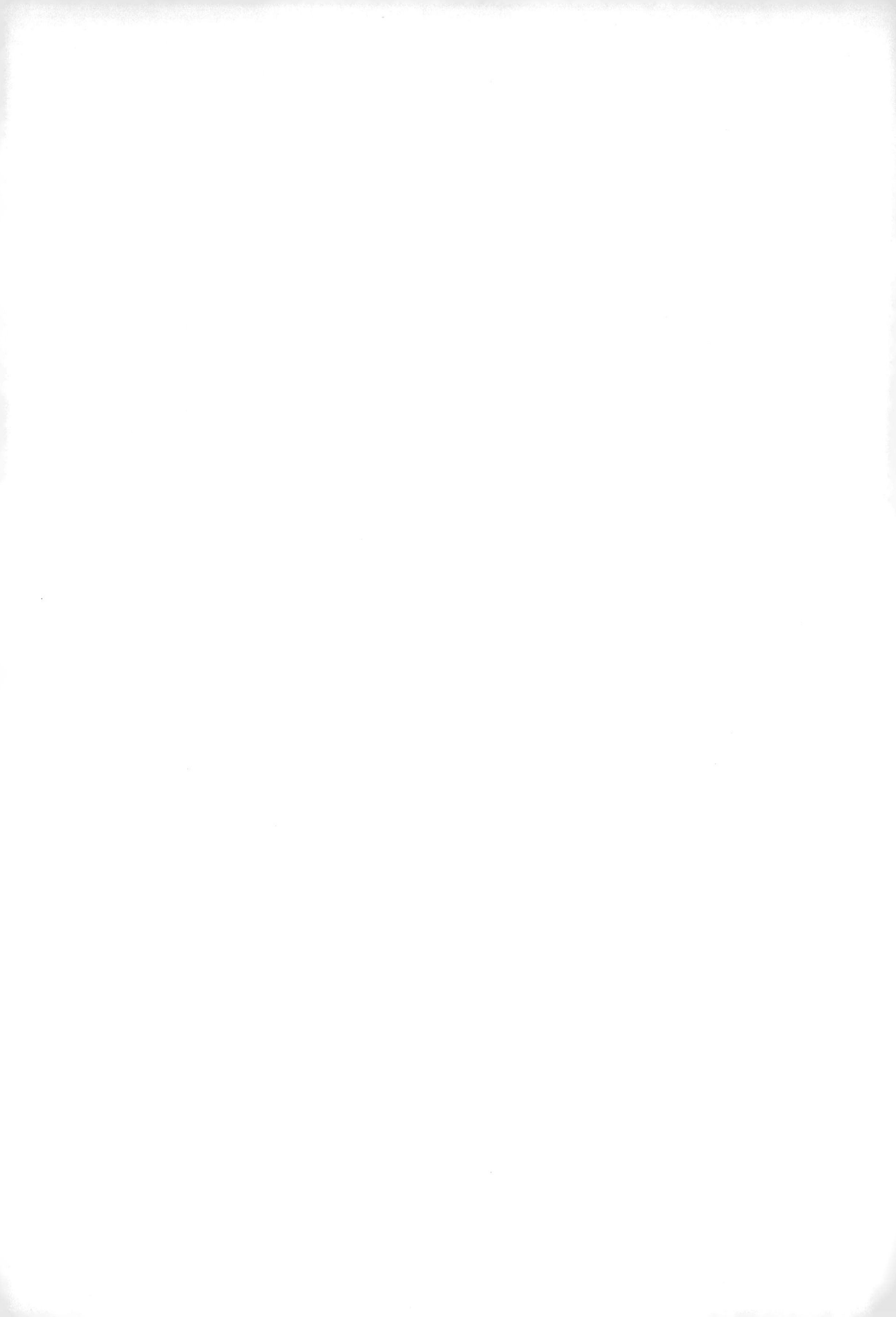

Introduction

Electrophysiological studies of afferent fibres in mesenteric nerves have demonstrated the occurrence of intestinal receptors that respond to chemical and mechanical stimuli (for reviews see Leek 1977; Jänig and Morrison 1986). However, the effects of drugs on these receptors have not been studied in great detail. One reason for this lack of information is that pharmacological studies conducted in vivo can be hard to interpret, since the compounds administered may have systemic effects reflected in the environment of the viscus under study. This problem can be overcome by recording intestinal motility as well as afferent nerve activity (see for example Cottrell and Iggo 1984). Recently we have developed an in vitro preparation of rat distal ileum with its associated mesenteric nerves which permits the recording of afferent impulses, tension in the longitudinal muscle, intraluminal pressure and electromyographic activity of the smooth muscle (Sharkey and Cervero 1986). Using this preparation we have studied the responses of intestinal receptors to mechanical and chemical stimulation of the gut.

Methods

A detailed description of the in vitro technique, including the organ bath and recording methods, has been previously published (for details see Sharkey and Cervero 1986 and Fig. 1). In the present study recordings were made from afferent fibres dissected from the mesenteric nerves about 20 mm from the gut wall. All afferent units had background activity under resting conditions (0.5 g longitudinal tension and 0–2 mmHg intraluminal pressure). Units were tested for mechanosensitivity by light stroking (along the longitudinal axis of the segment) and probing of the mucosa and serosa with a fine glass rod and by intraluminal distension (0–15 mmHg). Chemosensitivity was tested by application of 10 μl of a solution of bradykinin (10 μg) or acetylcholine (ACh; 100 μg) to the receptive field or on to the serosal surface of the segment. The spike shape of all single units was examined with an analog delay using the undelayed spike to trigger the oscilloscope sweep (Fig. 4 B).

The fibre composition of ten mesenteric nerves from the rat distal ileum was examined in two animals fixed by perfusion with 5% glutaraldehyde in 0.1 M phosphate buffer (pH 7.4) at room temperature. Mesenteric neurovascular bundles were dissected, pinned out onto cork and immersed in the same fixative overnight at 4 °C. The neurovascular bundles were then washed, post-fixed in osmium, stained in uranyl acetate, dehydrated in acetone and embedded in Epon. Thin sections were then stained with lead citrate and examined under an electron microscope.

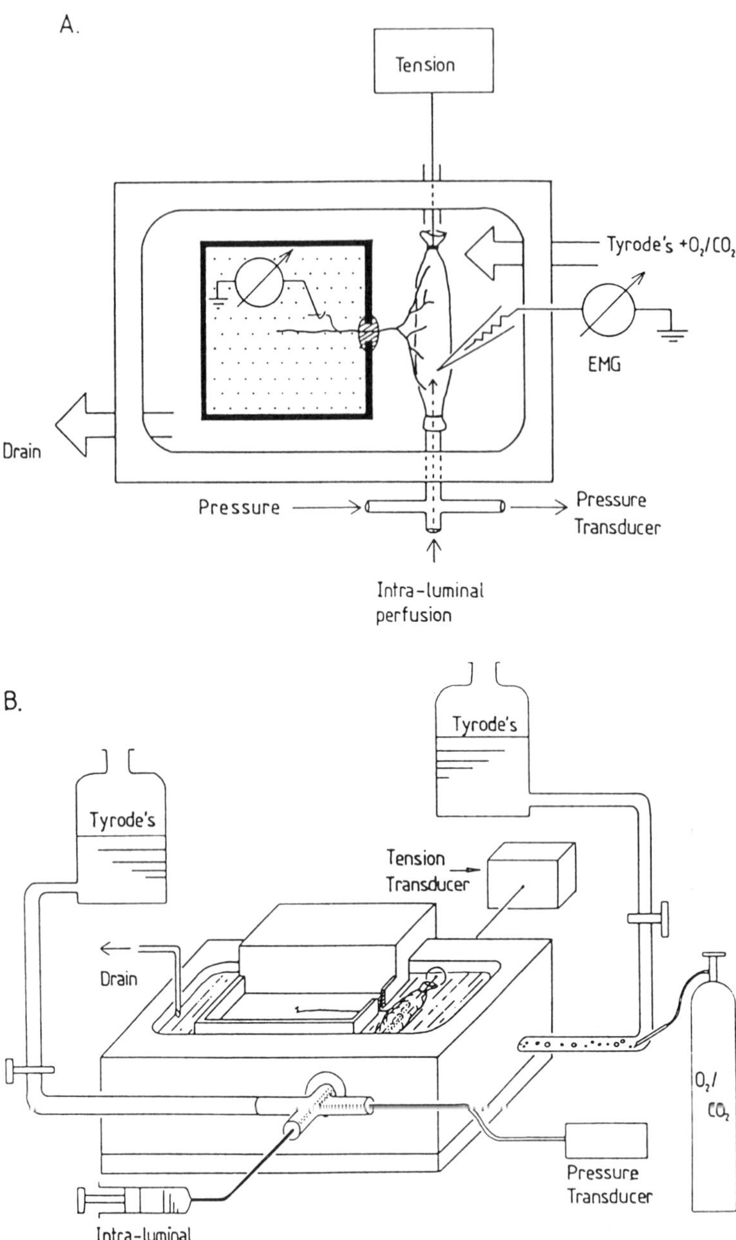

Fig. 1 A. Diagrammatic illustration of the experimental arrangement. Recordings of afferent nerve activity are made from fine filaments of the mesenteric nerves whilst simultaneously recording tension in the longitudinal muscle, intraluminal pressure and electromyographic activity. Changes in intraluminal pressure can be imposed and drugs can be applied to the serosal and mucosal surfaces. **B** Schematic diagram of the organ bath and dissection platform, showing the position of the ileal segment. Full details can be found in Sharkey and Cervero (1986) from which publication this figure was taken

Results

Single-unit activity was recorded from 56 afferent fibres (from 30 rats), all of which showed some background activity. The conduction velocities of 48 of these fibres were measured (Fig. 2) and were found to range from 0.3 to 1.6 m/s (mean 0.7 m/s). This range of conduction velocities indicates that all of these fibres were unmyelinated. Electron-microscopic examination of the mesenteric nerves confirmed that these nerves do not contain myelinated axons (see Fig. 3). Transverse sections through the neurovascular bundles consistently showed two nerve fascicles running between an arteriole and a venule. Each fascicle was 30–50 μm in diameter and contained between 600 and 1000 unmyelinated fibres.

The responses of intestinal afferent units to mechanical and chemical stimulation of the gut are summarized in Table 1. Most units (84 %) responded to both mechanical and chemical stimuli. A small proportion (14 %) responded only to mechanical stimuli and one unit responded only to bradykinin. An example of a unit responding to intraluminal distension is shown in Fig. 4. About half of the units tested responded to distension in a rapidly adapting manner and the other half were slowly adapting. Receptive fields were found on the serosal and mucosal surfaces of the intestine when examined by probing with a glass rod. They tended to be single mechanosensitive spots and those on the surface of the intestine were often associated with the course of a blood vessel.

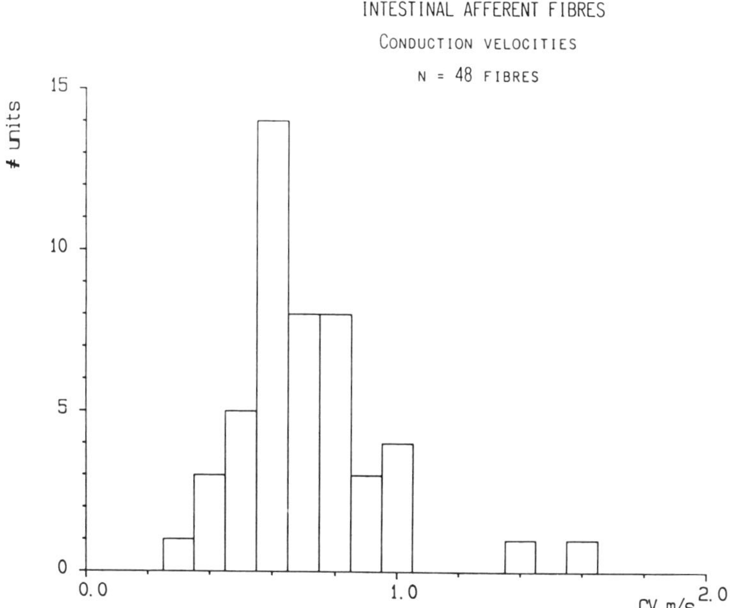

Fig. 2. Conduction velocities of 48 intestinal afferent fibres from rat mesenteric nerves

Table 1. Response of 56 intestinal afferent fibres to mechanical and chemical stimulation of the intestine. Values in parentheses are percentages

	Serosal probing	Distension	Mucosal stroking	Serosal stroking	ACh	Bradykinin
Mechanosensitive: n = 8	8 (100)	7 (87.5)	1 (12.5)	1 (12.5)	-	-
Chemosensitive: n = 1	-	-	-	-	-	+
Mechanochemosens.: n = 47	42 (89.4)	39 (83.0)	10 (21.3)	12 (25.5)	35 (74.5)	30 (63.8)

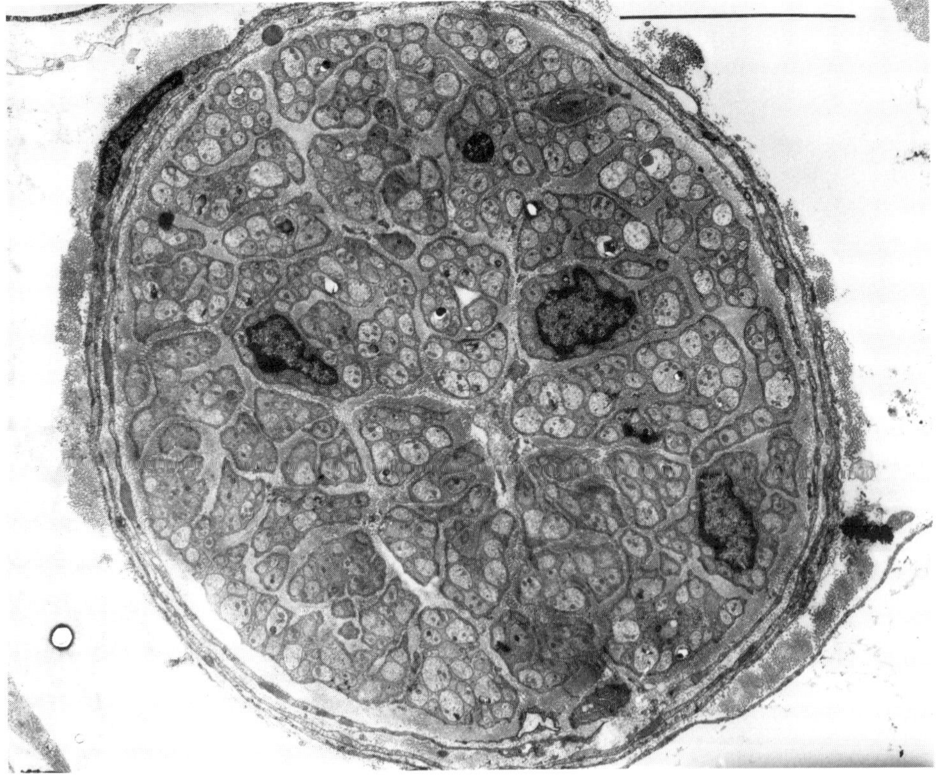

Fig. 3. Electron micrograph of a transverse section of a nerve fascicle from a mesenteric neurovascular bundle. Note the absence of myelinated fibres. Scale bar 10 μm

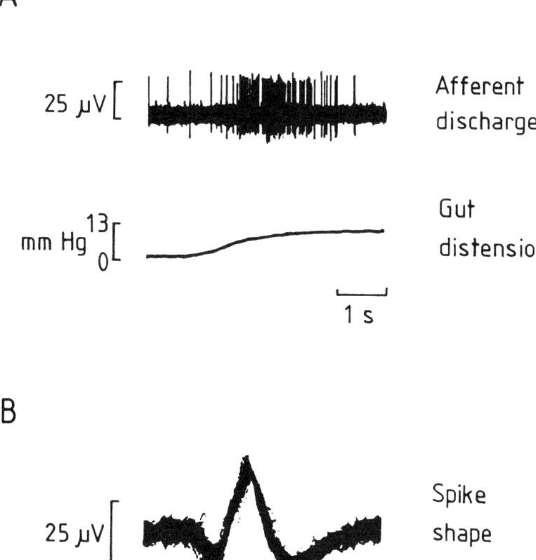

Fig. 4 A. Response of a single afferent unit to intraluminal distension of the intestine. **B** Ten superimposed action potentials from the same unit. The unitary nature of the recording was assessed by passing the signal through an analog delay, using the undelayed spike to trigger the oscilloscope

Discussion

Using a newly developed in vitro preparation we recorded single-unit afferent activity in mesenteric nerves of the rat distal ileum. We were able to measure changes in motility and afferent activity in a single preparation for up to 6 h and identified afferent units, all of which had background activity, that responded to chemical and mechanical stimulation of the gut. The presence of background activity was found in mesenteric nerves in in vivo preparations (see Jänig and Morrison 1986).

The mesenteric nerves from which activity was recorded consisted of two nerve fascicles containing 1500–2000 unmyelinated fibres, although it seems likely that some of these fibres will become myelinated more centrally. Mesenteric nerves at this level contain four types of fibres: (1) postganglionic sympathetic, (2) preganglionic parasympathetic, (3) visceral primary afferent and (4) a type of afferent with its cell body in the wall of the gut and projection to the abdominal prevertebral ganglia (Schofield 1968; Dalsgaard and Elfvin 1982). We are at present attempting to correlate afferent activity with the type of afferent fibre found in rat mesenteric nerves.

Mechanosensitive afferent endings in the intestine have been reported to respond to probing, distension and contraction of the gut wall and tension on the mesenteric attachments (Morrison 1977; Jänig and Morrison 1986). The same stimuli evoked afferent activity in our preparations. The receptive fields of the units in our study usually consisted of single mechanosensitive spots which were distributed on the serosal and mucosal surfaces of the segment. These results agree with those of in vivo studies of mechanosensitive intestinal afferent endings (Jänig and Morrison 1986). Afferent activity could be evoked in most mechanosensitive endings by intraluminal distension and by probing the serosal surface of the segment. Blumberg et al. (1983) reported that of the cat colonic afferent units with resting activity that they recorded from , only about half responded to mechanical probing, although virtually all responded to distension. The range of distension pressures used to activate afferents in the present study (0–15 mmHg) is low compared with those used by others in in vivo studies on larger animals (Morrison 1977; Jänig and Morrison 1986). This may be due to technical differences in our preparation or to species differences.

Both ACh and bradykinin caused excitation of the majority of afferent units tested in the present study. Longhurst et al. (1984) reported that most of the C fibres in the cat sympathetic paravertebral chain they recorded from were excited by bradykinin, although these fibres were apparently mechanically insensitive. In contrast, virtually all our fibres that responded to ACh and bradykinin were found to be mechanosensitive, a finding that is in line with previous in vivo studies (Cottrell and Iggo 1984; Jänig and Morrison 1986). In some cases we were able to see an increase in firing of a unit in response to ACh or bradykinin with no observable changes in tension or pressure of the segment, or well before any increases in tension took place. Although we cannot completely exclude the possibility of small, undetected movements in the preparation, this indicates a direct action of these drugs on afferent receptors in the wall of the ileum, in addition to their indirect actions through smooth muscle contractions.

Acknowledgements. This work was supported by a grant from the Wellcome Trust. We are very grateful to Andrew Amos and Steven Allen for expert technical assistance, Deborah Carter for electron microscopy and Perry Robbins for photography.

References

Blumberg H, Haupt P, Jänig W, Kohler W (1983) Encoding of visceral noxious stimuli in the discharge patterns of visceral afferent fibres from the colon. Pflugers Arch 398 : 33–40

Cottrell DF, Iggo A (1984) The responses of duodenal tension receptors in sheep to pentagastrin, cholecystokinin and some other drugs. J Physiol (Lond) 354 : 477–496

Dalsgaard C-J, Elfvin L-G (1982) Structural studies on the connectivity of the inferior mesenteric ganglion of the guinea pig. J Auton Nerv Syst 5 : 265–278

Jänig W, Morrison JFB (1986) Functional properties of spinal visceral afferents supplying abdominal and pelvic organs with special emphasis on visceral nociception. Prog Brain Res 67 : 87–114

LEEK BF (1977) Abdominal and pelvic visceral receptors. Br Med Bull 33 : 163–168

LONGHURST JC, KAUFMAN MP, ORDWAY GA, MUSCH TI (1984) Effects of bradykinin and capsaicin on endings of afferent fibers from abdominal visceral organs. Am J Physiol 247 : R552–R559

MORRISON JFB (1977) The afferent innervation of the gastrointestinal tract. In: BROOKS FP, EVERS PW (eds) Nerves and the gut. Slack, New Jersey, pp 297–322

SCHOFIELD GC (1968) Anatomy of muscular and neural tissues in the alimentary canal. In: CODE CF (ed) Handbook of physiology, sect 6, vol 4. American Physiological Society, Washington, pp 1579–1628

SHARKEY KA, CERVERO F (1986) An in vitro method for recording single unit afferent activity from mesenteric nerves innervating isolated segments of rat ileum. J Neurosci Methods 16 : 149–156

15 Modulations of Testicular Polymodal Receptor Activity: Implication of Receptors in Inflammatory Pain

T. Kumazawa, K. Mizumura, and J. Sato

Inflammation has classically been characterized by four signs: rubor, calor, tumor, and dolor. Nociceptors involved in the dolor would be sensitized by various changes associated with three other signs: liberation of chemical mediators, local temperature increase, and edema.

Our previous investigations (Kumazawa and Mizumura 1980; Kumazawa et al., in press) have revealed that the great majority of thin-fiber afferents in the superior spermatic nerve are of the polymodal receptor type signalling visceral pain. To test whether these testicular polymodal receptors are implicated in inflammatory pain, two features of their chemical responses have been investigated: (1) alteration by putative chemical modulators and (2) the effect of local temperature increases known to occur in inflamed tissues.

The experimental methods are basically the same as reported previously (Kumazawa et al., in press). The testis and epididymis with the spermatic cord attached were excised from dogs that were deeply anesthetized with pentobarbital and kept in an areflexic state. Single- or multifiber activities were recorded from the superior spermatic nerve placed in an oil pool, while the testis and epididymis, exposed at the tunica vaginalis visceralis, were immersed in a test pool of Krebs-Henseleit solution (Krebs solution) equilibrated with a gas mixture of 5 % CO_2 and 95 % O_2. The temperature of the solution bathing the scrotal contents was adjusted by regulating the temperature of the water circulating in the trough surrounding the test pool. After the temperature of the receptive field reached a preset level, chemical stimulation was applied by replacing the Krebs solution with a stimulus solution of the same temperature: hypertonic saline and high K^+ solution for 30 s or bradykinin (BK) for 1 min with an interval of 10 min between trials. Heat stimulation was carried out by raising the temperature of the Krebs solution from 34 °C to 50 °C at a rate of $0.18° \pm 0.02$ °C/s. The temperature of the oil pool was measured and the conduction velocity at the nerve trunk in the oil pool was corrected to the value at 37 °C, using the Q_{10} value reported by Paintal (1965). In multifiber recordings, the number of active units was estimated from the response to hypertonic saline. A normalized discharge rate was obtained for multifiber recordings by dividing the response to 0.6 M saline by the mean discharge rate obtained from the average response of 107 single units to the same solution.

Enhancement of Chemical Responses after "Heat Sensitization"

It is well known that repetitively applied heat stimulation to cutaneous polymodal nociceptors frequently causes enhancement of subsequent heat responses ("heat sensitization"; Bessou and Perl 1969), and similar phenomena have been found in testicular polymodal receptors (Kumazawa and Mizumura 1980; Kumazawa et al., in press). In the heat-sensitized state, an enhancement of the response to other types of stimulation is also expected. As shown in Fig. 1, BK responses tested at 34 °C after strong suprathreshold heat stimulation (53 °C), were enhanced in parallel with increases in the subsequent heat (45 °C) responses. In another series of experiments, threshold temperature was measured using a

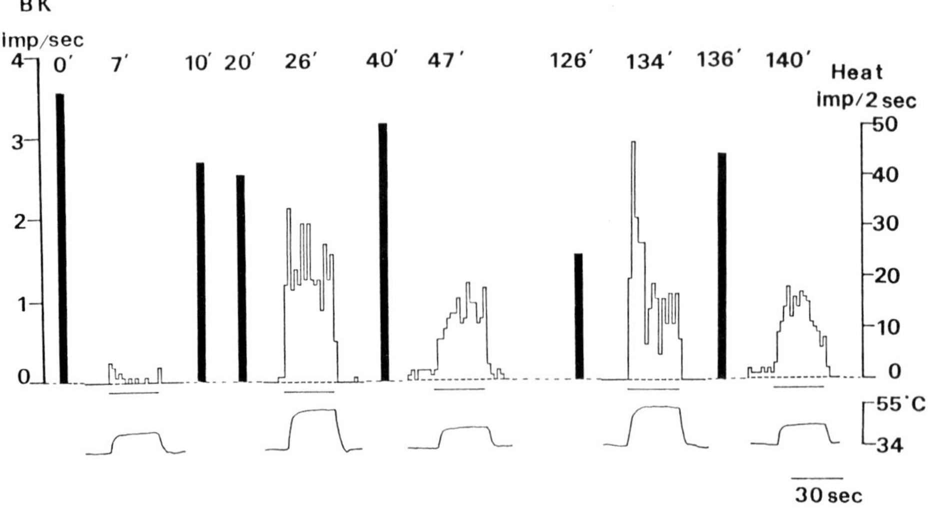

Fig. 1. Suprathreshold heat stimulation enhances subsequent responses to BK as well as to heat. White column: peristimulus time histogram of the response (scale at the right) induced by heat stimulation (shown at the bottom). Black column: discharge rates (scale at left) induced by 9×10^{-8} M BK stimulation. The time in minutes after the beginning of the first BK application is shown at the top

ramp heat stimulus. In eight polymodal receptor units in which threshold temperatures for the second heat stimulus were lower than those for the first (average threshold decrement from 48° to 44.2 °C), the mean increase in discharge rate to 0.6 M NaCl tested at 34 °C after the second heat stimulus was 2.85 imp/s, significantly greater than before heating (1.54 imp/s; $p<0.05$ by paired t-test). The enhancement effect was observed even 60 min after the end of heat stimulation in the few cases where observations were continued for a long time. In those units not sensitized by heat, there was no significant difference in the NaCl response before and after heat stimulation.

Effects of Subthreshold Temperature Rises on Chemical Responses

The threshold temperature for heat responses of the testicular polymodal receptors measured in similar in vitro preparations was 44.4° ± 0.4 °C (Kumazawa et al., in press). Temperature increments expected at the inflamed tissue never exceeded the threshold temperature of the receptor. The effects of temperature rise within the subthreshold range were tested on the responses for various concentrations of BK and hypertonic saline (Kumazawa et al. 1987). The average mean discharge rates during a 1-min stimulation

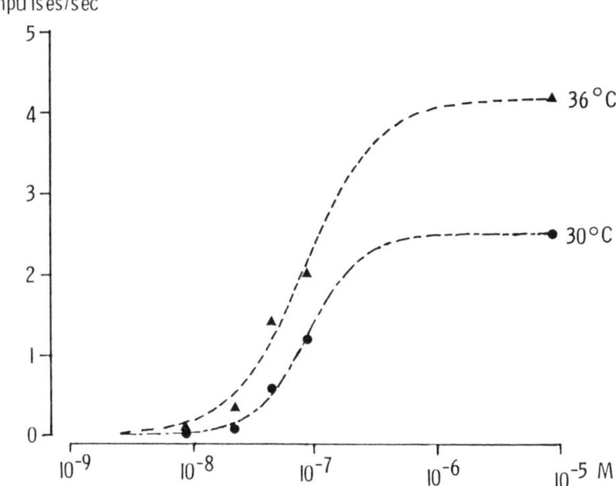

Fig. 2. Concentration-response relationship of BK at 30° and 36 °C. Ordinate: mean evoked discharge rate during 1-min period of BK application. Abscissa: concentration of BK. ●, response at 30 °C; ▲, response at 36 °C; interrupted lines, best-fitting lines of the response at each temperature (cited from Kumazawa et al. 1987)

period were plotted against the concentrations of BK at 30° and 36 °C and the best fitting lines of the responses at each temperature were drawn (Fig. 2). The responses were greater and the threshold concentrations lower at 36 °C than at 30 °C.

Responses to 0.77 M NaCl were tested at four temperatures in steps of 3 °C: 34 °, 37°, 40°, and 43 °C. At temperatures up to 43 °C, only a few units showed a slight increase in discharge rate (less than 0.6 imp/s) at a fixed temperature. Thus the temperature per se was usually subthreshold for most receptors tested. However, responses to 0.77 M NaCl increased linearly with increase in temperature.

The above results indicate that the response of testicular polymodal receptors to BK and algesic salt solutions are enhanced by an increase in the temperature of their receptive fields, at least in the range observed in inflamed tissues.

Enhancement of Chemical Responses by Prostaglandin E_2 and I_2 and Serotonin

An increase in the levels of several types of prostaglandins (PGs) and 5-hydroxytryptamine (5-HT, serotonin) are known to occur in inflamed tissues. The response of cutaneous nociceptors, muscular group IV, and joint afferents is augmented by 5-HT and/or PGE_2 (Handwerker 1976; Mense 1981; Schaible and Schmidt 1985). The direct effects of PGE_2

were tested at 34 °C on preparations previously unchallenged by BK. PGE_2 was added cumulatively every 2 min from 1.4 x 10^{-7} to 1.4 x 10^{-5} M. At 1.4 x 10^{-7} M, PGE_2 never provoked an increased discharge rate in 17 trials (nine single units and eight multifiber recordings). In contrast to the results in unchallenged preparations, when PGE_2 1.4 x 10^{-7} M was applied shortly (2–5 min) after the BK response, a clear increased discharge with a similar time course and pattern to the BK response appeared in five of 10 cases tested. At concentrations higher than 1.4 x 10^{-6} M, PGE_2 evoked a small increased discharge: the number of instances of response and the discharge rate tended to increase in

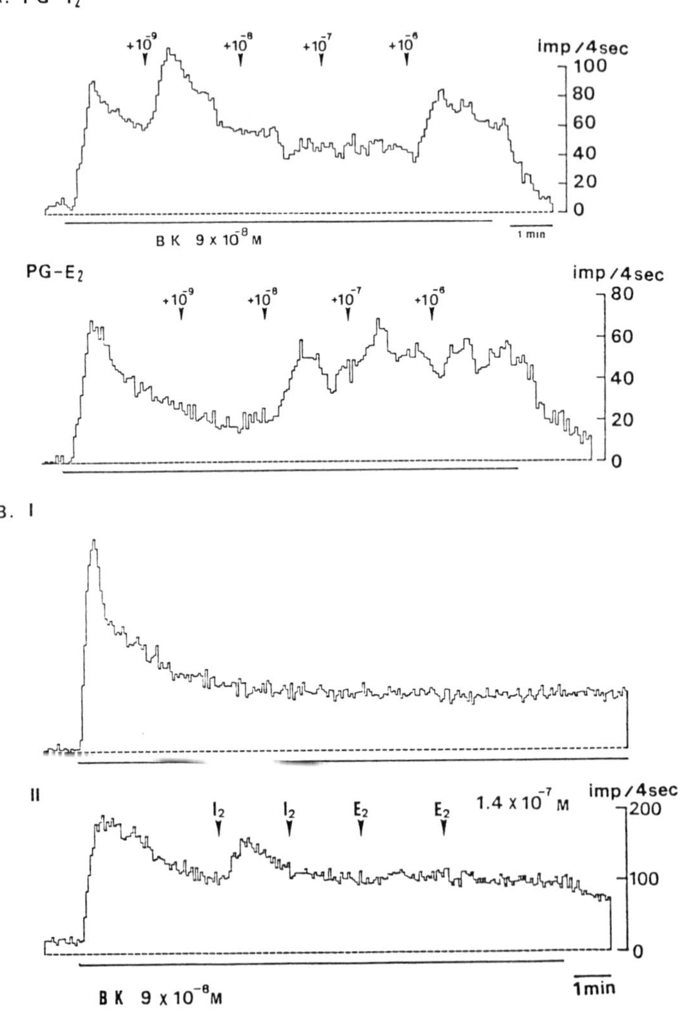

Fig. 3 A, B. Effects of prostaglandins applied during BK responses: threshold, tachyphylaxis, and cross-tachyphylaxis. During a steady state of the response to BK, as shown in **BI**, PGI_2 or PGE_2 of 10^{-9}–10^{-6} M were applied cumulatively at arrows in **A**, indicating threshold concentration and tachyphylaxis. **BII**, cross-tachyphylaxis between PGI_2 and PGE_2 (**BI** control)

parallel with an increase of concentration. When PGE_2 was applied with BK, it significantly enhanced the BK responses (1.75 imp/s in the PG group; 0.81 imp/s in the control group). PGE_2 also enhanced the responses to high K solutions and hypertonic saline, but at a higher concentration and longer application than needed for the effects on the BK responses. The threshold concentration of PGE_2 for its modifying effect was estimated during a steady state of BK response that was reached in about 3–4 min after BK application (Fig. 3BI). At this stage, PGE_2 was added cumulatively every 2 min from 1.4×10^{-9} M to 1.4×10^{-6} M in four steps (Fig. 3A). The first concentration inducing an increased discharge was 1.4×10^{-8} M (in seven multifiber recordings and in three of four single-unit recordings). One unit increased its discharge rate at 1.4×10^{-9} M. As shown in Fig. 3A, another cyclooxygenase product, PGI_2 also had similar enhancing effects, but the threshold concentration tended to be lower and the time course faster than with PGE_2. In pleural fluid of rat carrageenin-induced pleurisy, PGI_2 appears and also diminishes earlier than PGE_2 (Katori et al. 1980). The two types of PG might share an augmentation effect on the response to algesic substances.

Figure 3 shows another interesting feature of PGs, tachyphylaxis. Once the PGE_2- or PGI_2-induced enhancing effect on BK responses is reached, subsequent application of either substance becomes ineffective even at higher concentrations. However, it was found that the enhancing effects of both PGs were dose-dependently increased in another experimental series in which the effect of different concentrations of PGs was tested noncumulatively. Furthermore, as shown in Fig. 3BII, after tachyphylaxis for PGI_2 was established, PGE_2 also became ineffective or vice versa, i.e., there was cross-tachyphylaxis between PGI_2 and PGE_2.

When 5-HT was applied on the units unchallenged by BK every 5 min cumulatively from 1.1×10^{-6} to 1.4×10^{-4} M, it had only a weak excitatory, long latency effect, and this excitatory effect did not correlate clearly with the concentration of 5-HT. However, regardless of whether 5-HT itself induced activity, responses to BK and hypertonic saline were enhanced by 5-HT. As shown in Fig. 4A, 5-HT applied after three exposures to BK plus PGE_2 induced augmentation. The average response to BK after a 5-min application of 5-HT (1.1×10^{-6} - 5.6×10^{-5} M) was significantly ($\mathbf{p} < 0.005$) increased (Fig. 4B). The response to hypertonic saline (0.6 M) after 5-HT (5.6×10^{-6} - 2.8×10^{-5} M) for 5–20 min was significantly greater (2.07 ± 0.44 imp/s) than that before 5-HT (0.64 ± 0.16 imp/s; $\mathbf{p} < 0.005$ by paired-t test; $\mathbf{n} = 11$) (Mizumura et al., in press). Confirming the result of our previous report (Kumazawa and Mizumura 1979), synthetic substance P (SP) caused only quite weak excitation in some polymodal receptors. The incidence of weak excitation increased at higher concentrations. The latencies of SP excitation in unit recordings ranged between 48 and 125 s and the increased discharge lasted only for 1 or 2 min during a 5-min application period. The evoked discharge during 5 min of SP application was between 0.01 and 0.18 imp/s. Higher discharge rates were obtained in units with spontaneous discharges. Application of SP for 5 min did not affect subsequent BK responses. On average, the increase of the mean discharge rate during BK stimulation before SP (1.05 ± 0.26 imp/s) was not significantly different from that after SP (1.01 ± 0.26 imp/s). Since even at concentrations as high as 6×10^{-5} M no clear sensitization was observed, any possible sensitizing effect of SP must be weak. Fitzgerald and Lynn (1979) also failed to detect any enhancing effect on responses to heat and pressure of polymodal receptors of cats and rabbits. This raises some doubt about the proposal that SP is the mediator of hyperalgesia induced by antidromic stimulation of afferent nerves.

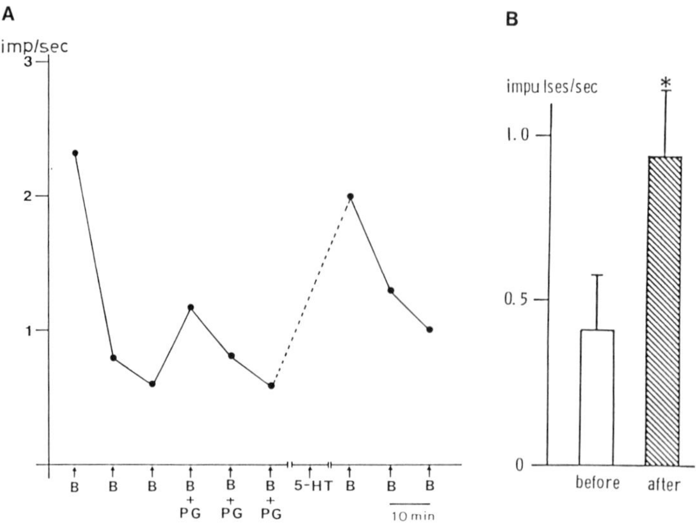

Fig. 4 A, B. Augmenting effect of 5-HT on BK response. **A** Effect on the response to BK (9×10^{-8} M) of a unit. Ordinate: mean discharge rate during a 1-min stimulation period. Abscissa: trial sequence. 5-HT (5.6×10^{-5} M) was applied after three testings of BK plus PGE_2 (1.4×10^{-7} M), and further augmentation by 5-HT was observed. **B** Mean responses to BK of 15 units just before and after applying 5-HT

Effects of Aspirin and Opioids on Chemical Responses

A hyperalgesic effect for PGs is suggested by the fact that inflammatory pain is suppressed by acetylsalicylic acid (ASA), which is known to inhibit PG biosynthesis (Moncada et al. 1975). ASA at concentrations of 5.5×10^{-3} and 5.5×10^{-4} M suppressed the response to BK of all 11 units tested. As shown in Fig. 5A, the response to BK of this unit became smaller after 4 min of ASA application and 14 min later had almost disappeared. The suppressive effect of ASA continued more than 20 min after its removal, with full recovery after about 30 min. In six of 11 units on which ASA was tested, attempts were made to reverse the ASA effects by PGE_2. After 16 min under ASA 5.5×10^{-4} M, the BK response had decreased to 0.27 ± 0.12 imp/s, significantly ($\mathbf{p}<0.001$) lower than before ASA application (2.47 ± 0.19 imp/s; Fig. 5B). The addition of PGE_2 caused recoverys of the BK responses to 1.87 ± 0.54 imp/s, significantly ($\mathbf{p}<0.05$) larger than the response during ASA administration. In contrast, ASA did not suppress the responses to hypertonic saline of testicular polymodal receptors. The responses to 0.6 M NaCl tested in nine units for 10–25 min ASA exposure were not significantly suppressed (Fig. 5B). In one unit, ASA was applied for more than 50 min with no effects. These results would support the hypothesis

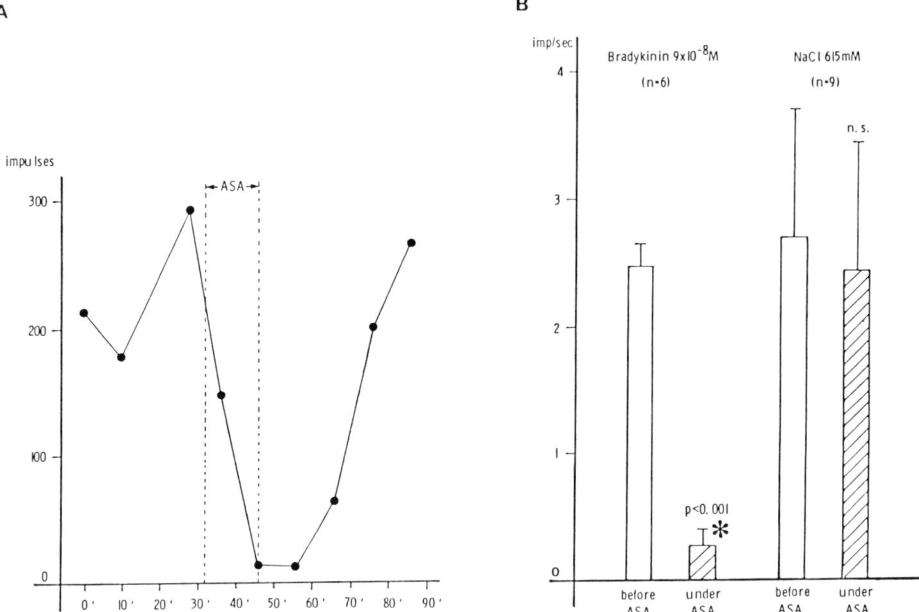

Fig. 5 A, B. Effects of aspirin on responses to BK and hypertonic saline. **A** Time course of suppressive effect of ASA on BK response of a polymodal receptor. Ordinate: total number of impulses evoked by a 1-min application of BK (9×10^{-8} M). Abscissa: time after the beginning of the first BK application. The period of ASA (5.5×10^{-4} M) application is marked by broken lines. **B** Comparison of responses to BK (left) and to hypertonic saline (right) before and during administration of ASA. Ordinate: net mean discharge rate during 60 s BK and 30 s hypertonic saline stimulation

that ASA suppresses the response of polymodal receptors to BK by reducing BK-stimulated production of PGs (Lembeck et al. 1976).

The analgesic effects of morphine have long been known to be induced by its central action. Peripheral analgesic effects of opioids, using the Randall-Selitto test in rats and the acetic acid writhing test in mice (Ferreira and Nakamura 1979), have also been reported. Although these studies have suggested that the opioid effect is caused by a direct action of opioids on the sensory receptors transmitting pain, there is no direct experimental evidence on unit discharges of nociceptor afferents. Contrary to our expectation, morphine hydrochloride caused excitation of polymodal receptors (Fig. 6): one of nine cases tested with 1 μM; 12 of 31 with 10 μM; 17 of 30 with 100 μM; and three of seven with 300 μM. The effects of morphine were also tested during a steady state of BK or BK mixed with PGE_2 (Fig. 6A). Whenever morphine had any effect, it enhanced but never suppressed the BK responses. Similar effects of D-Ala^2-D-Leu^5 enkephalin (DADL, δ-agonist) and dynorphin (ϰ-agonist) were observed. DADL and dynorphin at 10 μM caused excitation in seven of 29 and seven of 17 cases tested respectively (Fig. 6B and C). These results indicate that opioids tested in the present experiment do not inhibit discharges of polymodal receptors evoked by BK or BK plus PGE_2, but do frequently elicit their excitation. The excitatory effects of these opioids are characterized by a strong tendency for tachyphylaxis. The effects of naloxone on these opioid responses were tested in some units, but due to inconsistency and also a strong tachyphylaxis of these responses, the results are inconclusive at present.

In summary, the present results provide quantitative data on modulations of the responses of the testicular polymodal receptors by chemical and thermal changes, which are expected to occur in inflamed tissues. These data strongly support involvement of the testicular polymodal receptors in signalling inflammatory pain.

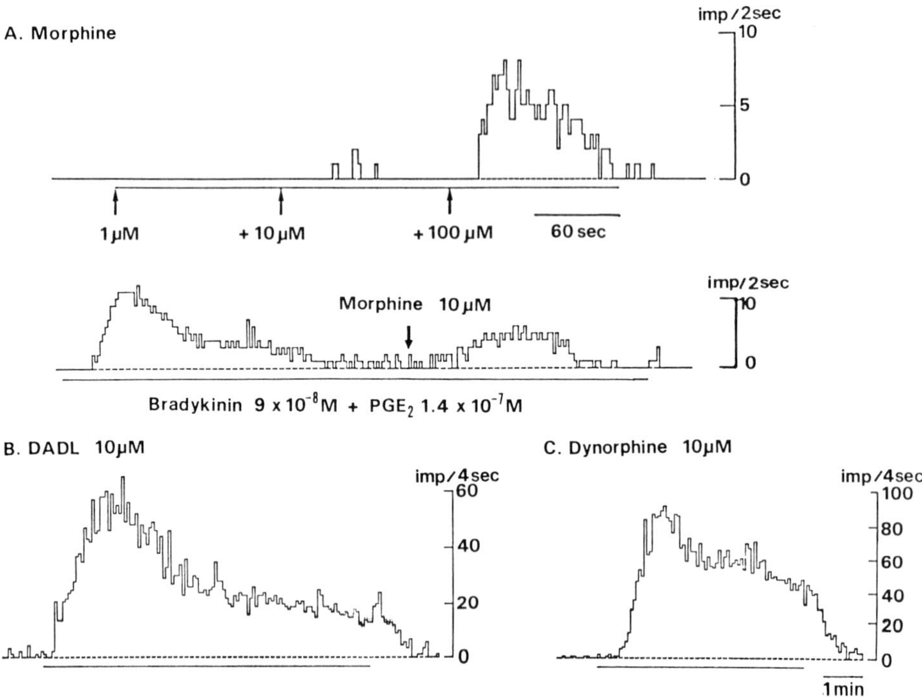

Fig. 6A–C. Opioids produced excitation in testicular polymodal receptors. **A** Above: Morphine (1–100 μM) cumulatively applied to a polymodal receptor; below: morphine applied (arrow) during the steady state of the response to BK plus PGE_2. **B** Excitation effect of DADL. **C** Excitation effect of dynorphin. **A:** single unit recordings; **B, C:** multifiber recordings

References

Bessou P, Perl ER (1969) Response of cutaneous sensory units with unmyelinated fibers to noxious stimuli. J Neurophysiol 32 : 1025–1043

Ferreira SH, Nakamura M (1979) II. Prostaglandin hyperalgesia: the periphal analgesic activity of morphine, enkephalins and opioid antagonists. Prostaglandins 18 : 191–200

Fitzgerald M, Lynn B (1979) The weak excitation of some cutaneous receptors in cats and rabbits by synthetic substance P. J Physiol (Lond) 293 : 66–67

Handwerker HO (1976) Pharmacological modulation of the discharge of nociceptive C-fibres. In: Zotterman Y (ed) Sensory functions of the skin in primate. Pergamon, Oxford, pp 427–439

Katori M, Harada Y, Tanaka K, Miyazaki H, Ishibashi M, Yamashita Y (1980) Changes of prostaglandin and thromboxane levels in pleural fluid of rat carrageenin-induced pleurisy. Adv Prostaglandin Thromboxane Res 8 : 1722–1737

Kumazawa T, Mizumura K (1979) Effects of synthetic substance P on unit discharges of testicular nociceptors of dogs. Brain Res 170 : 553–557

Kumazawa T, Mizumura K (1980) Mechanical and thermal responses of polymodal receptors recorded from the superior spermatic nerve of dogs. J Physiol (Lond) 299 : 233–245

Kumazawa T, Mizumura K, Sato J (1987) Thermally-potentiated responses to algesic substances of visceral nociceptors. Pain 28 : 255–264

Kumazawa T, Mizumura K, Sato J (in press) Response properties of polymodal receptors studied using in vitro testis-superior spermatic nerve preparations of dogs. J Neurophysiol

Lembeck F, Popper H, Juan H (1976) Release of prostaglandins by bradykinin as an intrinsic mechanism of its algesic effect. Naunyn Schmiedebergs Arch Pharmacol 294 : 69–73

Mense S (1981) Sensitization of group IV muscle receptors to bradykinin by 5-hydroxytryptamine and prostaglandin-E_2. Brain Res 225 : 95–105

Mizumura K, Sato J, Kumazawa T (in press) Effects of prostaglandins and other putative chemical intermediaries on the activity of canine testicular polymodal receptors studied in vitro. Pflügers Arch

Moncada S, Ferreira SH, Vane JR (1975) Inhibition of prostaglandin biosynthesis as the mechanism of analgesia of aspirin-like drugs in the dog knee joint. Eur J Pharmacol 31 : 250–260

Paintal AS (1965) Effects of temperature on conduction in single vagal and saphenous myelinated nerve fibres of the cat. J Physiol (Lond) 180 : 20–49

Schaible HG, Schmidt RF (1985) Coding of pain information from joint. In: Rowe MH, Willis WD (eds) Development, organization, and processing in somatosensory pathways. Liss, New York, pp 309–316

16 Appearance of Cold Sensitivity in Testicular Polymodal Receptors After Treatment with Clioquinol

K. Mizumura, J. Sato, and T. Kumazawa

Introduction

Painful dysesthesia is often observed in patients suffering from subacute myelo-optico-neuropathy (SMON), a condition that is aggravated by cold weather (Sobue 1979). In order to study a possible participation of activity of polymodal receptors, which are known to transmit nociceptive information (Kumazawa and Mizumura 1980a,b), in this painful sensation, we have tested the responses of polymodal receptors to clioquinol (QF), the causal agent of SMON. QF (1–500 μM) induces intermittent bursting discharges lasting for a long time (up to 3 h) after rinsing, and the response to hypertonic saline can be augmented following QF application (Kumazawa and Mizumura 1984). During these studies, we observed that polymodal receptors, normally insensitive to cold, responded to cold. In this report, characteristics of this cold sensitivity and the effects of ouabain were studied in vitro using canine testis superior spermatic nerve preparations; more than 90 % of these afferents are of the polymodal type (Kumazawa and Mizumura 1980b).

Methods

Male mongrel dogs were anesthetized with sodium pentobarbital (initial dosage 30 mg/kg i.v.), and a venous cannula was inserted into the cephalic vein of one side. A supplemental dose of pentobarbital was injected via this cannula, when necessary, to maintain the animal in an areflexic state. The testis and epididymis were exposed at the tunica vaginalis visceralis and excised from the animal, with the spermatic cord attached. They were held in a pool containing Krebs-Henseleit solution (test pool) equilibrated with 5 % CO_2, 95 % O_2 gas mixture. Single- or multiunit activity was recorded from the superior spermatic nerve immersed in an oil pool that was separated from the test pool by vaseline. In multifiber recordings, the number of active units was estimated from the response to hypertonic saline (Kumazawa and Mizumura 1984). Cold stimulation was carried out by replacing the Krebs solution (34° or 36°C) with precooled Krebs solution, and the temperature of the bathing solution was measured with a thermocouple. QF was dissolved in dimethylsulfoxide (DMSO) and diluted with Krebs solution to 100 or 500 μM, final concentration of DMSO being 0.2 %–1 %.

Response to cold stimulation up to 15°C was studied in more than 40 multifiber and 15 single-unit recordings. As in cutaneous polymodal receptors (Kumazawa and Perl 1977), cold stimulation seldom induced increased discharges in testicular polymodal receptors (Figs. 1A [lower histogram] and 2A), although spontaneous discharges were suppressed in some cases. The slight increase in discharges observed in a few cases displayed clear temperature dependency and its time relation to cooling was obscure. Thus, testicular polymodal receptors are considered to be normally insensitive to cold. As clearly shown in Fig. 1B (including two units), QF induced intermittent bursting discharges (QF discharges)

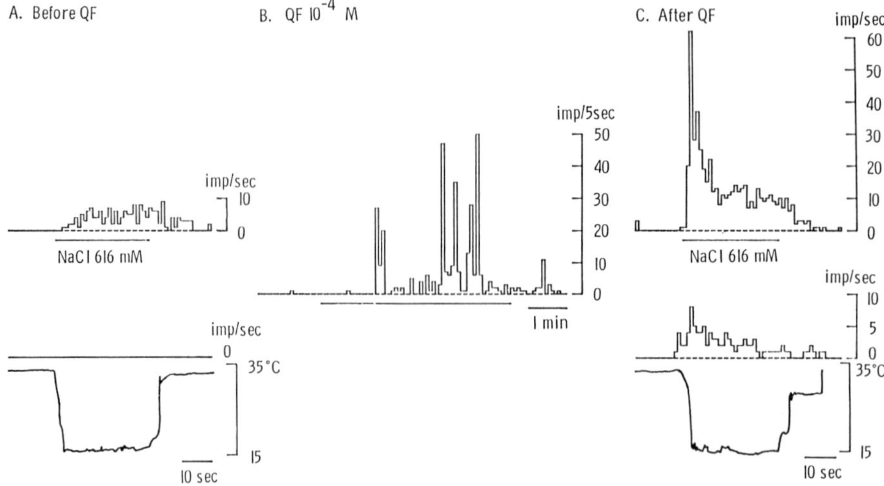

Fig. 1 A–C. Three kinds of changes in canine testicular polymodal receptor activities induced by clioquinol (QF). Peristimulus-time histograms are shown, 1 bin being 1 s in **A** and **C**, 5 s in **B**. These results were obtained from a nerve strand containing two units. Stimulation periods are indicated either with lines under histograms or with temperature recordings. **A, C** Responses to hypertonic saline (616 mM) and cold stimulation before (**A**) and after (**C**) application of QF. **B** Response to QF 10^{-4} M

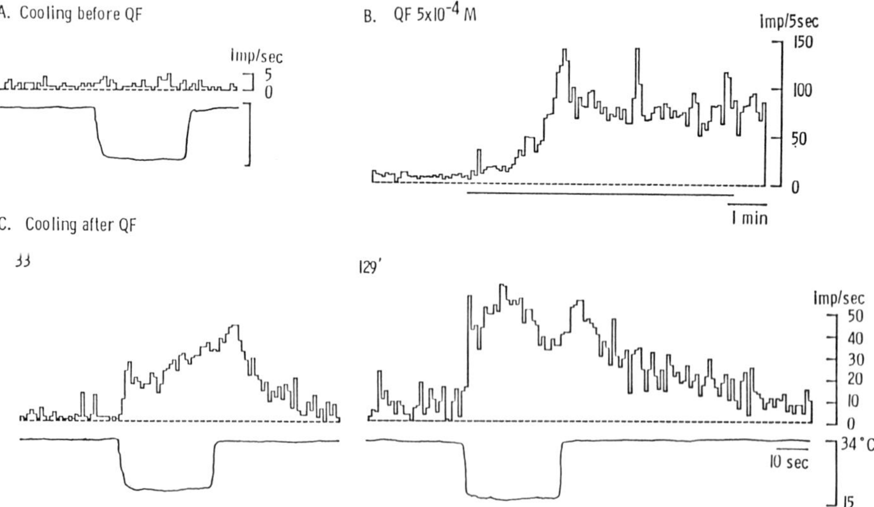

Fig. 2 A–C. Time course of cold discharges. **A, C** Response to cooling **A** before clioquinol (QF) and **C** after QF. **B** Response to QF 5×10^{-4} M. Cold discharges were not suppressed on rewarming and they could still be induced long after QF had been rinsed off

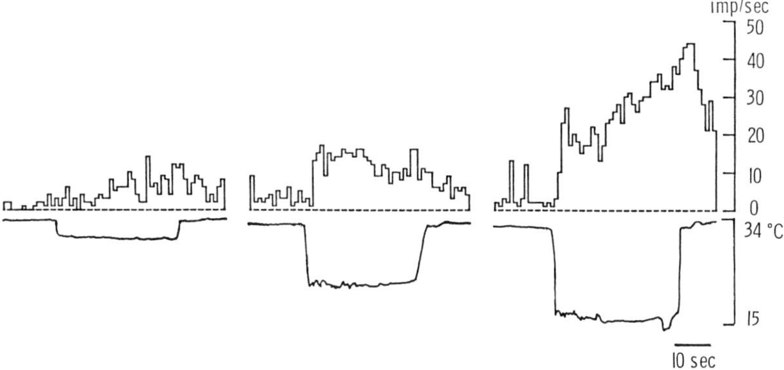

Fig. 3. Temperature dependency of cold discharges: an example of a multifiber recording. Testing carried out about 30 min after QF had been rinsed off

with about 2 min latency, and these discharges continued long after rinsing away the QF. As in our previous observation (Kumazawa and Mizumura 1984), the response to hypertonic saline was augmented after appearance of QF discharges (Fig. 1C).

Cold stimulation up to 15°C was tested in 51 cases after appearance of a QF discharge, and all except five cases responded with increased discharges (cold discharges). In the five cases without a cold response, the QF discharges were weak. Examples of cold responses are shown in Figs. 1C, 2C, and 3. A phasic increased discharge at the onset of stimulation was seldom seen. Increased discharges were not suppressed on rewarming, and often continued for several minutes after rewarming (Figs. 2C, 3). This cold sensitivity existed long after the QF was rinsed away (Fig. 2C), the longest effect lasting for more than 3 h. Cold discharges were not always maximal shortly after the rinsing of QF; they sometimes became greater in later tests (Fig. 2C). The increase in discharges were temperature-dependent (Fig. 3C): 30°C stimulation weakly increased discharges in this case, and temperature decrease to less than 25 °C consistently induced discharges, the discharge rates increasing roughly in parallel with the temperature decrease. Spontaneous fluctuation of excitability after QF sometimes obscured the temperature dependency. Threshold temperatures were between 25 ° and 30 °C in most cases tested.

It is proposed that temperature sensitivity of neurons is based on temperature dependency of electrogenic Na-K pump activity and conductances of Na and K channels (Carpenter 1981). In order to determine whether this hypothesis can explain the cold discharges described above, the effects of ouabain, an inhibitor of the Na-K pump, were studied. Ouabain (5 and 10 μM) induced discharges in polymodal receptors (untreated with QF) with a latency of several minutes (Mizumura et al. 1986), and these ouabain discharges were suppressed by cooling (to 15 °–25 °C) and augmented by warming (to 40 °C). When ouabain was applied after treatment with QF, it induced an increase in discharges similar to that seen in preparations not treated with QF. Cold discharges were no longer observable after ouabain, and abnormal bursting discharges were suppressed somewhat by cold.

These results clearly indicate that QF treatment can change the sensitivity of polymodal receptors to cold. The cold discharges elicited after QF treatment were roughly temperature-dependent, but they differed from the response of true cutaneous cold receptors (Hensel and Boman 1960) in that they had no clear phasic component at the onset of cooling and rewarming. In addition, they often continued for several minutes, even after rewarming. Nevertheless, these cold discharges were reversed by application of ouabain. The mechanism of cold discharge is an open question, but this result might suggest a contribution of Na-K pump activity to cold discharges after QF. Further experiments are needed to clarify the mechanism.

Aggravation of dysesthesia or paresthesia in cold weather is a well-known feature in some peripheral neuropathies, and impairment of peripheral circulation is often considered to be responsible for this change. The results reported here might suggest an alternative explanation for this clinical observation, i.e., cold sensitivity of polymodal receptors.

References

Carpenter DO (1981) Ionic and metabolic bases of neuronal thermosensitivity. Fed Proc 40 : 2808–2813

Hensel H, Boman KA (1960) Afferent impulses in cutaneous sensory nerve in human subjects. J Neurophysiol 23 : 564–578

Kumazawa T, Mizumura K (1980a) Chemical responses of polymodal receptors of the scrotal contents in dogs. J Physiol 299 : 219–231

Kumazawa T, Mizumura K (1980b) Mechanical and thermal responses of polymodal receptors recorded from the superior spermatic nerve of dogs. J Physiol (Lond) 299 : 233–245

Kumazawa T, Mizumura K (1984) Abnormal activity of polymodal receptor induced by clioquinol (5-chloro-7-iodo-8-hydroxyquinoline). Brain Res 310 : 185–188

Kumazawa T, Perl ER (1977) Primate cutaneous sensory units with unmyelinated (C) afferent fibers. J Neurophysiol 40 : 1325–1338

Mizumura K, Sato J, Kumazawa T (1986) Effects of ouabain on the activities of canine testicular polymodal receptors. Proc Int Union Physiol Sci 16 : 73

Sobue I (1979) Clinical aspects of subacute myelo-optico neuropathy (SMON). In: Vinken J, Bruyn GW (Eds) Handbook of clinical neurology, vol 37. North Holland, Amsterdam, pp 115–139

17 Fine Muscle Afferent Fibres and Inflammation: Changes in Discharge Behaviour and Influence on Gamma-Motoneurones

P. Berberich, U. Hoheisel, S. Mense, and P. Skeppar

Influence of an Artificial Myositis on the Discharge Behaviour of Muscle Group III and IV Afferent Units

Introduction and Methods

Inflammatory alterations of muscle tissue (e.g. in the course of rheumatic diseases) are associated with the subjective symptoms of spontaneous pain and/or tenderness of the affected muscle. Changes in the responsiveness of muscular nociceptors have been assumed to be - at least partly - responsible for these symptoms, but the exact nature of these changes has not yet been determined.

The present study was undertaken in order to find out how an artificial myositis affects the response behaviour of slowly conducting afferent units from a skeletal muscle. In cats anesthetized with chloralose (80 mg/kg i.p.) and rats anesthetized with Inactin (100 mg/kg i.p.) an inflammation of the gastrocnemius-soleus (GS) muscle was induced by infiltrating it with a solution of 2% carrageenan or 2% carrageenan plus 4% kaolin. The discharges of single group III and IV afferent fibres were recorded from thin filaments of the muscle nerve dissected by hand. The afferent units were classified as group III or IV according to their conduction velocity (group III 2.5–30 m/s, group IV below 2.5 m/s). Depending on their responsiveness to local pressure stimulation of the exposed GS muscle, the endings were sorted into one of the following categories: (1) "touch units" responding to touching the tissue with an artist's brush; (2) "moderate pressure units" giving clear responses to innocuous deformation of the tissue but not to the touch stimulus; (3) "noxious pressure units" requiring damaging intensities of stimulation for their activation. The last type corresponds to the nociceptive units of a previous and more detailed classification (Mense and Meyer 1985) while the first two categories - except for being mechanosensitive and non-nociceptive - have not been characterized further.

Background Discharge

Under control conditions (in cats without a myositis) and in the absence of intentional stimulation, about 30% of the fine muscle afferents had a background discharge, and the mean frequency was less than 1 imp/min (n = 15). The proportion of active units rose to nearly 60% and the mean frequency to about 11 imp/min (n = 36) in animals with an inflammation of the GS muscle. Cat group III units showed a statistically significant increase in mean background discharge from 1.1 (n = 6) to 20.7 (n = 10) imp/min, whereas group IV units did not [from 0.3 (n = 9) to 7.3 (n = 26) imp/min]. A characteristic feature of the background activity in many fibres from the inflamed muscle was its intermittent nature, with periods of silence alternating with phases of relatively high discharge frequency.

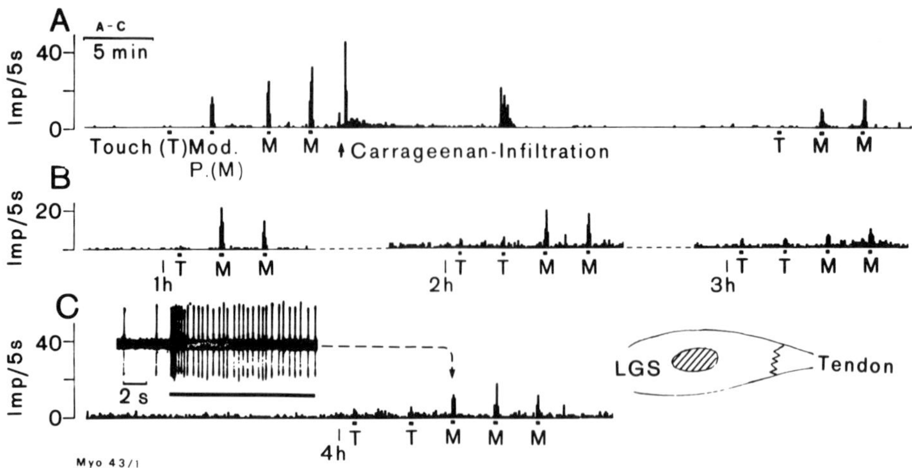

Fig. 1. Histogram (bin width 5 s) of the impulse activity of a cat non-nociceptive group IV muscle receptor (conduction velocity of afferent fibre: 0.84 m/s) during the transition from the normal state to an inflammation. The bars underneath the histogram indicate the period of mechanical stimulation. T, touching the receptive field; M, moderate (innocuous) local pressure; LGS, lateral gastrocnemius-soleus muscle. The hatched area on the LGS outlines the receptive field. 1 h, 2 h, 3 h, 4 h, hours after the infiltration of the muscle with carrageenan

Both nociceptive endings (noxious pressure units) and non-nociceptive endings (touch units and moderate pressure units) exhibited an increase in background activity after induction of the inflammation. Figure 1 shows a moderate pressure unit with a group IV afferent fibre, the discharges of which were recorded for a period of more than 4 h. Fifteen minutes after the beginning of panel A, carrageenan was injected into the muscle, causing a transient phase of high activity. The background activity started to increase about 1 h after the injection of carrageenan (Fig. 1B) and remained at an elevated level for the rest of the recording period. The first signs of a lowered mechanical threshold likewise occurred 1–2 h after the onset of the inflammation. At this time the touch stimulus, which was ineffective before (cf. Fig. 1A), started to elicit responses. It has to be pointed out, however, that not in all cases did the rise in background activity and the lowering of the mechanical threshold occur simultaneously. There were also units developing a higher background activity without a detectable lowering of the mechanical threshold.

In inflamed muscles, the level of background activity in the three response types (noxious and moderate pressure units, touch units) was of a similar magnitude (around 10 imp/min). This does not mean, however, that nociceptive and non-nociceptive units exhibit a similar increase in background discharge, since in an inflamed muscle a true touch unit cannot be distinguished from a sensitized nociceptor with a low mechanical threshold (see below).

Mechanical Excitability

Unlike the units in a normal muscle which had a quite well defined mechanical threshold and showed well-reproducible responses upon local pressure stimulation, the afferents from the inflamed muscle were less consistent in their response behaviour. A given unit could show marked fluctuations in its mechanical threshold, and the reproducibility of the responses was often poor. When tested repeatedly with mechanical stimuli many units exhibited long-term changes in the frequency of the background activity. Thus, noxious local pressure was often followed by a shift to a higher level of background activity, while stimulation with innocuous pressure in some units resulted in a reduction of the background discharge (Hoheisel and Mense 1986). The whole sample of the slowly conducting afferent units showed a shift of the response types from noxious pressure units to moderate pressure units and touch units under the influence of an inflammation, but the differences were not statistically significant. When cat group III and IV units were evaluated separately, the decrease in number of the noxious pressure units and the increase in the moderate pressure units became significant for group IV units, while the inflammation-induced changes in response behaviour remained non-significant for group III units.

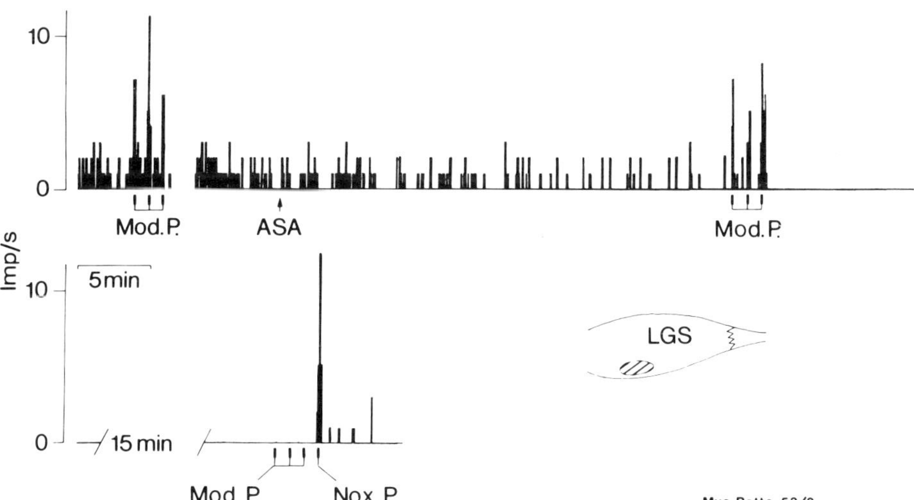

Fig. 2. Reduction of resting discharge and increase in mechanical threshold of a rat group IV muscle receptor from an inflamed muscle after intravenous injection of acetylsalicylic acid (ASA; 100 mg/kg). Mod. P., moderate (innocuous) local pressure applied to the receptive field outlined in the inset; Nox. P., noxious pressure. Conduction velocity of afferent fibre: 1.2 m/s

Effects of Acetylsalicylic Acid

In order to find out how the increased background discharge in group IV units is influenced by a typical non-steroidal anti-inflammatory substance, acetylsalicylic acid (ASA; 100 mg/kg) was injected intravenously in rats with an artificial myositis of the GS muscle. For the experiments rats were preferred over cats since only one receptor per animal could be tested with systemic application of the analgetic. Of the eight units tested, three showed a clear decrease in background activity which began 10–20 min after the injection of ASA. In one case an increase in mechanical threshold causing the transition from a moderate pressure unit to a noxious pressure unit was observed in parallel to the reduction in background activity (Fig. 2).

The observation that in about half of the tested units the background discharge was not influenced by ASA might indicate that some group IV units develop a background discharge without the involvement of prostaglandins, the synthesis of which had probably been blocked by the ASA concentration used.

Excitability Changes in Gamma-Motoneurones During Inflammation of Their Target Muscle

Introduction and Methods

In the clinical literature both decreases and increases of muscle tone have been reported to occur in the course of painful alterations of deep tissues such as muscles and joints. The change in muscle tone is perceived as painful and tends to become chronic (Brügger 1984). One possible explanation for the long-term increase in muscle tone is that the stimulation of muscle or joint nociceptors leads to an excitation of gamma-motoneurones which in turn produce an increase in muscular tension by activating the gamma loop (Fig. 3). The muscular hypertonus impairs the blood supply of the muscle; the resulting ischemia enhances the excitation of the nociceptors and thus perpetuates the pain (vicious circle; cf. Travell and Simons 1983).

The present experiments were designed to test whether gamma-mononeurones of the cat behave in accordance with this model if an artificial myositis is induced in the muscle they project to. The animals were deeply anesthetized with chloralose; the lateral head of the gastrocnemius-soleus (LGS) muscle was injected with carrageenan plus kaolin and recordings of the impulse activity of single fusimotor fibres were made from thin filaments of the nerve to the medial head of the gastrocnemius (MG) muscle. The fusimotor fibres were identified by their reflex excitability following stimulation of the LGS nerve and by their conduction velocity (12–48 m/s) following stimulation of the sciatic nerve. No attempts were made to differentiate between dynamic and static gamma-mononeurones.

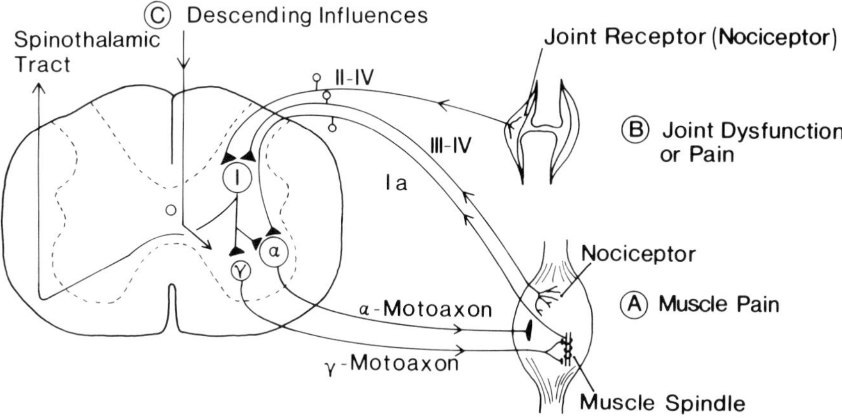

Fig. 3. Hypothetical model of the mechanisms leading to a muscular hypertonus. I, interneurone(s). See text

Effect on Background Activity

The above-described concept of a vicious circle implies that the activity in fusimotor neurones to a lesioned muscle is increased. The results of our study do not support such an assumption. Under control conditions about 75 % of the 42 gamma-motoneurones studied showed a background discharge; after induction of an inflammation this proportion decreased to about 41 % (n = 27). As can be seen from Fig. 4, this decrease in the number of active units was associated with a reduction of the mean background discharge to about half of the control value.

Changes in Electrical and Mechanical Reflex Excitability

The fusimotor units in the MG nerve had quite well defined electrical thresholds in the group II–III range following electrical stimulation of afferent fibres in the LGS nerve. Under the influence of a myositis of the LGS muscle, the reflex thresholds were shifted into the group III–IV range.

Similar results were obtained when the mechanical reflex excitability (by local pressure stimulation of the LGS muscle) of fusimotor neurones was tested. Under control conditions, most of the units gave clear responses to the "moderate pressure" stimulus, which consisted in an innocuous deformation of the muscle. In animals with an inflamed LGS muscle the fusimotor fibres showed a decrease in responsiveness to mechanical stimuli which was characterized by the absence of high-frequency responses. In a few cases the time-course of the influence of the inflammation on gamma-motoneurones could be studied by injecting carrageenan during the recording period. The preliminary data suggests that the depression of the gamma-neurones occurs already in an early phase of the inflammation, i.e. about 30–60 min after the injection of carrageenan.

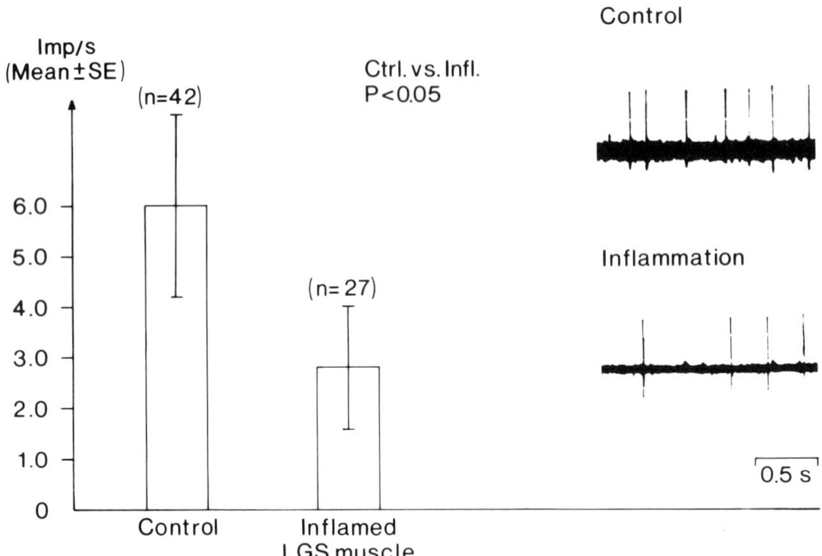

Fig. 4. Reduction of the resting activity of fusimotor fibres supplying the medial gastrocnemius muscle (MG) by an inflammation of the lateral gastrocnemius-soleus muscle (LGS). The original registrations show examples of the activity in single fusimotor fibres under control conditions (upper) and after induction of the myositis (lower)

Discussion and Conclusions

Group III and IV Primary Afferent Units

The study showed that the slowly conducting afferent fibre system is more active during an artificial myositis. This is expressed in an increase of the background activity in many nociceptive units – which could account for the spontaneous pain accompanying many forms of myositis – and in a decrease in mechanical threshold – which could be the neurophysiological correlate of the tenderness of an inflamed muscle. Since in the cat the background activity rose significantly in group III afferents only, while the lowering in threshold was significant in group IV units only, the two fibre groups may be involved in the mediation of spontaneous pain and tenderness respectively.

However, not only nociceptive but also non-nociceptive endings (touch units and moderate pressure units) showed an increase in background activity and/or a lowering in mechanical threshold during an inflammation. The significance of this finding is not clear; similar results have been reported for group III and IV afferents from arthritic joints in the cat and rat (Schaible and Schmidt 1985; Iggo et al. 1984). After injection of carrageenan the muscle became oedematous. The elevated intramuscular pressure could contribute to the increased activity in non-nociceptive units; it should, however, dampen the effects of mechanical stimuli and thus cannot account for the decrease in mechanical threshold.

The sensitization of receptive endings produced by an inflammation seems to be more effective than that following intramuscular injections of bradykinin, which sensitizes almost exclusively nociceptors (Mense and Meyer 1981). These data agree with the notion that bradykinin is only one of many sensitizing factors that are released from carrageenan-inflamed tissues (Di Rosa et al. 1971).

In spite of the fact that the whole muscle was infiltrated with the carrageenan solution a great proportion of the receptors appeared to be unchanged in their response behaviour. For instance, in the inflamed muscle many units exhibited neither a background activity nor a lowered mechanical threshold, i.e. they behaved like nociceptors in a normal muscle. In addition, some nociceptive units with an increased background activity did not react to ASA. These findings may indicate that different types of group III and IV nociceptors exist which are differently affected by an inflammation and by analgesic drugs. On the other hand, many units in an inflamed muscle showed a combination of a high resting discharge with a mechanical threshold in the noxious range. Apparently, changes in background discharge can occur without concomitant changes in the mechanical threshold.

Since some of the afferent units possessed double receptive fields – in our sample five of 45 units studied in normal muscle – one could speculate that this feature is the basis for the independence of background activity and mechanical threshold. However, the combination of a high background discharge with an apparently unchanged (high) mechanical threshold was also observed in units with single receptive fields.

Gamma-Motoneurones

The main effect of an artificial myositis on the fusimotor neurones supplying the inflamed muscle (or synergistic parts of it) seems to be a depression of activity in these neurones. This was true not only for the background discharge but also for their reflex excitability by electrical and mechanical stimuli. A possible explanation for this behaviour would be that the fusimotor neurones are subject to an inhibitory influence from homonymous muscle nociceptors which are tonically active during an inflammation. There is some evidence supporting this assumption: in our study the discharges of gamma-mononeurones in response to electrical and mechanical stimulation via the reflex arc could be reduced by increasing the stimulus intensity to noxious levels. Other authors have described both excitatory and inhibitory effects in extensor gamma-motoneurones upon electrical stimulation of muscle afferents at group III strength (Appelberg et al. 1983). The excitation might be due to activation of group III afferents from low-threshold mechanosensitive receptors which are known to have a strong excitatory influence on gamma-motoneurones (Ellaway et al. 1982), while the inhibition could be caused by group III nociceptors. Thus, the state of activity in gamma-motoneurones might depend on the balance between the nociceptive and non-nociceptive input via slowly conducting muscle afferents. Stimuli which elicit an input in nociceptive and non-nociceptive afferent fibres, such as injection of pain-producing substances, will produce an excitatory response (Hong et al. 1978) if the input via non-nociceptive units is more effective, whereas a predominant input via nociceptive muscle afferents will lead to a depression.

The data suggests that - in contrast to the widely held concept of a positive feedback mechanism - the gamma-motoneurones of a given muscle are depressed if the muscle is inflamed. This does not mean that the vicious circle does not exist. In the present study, only the gamma-motoneurones supplying an inflamed extensor muscle were examined. It is conceivable that the type of the target muscle (e.g. extensor vs flexor, postural vs locomotor) and the form and location of the lesion (e.g. arthritis vs myositis) are important factors governing the reaction of gamma-motoneurones to a painful tissue alteration.

References

Appelberg B, Hulliger M, Johansson H, Sojka P (1983) Actions on gamma-motoneurones elicited by electrical stimulation of group III muscle afferent fibres in the hind limb of the cat. J Physiol (Lond) 335 : 275–292

Brügger A (1984) Neurologische und morphologische Grundlagen der sogenannten rheumatischen Schmerzen - ein Beitrag zum Verständnis der Funktionskrankheiten. In: Berger M, Gerstenbrand F, Lewit K (eds) Schmerz bei Funktionsstörungen des Bewegungssystems. Fischer, Stuttgart New York, pp 56–79

Di Rosa M, Giroud JP, Willoughby DA (1971) Studies of the mediators of the acute inflammatory response induced in rats in different sites by carrageenan and turpentine. J Pathol 104 : 15–29

Ellaway PH, Murphy PR, Tripathi A (1982) Closely coupled excitation of gamma-motoneurones by Group III muscle afferents with low mechanical threshold in the cat. J Physiol (Lond) 331 : 481–498

Hoheisel U, Mense S (1986) Modulation of background activity in rat Group IV afferent units from inflamed muscle by mechanical stimuli and acetylsalicylic acid. Pflügers Arch [Suppl] 406 : R 21

Hong SK, Kniffki K-D, Schmidt RF (1978) Reflex discharges of extensor and flexor gamma motoneurones by chemically induced muscle pain (Abstr). Pain 1 : 58

Iggo A, Guilbaud G, Tégner R (1984) Sensory mechanisms in arthritic rat joints. In: Kruger L, Liebeskind JC (eds) Advances in pain research and therapy, vol 6. Raven, New York, pp 83–93

MENSE S, MEYER H (1981) Bradykinin-induced sensitization of high-threshold muscle receptors with slowly conducting afferent fibres. Pain [Suppl] 1 : 204

MENSE S, MEYER H (1985) Different types of slowly conducting afferent units in cat skeletal muscle and tendon. J Physiol (Lond) 363 : 403–417

SCHAIBLE H-G, SCHMIDT RF (1985) Effects of an experimental arthritis on the sensory properties of fine articular afferent units. J Neurophysiol 54 : 1109–1122

TRAVELL JG, SIMONS DG (1983) Myofascial pain and dysfunction. The trigger point manual. Williams & Wilkons, Baltimore London

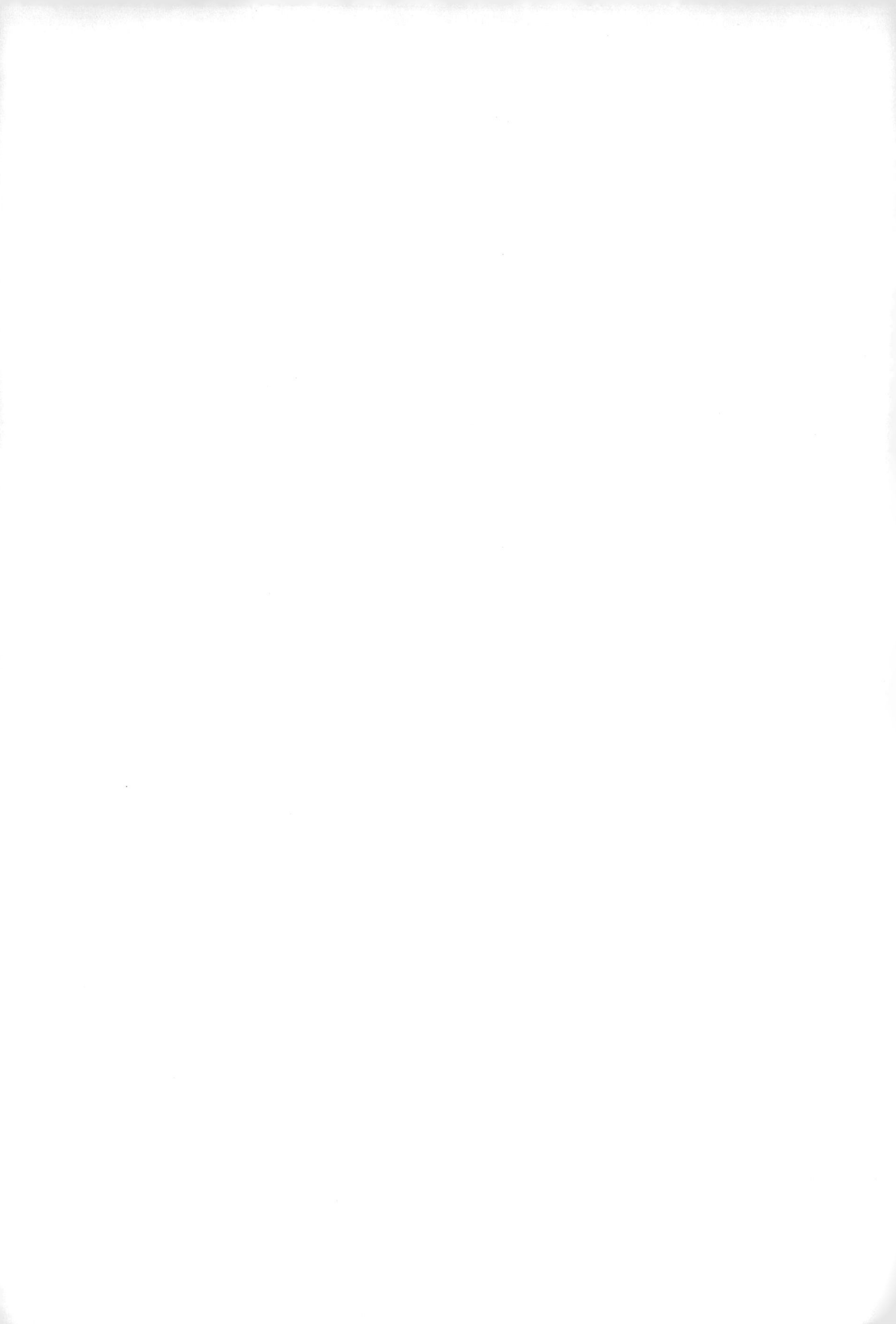

18 Effects of Opiates on Inflammation-Evoked Activity in Small Afferents Supplying the Knee Joint of the Cat

N.J. W. Russell, H.-G. Schaible, and R.F. Schmidt

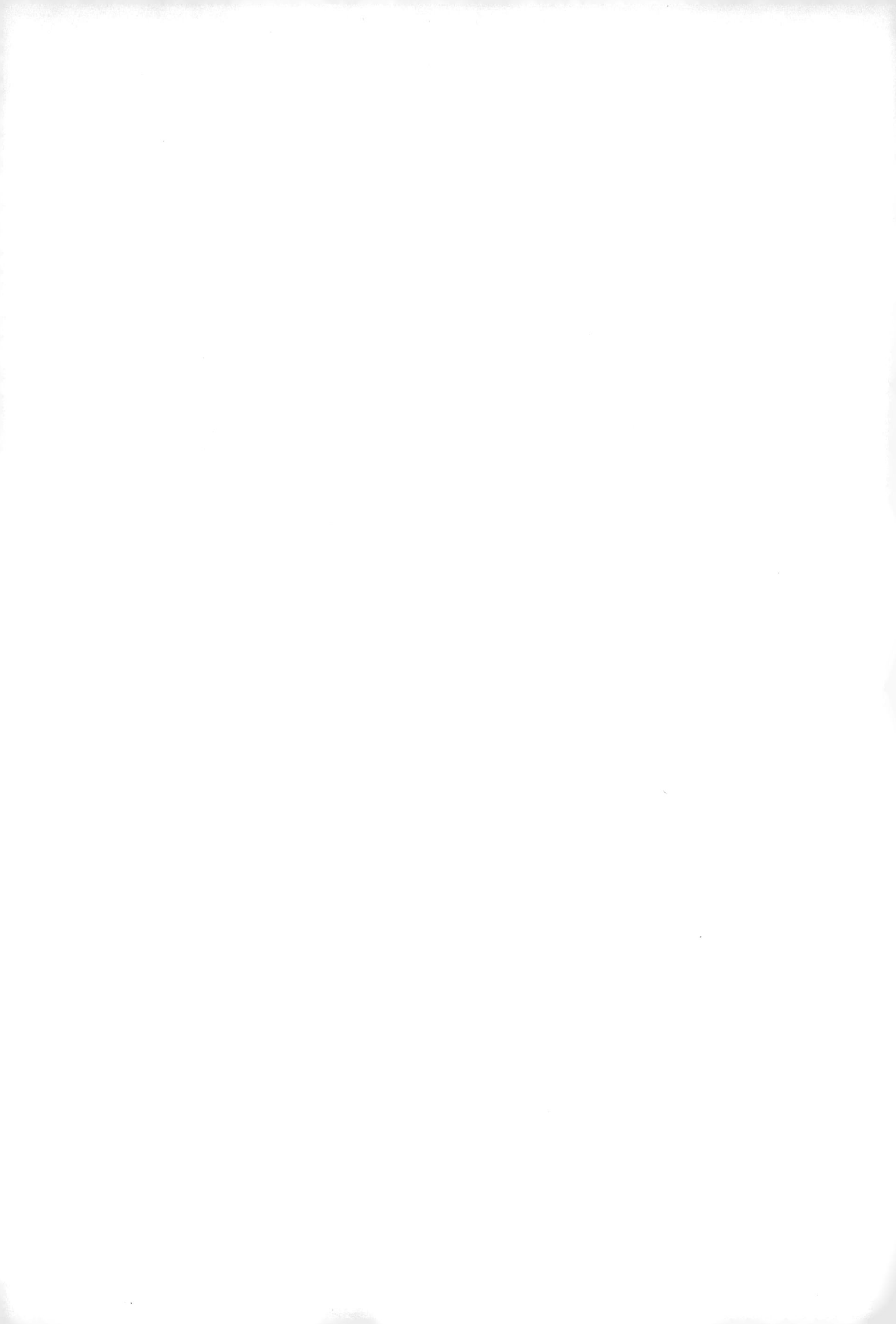

Several lines of evidence suggest that the activity of primary afferent neur… modulated by opiates acting at a peripheral site (for a recent summary of the … Russell et al. 1987 in press). Against this background the object of the present … riments was to study the peripheral effects of a range of opiate agonists on th… impulse traffic in small-diameter afferents from the acutely inflamed joint. This model … been chosen because studies of the receptive properties of fine afferent fibers in the medial articular nerve (MAN) of the cat have revealed that acute inflammation of the knee joint leads to the appearance or increase of spontaneous impulse activity and to increased sensitivity to movement (Schaible and Schmidt 1985), and that these symptoms of inflammation can be clearly reduced by cyclo-oxygenase inhibitors (Heppelmann et al. 1986) or partly mimicked by prostaglandins E_1 and E_2 (Heppelmann et al. 1985). In this model an antinociceptive effect of opiates should also be reflected in a depression of the spontaneous discharges of individual fine primary afferent fibers.

A more detailed report on the experiments described here is in press (Russell et al. 1987 in press).

Remarks on Methods

Recordings were made from functionally single units in filaments of the right MAN in a series of 12 chloralose-anaesthetised cats. For details of the anaesthesia and preparation see Schaible and Schmidt (1983a,b). Acute inflammation of the right knee joint was induced by intra-articular injection of kaolin (4 %) and carrageenan (2 %) at least 4 h prior to recording.

For each of the single units isolated, local probing confirmed that it had a receptive field on the joint, and that it was accessible to drugs injected intra-arterially (positive response to KCl). The 19 spontaneously discharging units in this series of 12 experiments had conduction velocities in the range 0.4–6.9 m/s.

Test compounds were administered by a retrograde bolus unjection (< 2 ml) into the right saphenous artery, which meant that compounds reached the knee joint via the genicular artery, a branch of the saphenous artery.

Test Protocol and Test Drugs

Impulse activity of single units with stable resting discharges was recorded for several minutes, up to 30 min. Thereafter, the test substances were injected in three portions all within 30 s followed by an injection of 1 ml Tyrode. An effect was considered inhibitory if the average discharge frequency (measured as impulses per minute) was significantly lower during the period after drug application than during the preceding control period. All except one unit were exposed to more than one of the test substances.

The opiates used in this study and the dose ranges employed were U50488 (1–10 mg/kg i.a.), ethylketocyclazacine (EKC; 0.5–4 mg/kg i.a.), morphine (1–5 mg/kg i.a.) and (D-Ala2, MePhe4, Gly-05) enkephalin (glyol; 0.5–5 mg/kg i.a.). Naloxone was used at a dose of 1 mg/kg i.a.. These compounds were chosen because it is known that U50488 and EKC have relatively selective agonist affinities for the kappa opiate receptor subtype, whereas morphine and glyol are mu opiate receptor agonists.

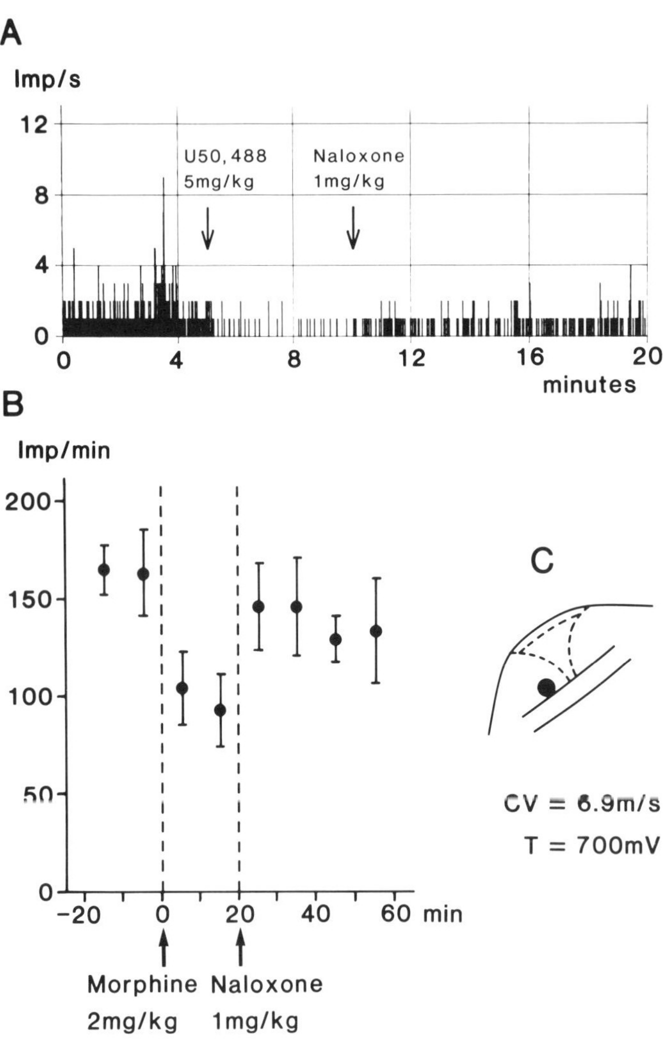

Fig. 1 A–C. Effects of intra-arterial injection of opiates U50488 (**A**) and morphine (**B**) on the spontaneous discharge of a single Group III afferent in the MAN. The actions of both drugs were reversed by naloxone. **C** The location of the receptive field of this unit on the medial aspect of the knee joint. T, electrical threshold of the fiber under observation; CV, conduction velocity

Actions of Mu and Kappa Agonists

The test procedures and the results are shown in Fig. 1. A group III afferent fiber (conduction velocity 6.9 m/s) with one receptive field (Fig. 1C) and showing spontaneous activity was exposed to U50488 (Fig. 1A, kappa agonist) and to morphine (Fig. 1B, mu agonist). In both cases the applications led to a significant inhibition of activity which was reversed by naloxone (specific opiate receptor antagonist).

Figure 2 shows the effects observed on the whole sample of articular afferents testing the four opioids. Ten units were tested with glyol. For five of these, glyol produced statistically significant inhibition. Morphine produced inhibition in three of nine units. Fourteen units were tested with EKC and inhibition was observed with nine of them. The effect of U50488 was tested on seven units, six of which showed inhibition (see Fig. 1.)

In almost all cases where an inhibitory effect of the test drugs was observed, its reversibility was also tested with naloxone (1 mg/kg i.a.). In the majority of cases a reversal could be seen.

Finally, an interesting aspect of opiate action on fine articular afferents is revealed in Fig. 3. The figure shows, for this sample of afferents, different combinations of responses to the two classes of opiate agonists. Some units were sensitive to either mu or kappa agonists only, and quite a few responded to both. This finding may be compared with observations on cell bodies of mouse dorsal root ganglia in culture (Werz and MacDonald 1982, 1984), where a similar spectrum of opiate effects was observed with mu, delta and kappa agonists.

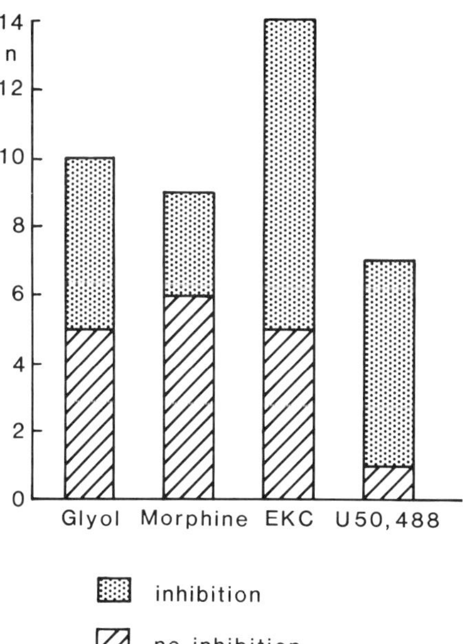

Fig. 2. Number of units which showed inhibition of spontaneous activity in response to opiate administration. The inhibitory actions were statistically significant at a level of $p < 0.01$ or better (for method of evaluation see Russell et al. 1987 in press)

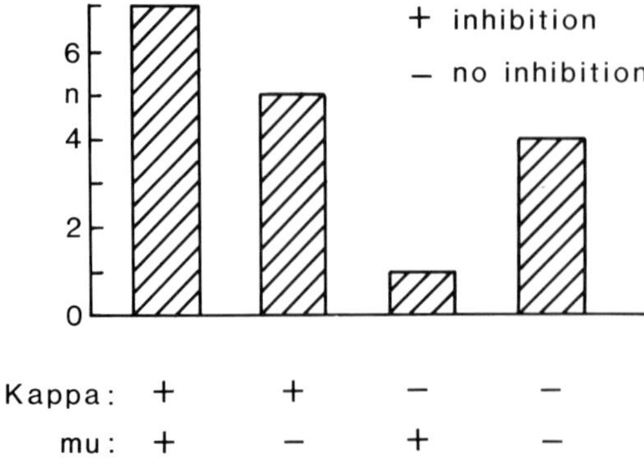

Fig. 3. Summary of the responses to kappa agonists (U50488, EKC) and mu agonists (glyol, morphin) in those fine afferents of our sample where at least on opiate of each type had been tested. Inhibition was again measured as a statistically significant reduction of the spontaneous impulse activity

Conclusion

These results show that opiates can exert inhibitory effects on spontaneous discharges in small-diameter afferents from inflamed knee joints in the cat. It is reasonable to assume, on the grounds of its reversibility with naloxone and its dose dependence, that the inhibition is due to the activation of specific opiate receptors in the terminal regions of the fibers (Russell et al. 1987 in press).

The increased sensory inflow from fine articular afferents during an acute inflammation is thought to be responsible for pseudaffective responses in animals and for pain (Schaible and Schmidt 1985). Correspondingly, the inhibitory effect of opiates on such resting discharges has to be considered as a peripheral analgesic action of these drugs. This conclusion is consistent with the peripheral analgesic action of opiates reported by others (Ferreira et al. 1984; Smith et al. 1982).

References

FERREIRA SH, LORENZETTI BB, RAE GA (1984) Is methylnalorphinium the prototype of an ideal peripheral analgesic? Eur J Pharmacol 99 : 23–29

HEPPELMANN B, SCHAIBLE H-G, SCHMIDT RF (1985) Effects of prostaglandins E_1 and E_2 on the mechanosensitivity of group III afferents from normal and inflamed cat knee joints. In: FIELDS HL, DUBNER R, CERVERO F (eds) Advances in pain research and therapy. Raven, New York, pp 91–101

HEPPELMANN B, PFEFFER A, SCHAIBLE H-G, SCHMIDT RF (1986) Effects of acetylsalicylic acid and indomethacin on single groups III and IV sensory units from acutely inflamed joints. Pain 26 : 337–351

RUSSELL NJW, SCHAIBLE H-G, SCHMIDT RF (1987) Effects of opiates on the discharges of fine afferent units from inflamed knee joint. (in press)

SCHAIBLE H-G, SCHMIDT RF (1983a) Activation of groups III and IV sensory units in medial articular nerve by local mechanical stimulation of knee joint. J Neurophysiol 49 : 35–44

SCHAIBLE H-G, SCHMIDT RF (1983b) Responses of fine medial articular nerve afferents to passive movements of knee joint. J Neurophysiol 49 : 1118–1126

SCHAIBLE H-G, SCHMIDT RF (1985) Effects of an experimental arthritis on the sensory properties of fine articular afferent units. J Neurophysiol 54 : 1109–1122

SMITH TW, BUCHAN P, PARSONS DN, WILKINSON S (1982) Peripheral antinociceptive effects of N-methyl-morphine. Life Sci 31 : 1205–1208

WERZ MA, MCDONALD RL (1982) Heterogeneous sensitivity of cultured dorsal root ganglion neurones to opioid peptides selective for mu- and delta-opiate receptors. Nature 229 : 730–733

WERZ MA, MCDONALD RL (1984) Dynorphin reduces voltage-dependent calcium conductance of mouse dorsal root ganglion neurones. Neuropeptides 5 : 253–256

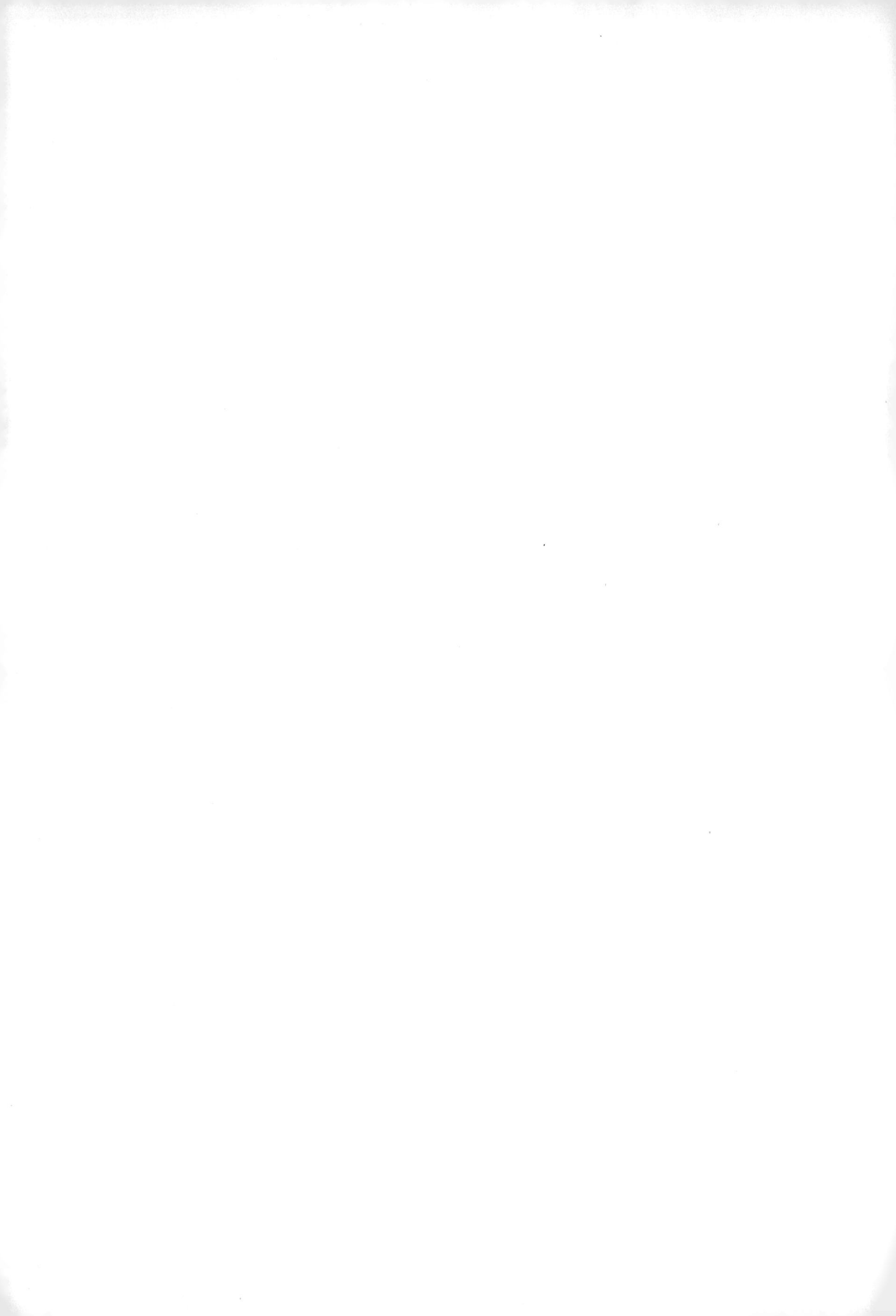

19 Vasodilation of Articular Blood Vessels Induced by Antidromic Electrical Stimulation of Joint C Fibres

W.R. Ferrell and R. Cant

Introduction

In previous experiments it was observed that electrical stimulation of the posterior articular nerve (PAN) of the cat knee joint above C fibre threshold resulted in plasma protein extravasation into the synovial cavity (Ferrell and Russell 1985). In other sites, such as skin, it has been observed that this neurogenically mediated increase in blood vessel permeability is accompanied by dilation of these vessels (Couture and Cuello 1984). The present experiments were performed to establish whether such neurogenic vasodilation also occurs in articular blood vessels.

These vessels are known to be innervated by sympathetic vasoconstrictor fibres, as Cobbold and Lewis (1956) observed that stimulation of the sympathetic chain resulted in reduction of blood flow to the cat knee joint. Vasoconstriction also occurred when the distal portion of the cut medial articular nerve (MAN) was electrically stimulated. Although the electrical stimulus parameters used by Cobbold and Lewis (1956) were not stated, the stimuli must have been sufficient to activate C fibres, as sympathetic efferent fibres in articular nerves are known to be unmyelinated (Langford and Schmidt 1983). Electrical stimulation of the joint nerve at intensities sufficient to activate these fibres would also recruit unmyelinated afferent fibres, which constitute about half of the total population of unmyelinated fibres in articular nerves (Langford and Schmidt 1983). It would be expected that electrical stimulation of these fibres should result in dilation of articular blood vessels, yet Cobbold and Lewis (1956) described only vasoconstriction of joint blood vessels in response to electrical stimulation of articular nerves. Thus, the present experiments were performed to re-examine this.

Methods

Adult cats deeply anaesthetised with intraperitoneal pentobarbitone (45 mg/kg) were used in these experiments. Anaesthesia was maintained by additional intravenous doses as required. Arterial blood pressure was continuously monitored via a cannula inserted into the carotid artery.

Changes in blood flow to the knee joint were indirectly assessed by monitoring alterations in intra-articular temperature. This was achieved by insertion of a 23G hypodermic thermocouple into the joint space by an anterolateral approach (Fig. 1). This thermoprobe was connected to an amplifier (Harvard Thermalert model TH-6D) having resolution to 0.01 °C. The analog output of the amplifier was then further amplified, inverted and filtered (bandwidth D.C. to 0.1 Hz), with this signal being recorded on one channel of a pen recorder whilst blood pressure was recorded on the other channel. Providing that blood pressure remained stable (ensured by maintenance of a deep level of anaesthesia), rectal temperature was kept at 37° ± 0.5 °C (mean ± SE) by a thermistor-controlled heating element, and

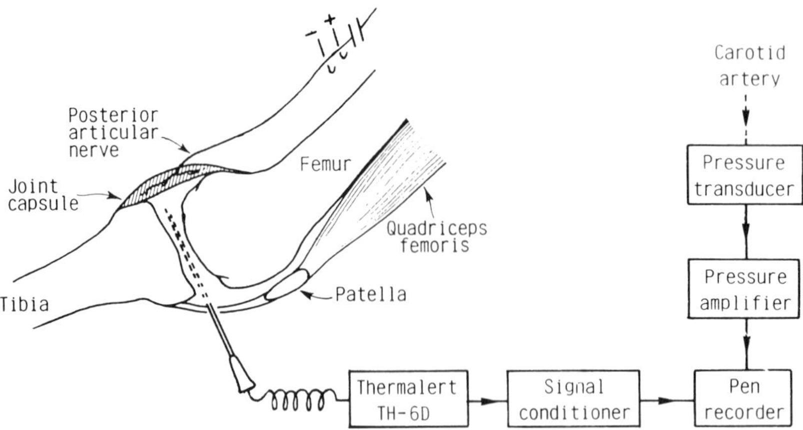

Fig. 1. Diagram of the experimental arrangement

care was taken to minimise heat losses from the knee (fur not shaved from the hindlimb and the sciatic nerve stimulated rather than PAN, as described below), intra-articular temperature remained stable for protracted periods in the absence of any experimental procedures. Mean intra-articular temperature was 33° ± 0.62 °C.

In early experiments antidromic activation of knee joint C fibre afferents was achieved by direct electrical stimulation of PAN directly. Subsequently it was found that more reliable results could be obtained by electrical stimulation of the sciatic nerve just beyond the hip with all branches of this nerve except PAN being sectioned. In all instances PAN or the sciatic nerve was sectioned proximally so that action potential propagation only occurred peripherally. This could easily be checked by the absence of any effect on arterial blood pressure of high-intensity stimulation of these nerves. The electrical stimuli consisted of a 1-min train of square wave pulses of width 1 ms, frequency 10 Hz and amplitude 15 V, this last being ample to activate articular C fibres (Sato et al. 1983). These pulses were delivered by silver chloride hook electrodes placed over the nerve in a pool of warmed mineral oil.

Results

In nine of a series of 11 animals it was observed that stimulation of unmyelinated articular nerve fibres produced a characteristic pattern of initial fall in the temperature of the joint innervated by these fibres during the period of stimulation followed by a prolonged rise in intra-articular temperature on cessation of stimulation (Fig. 2). The magnitude of the rise in temperature ranged from 0.15° to 0.73 °C, with a mean of 0.28° ± 0.06 °C (n = 11). The time taken for the temperature to rise above and then return to control values ranged from 8 to

30 min with a mean of 12.9 ± 3 min (n = 11). The magnitude and duration of the initial fall in intra-articular temperature was limited by the period of stimulation, but the maximum temperature fall observed at the end of the 1-min stimulus train ranged from 0.04° to 0.25 °C with a mean of 0.1° ± 0.02 °C (n = 11). In two animals it was found that no rise in intra-articular temperature occurred on PAN stimulation although the initial fall in temperature was present.

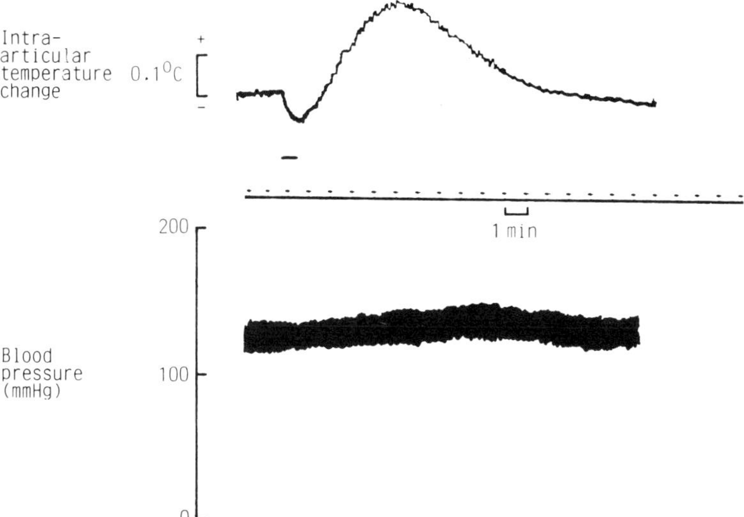

Fig. 2. Effect of electrical suprathreshold stimulation of knee joint C fibres (black bar) on the temperature of the knee joint cavity. A fall in temperature occurs during the 1-min stimulation period, followed by a long-lasting elevation of temperature

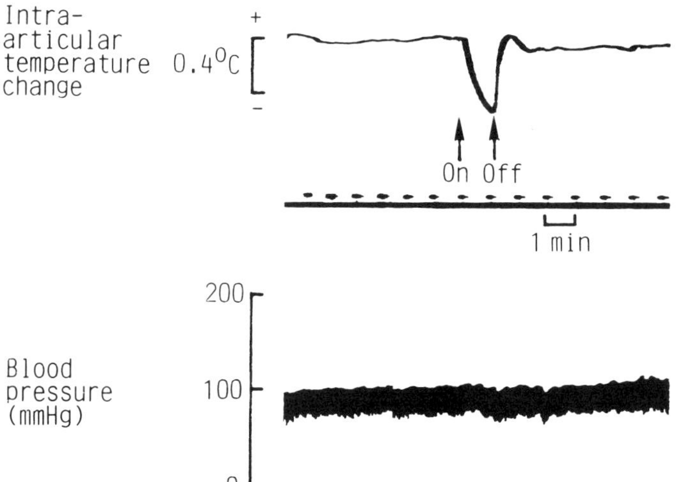

Fig. 3. Knee joint temperature change in response to a 1-min period of occlusion of its arterial blood supply (arrows). Only a small and short-lasting dilation occurs on release

The initial fall in temperature is consistent with the vasoconstriction of articular blood vessels originally described by Cobbold and Lewis (1956). The subsequent rise in temperature suggests that dilation of these vessels then occurs. As no such dilation was observed by Cobbold and Lewis (1956), the present experiments were directed at establishing the mechanisms underlying this dilator response.

It could be argued that this dilation represents reactive hyperaemia resulting from the preceding period of vasoconstriction. To test this hypothesis, the arterial blood flow to the hindlimb was interrupted by placing weights on a length of stout thread which was looped around the femoral artery high up in the groin. As shown in Fig. 3, occlusion of the blood supply to the joint, although providing a much more intense hypoxic stimulus than vasoconstriction, produces only a very small and short-lasting "rebound" dilation. This was tested in two other animals, and in each case a similar pattern to that illustrated in Fig. 3 was observed.

Another possible cause of the dilator response is that articular nerves contain not only sympathetic adrenergic vasoconstrictor fibres, but perhaps also sympathetic cholinergic vasodilator fibres. Two lines of evidence argue against this concept. Firstly, electrical stimulation of the cut peripheral ends of the dorsal roots L7 and S1 (containing the majority of PAN afferents but no sympathetic efferent fibres) results in dilation without preceding constriction (Fig. 4). This response was consistently observed in all four animals examined. The time course of this dilation is roughly comparable to that occurring during peripheral nerve stimulation.

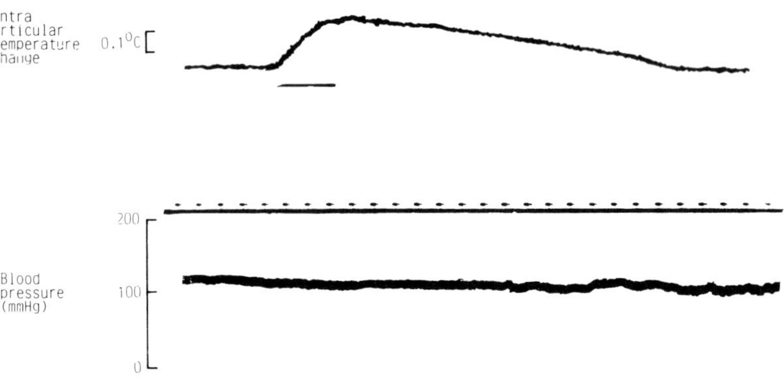

Fig. 4. Electrical stimulation of articular C fibre afferents in dorsal roots L7 and S1 (black bar) only produces a rise in knee joint temperature

The second line of evidence is that the dilator response can be abolished by intra-articular injection of the substance P antagonist (D-Pro4, D-Trp7, 9, 10)-SP(4–11) before electrical stimulation of the joint nerve (Fig. 5). The constrictor response is enhanced when the dilator response is abolished (Fig. 5B), probably because it is now completely unopposed. The dilator response can be restored (Fig. 5C) by removing the substance P antagonist and allowing 20 min to elapse. Figure 5 represents data from one cat, but essentially similar results were obtained in a further two animals.

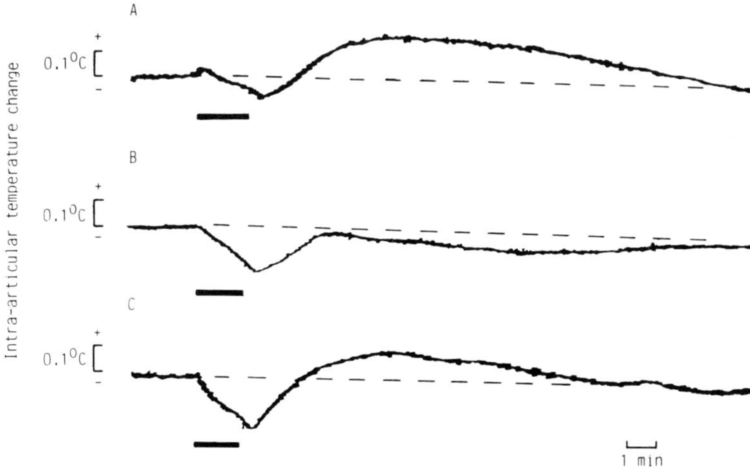

Fig. 5 A. Control trace: electrical stimulation of articular C fibres (black bar) produces fall followed by rise in intra-articular temperature. **B** Intra-articular injection of 100 μg of the substance P antagonist (D-Pro4, D-Trp7,9,10)-SP(4–11) just prior to stimulation abolishes the dilator response. **C** Removing the antagonist, washing out the synovial space and allowing 20 min to elapse restores the response almost to control values

Discussion

The results of the present experiments indicate that, consistent with the findings of Cobbold and Lewis (1956), articular nerves contain sympathetic efferent fibres which are vasoconstricting in nature. The main difference is the obvious dilator response observed in the present experiments. The lack of such a response in the experiments of Cobbold and Lewis is perhaps due to differences in the nerve used (MAN vs PAN) or, more likely, differences in the species of animal used (dogs vs cats).

The dilator response was demonstrated to arise from afferent fibres, as it could be elicited on electrical stimulation of the appropriate dorsal roots. Assuming that (D-Pro4 D-Trp7,9,10)-SP(4–11) is a specific substance P antagonist, it would appear that the dilator response is mediated by articular afferents which release substance P from their terminals when depolarised. It is unlikely that the substance P antagonist has a direct effect on the blood vessels of the knee joint, as any intra-articular temperature changes occurring on its injection differ little from those observed when saline (at the same temperature as the substance P antagonist) is injected.

The findings from these experiments, taken together with the results of previous experiments (Ferrell and Russell 1985), indicate that the two components of neurogenic inflammation – vasodilation and increased permeability of blood vessels – occur on antidromic activation of articular C fibre afferents. It is possible that in naturally occurring joint disease, these afferents could, by means of the "axon reflex", contribute to the initiation or maintenance of the inflammatory process. Thus, the potential for a neurogenic component of joint inflammation exists, particularly in view of the finding that the spontaneous activity of C fibres is greatly enhanced in acutely inflamed joints in cats (Coggeshall et al. 1983) and rats (Guilbaud et al. 1985).

Therefore, in addition to their recognised role in nociception, articular C fibre afferents could also have an important role to play in acute inflammatory diseases of joints.

References

Cobbold AF, Lewis OJ (1956) The nervous control of joint blood vessels. J Physiol (Lond) 133 : 467–471

Coggeshall RE, Hong KAP, Langford LA, Schaible H-G, Schmidt RF (1983) Discharge characteristics of fine medial articular afferents at rest and during passive movements of inflamed knee joints. Brain Res 272 : 185–188

Couture R, Cuello AC (1984) Studies on the trigeminal antidromic vasodilatation and plasma extravasation in the rat. J Physiol (Lond) 346 : 273–286

Ferrell WR, Russell NJW (1985) Plasma extravasation in the cat knee-joint induced by antidromic articular nerve stimulation. Pflugers Arch 404 : 91–93

Guilbaud G, Iggo A, Tegner R (1985) Sensory receptors in ankle joint capsules of normal and arthritic rats. Exp Brain Res 58 : 29–40

Langford LA, Schmidt RF (1983) Afferent and efferent axons in the medial and posterior articular nerves of the cat. Anat Rec 206 : 71–78

Sato Y, Schaible H-G, Schmidt RF (1983) Types of afferents from the knee joint evoking sympathetic reflexes in cat inferior cardiac nerves. Neurosci Lett 39 : 71–75

20 A Comparison of the Electrophysiological and Immunocytochemical Properties of Rat Dorsal Root Ganglion Neurones with A and C Fibers

S. N. Lawson, P. J. Waddell, and P. W. McCarthy

Introduction

There are a number of differences in electrophysiology, immunocytochemistry and cytology between groups of dorsal root ganglion (DRG) neurones. In this paper we look at some of these differences in the rat and ask if there is any evidence that they are directly related to whether the neurones have myelinated (A) or unmyelinated (C) peripheral fibers.

Electrophysiological Differences Between A and C Neurones

The most obvious electrophysiological difference between the somata of A and C fibers is in the mean duration of the action potential (AP). The C-cell APs are longer, as they have a marked inflection or "hump" on their falling phase. This has been shown in several species, including the pigeon (Görke and Pierau 1980) and the rat (Harper and Lawson 1985b). The presence of a hump in DRG neurone APs has been correlated with the existence of an inward Ca^{++} current (in addition to the Na^{+} current) in the pigeon (Görke and Pierau 1980) and in cultured DRG neurones of the mouse (e.g. Heyer and Macdonald 1982) and chick (Dichter and Fischbach 1977). However, it is not only the C cells which display such a hump. A proportion of A neurones in both pigeon and rat also have an inflection on their repolarisation phase although much less marked than in C neurones, (Görke and Pierau 1980; Harper and Lawson 1985b).

Another consistent finding has been that the mean duration of the after-hyperpolarisation (AHP) is longer in C cells than in A cells (Görke and Pierau 1980; Harper and Lawson 1985b).

In the present paper we examine the electrophysiological differences between cells with and without humps from all conduction velocity (CV) groups to see whether these differences are more closely related to myelination or to the presence of a hump.

Immunocytochemical Markers for Neuronal Subgroups

Rat DRG neurones have been subdivided into large light or A neurones and small dark (SD) or B neurones according to their cytology, the abundance of neurofilaments and their size (Andres 1961; Lawson et al. 1984). These populations have overlapping distributions of cell size, the large light neurones spanning the entire size range of DRG neurones while the SD cells are confined to the lower end of the range (see Lawson et al. 1984). In this paper the previously used term "large light" has been replaced by "light" (L) in view of the fact that this population includes small, medium and large-sized neurones. The antineurofilament antibody RT97 labels the L cell bodies while leaving the SD cell bodies unlabelled (Lawson et al. 1984), presumably because of the abundance of neurofilaments in L cells.

Although it is generally assumed that SD neurones in the rat have predominantly unmyelinated fibers while L cells have myelinated fibers, direct evidence is needed to test this assumption. Recently cell size measurements of neurones with known conduction velocities (CVs) supported this assumption, since cells with C fibers fell within the SD size range while the size range of A fiber cells extended beyond it (Harper and Lawson 1985a). In this paper we provide evidence that RT97 acts as a specific label for neurones whose CVs indicate that they have myelinated fibers (also see Lawson and Waddell 1985).

Many other antibodies label subgroups of DRG neurones, particularly of the smaller neurones. Since the size distributions of L and SD neurones overlap considerably, it is not clear to what extent each of these subgroups might include L as well as SD cells. We have therefore examined the size distributions and the RT97 immunoreactivity of neurones labelled with a variety of antibodies.

We have examined the following antibodies: (1) anti-substance P (SP), since SP-like immunofluorescence (SPLI) is displayed by 20 % of neurones in rat DRGs which are in the small size range (Hökfelt et al. 1980). (2) Monoclonal antibody 2C5, which also labels a subpopulation of small neurones comprising 20 %–25 % of DRG neurones in L4 (Lawson et al. 1985). The epitope for 2C5 is a lactoseries carbohydrate chain (for details see Dodd and Jessell 1985). It has been reported that there is virtually no overlap between the population labelled with 2C5 and that displaying SPLI (Dodd and Jessell 1985). These two populations taken together should be equivalent in size to about 80 % of the SD population, since the SD population makes up about 50 %–55 % of the neurones. (3) anti-CGRP (calcitonin gene-related peptide). It has been reported that CGRP-like immunoreactivity (CGRPLI) is seen mainly in small DRG neurones with less intense staining in medium-sized neurones, and many neurones showing SPLI also display CGRPLI (Gibson et al. 1984; Skofitsch and Jacobowitz 1985).

Methods

Intracellular Recordings

Female rats aged 6–8 weeks were anaesthetised with sodium pentobarbitone. The L4, L5 and L6 DRGs with their dorsal roots and peripheral nerves were dissected out, placed in an in vitro chamber and superfused with oxygenated balanced salt solution maintained at 37 °C. For more details of the method see Lawson and Waddell (1985). Intracellular recordings were made from the DRG somata with electrodes containing 3 M KCl or dye, either Lucifer yellow CH in 0.1 M LiCl or ethidium bromide in 1 M KCl. CVs were measured from sites on the peripheral nerve and dorsal root to the cell body over distances of about 10–40 mm. AP and AHP characteristics were measured, and in some cells dye was then injected into the cell. During some recordings TTX (10^{-6} g/ml) was applied in the superfusate for 3 min and then washed off.

Neurones were classified into different CV groups as follows: C fibers < 1.3 m/s; A fibers > 1.5 m/s, subdivided into Aδ fibers 1.5–12 m/s and Aα/β fibers > 12 m/s. The boundary between C and A fiber groups was based on clear populations visible in the frequency distribution histogram of CVs in a much larger group of units than those reported here (n = 505). The boundary between Aδ and Aα/β is based on the same data but its exact position is not so clear. The boundary was set at 12 m/s for the purpose of comparing the slow A fiber group with the fast A fiber group. These CV groups are consistent with those previously reported for female rats of the same age (Harper and Lawson 1985a) but the CVs for each group are slower than those reported by Lynn and Carpenter (1982) in older rats (their Aδ fiber CVs ranged from 5 to 15 m/s). This difference is to be expected, since CV increases with age in the rat for both myelinated and unmyelinated fibers (Birren and Wall 1956; Hopkins and Lambert 1973).

RT97 Indirect Immunoperoxidase Method

DRGs containing a dye-labelled neurone of known CV were fixed overnight in Bouin's fixative, embedded in wax and 7 μm sections were cut. The fluorescent cell was located, drawn and measured under interference contrast with a camera lucida attachment to the fluorescent microscope. The indirect immunoperoxidase method was used to demonstrate RT97 immunoreactivity (see Lawson et al. 1984). The labelled cells were relocated and the relative intensity of the immunoreactivity was measured.

Double Immunofluorescence Labelling

Population Studies

Rats aged 8–12 weeks were anaesthetised with sodium pentobarbitone and perfused through the heart with isotonic saline, followed by 500 ml of either ice-cold paraformaldehyde or room-temperature Zamboni's fixative. The L4 DRGs were removed and left in fixative for 1–2 h then overnight in 30% sucrose in phosphate buffer. Multiple series of 7-μm-thick frozen sections were taken from each DRG. Each series comprised one section taken at regular intervals (usually 400 μm) throughout the ganglion. Each series of sections was incubated in the first layer of antibody (containing two primary antibodies) for 24–48 h at 4 °C and in the second antibody layer for 30–60 min at room temperature. For further details and references of primary antibodies see Lawson et al. (1984) for RT97, Lawson et al. (1985) for 2C5, Harmer and Keen (1986) for anti-SP and Gibson et al. (1984) for anti-CGRP. Second-layer antibodies used were FITC-conjugated goat anti-mouse IgG to react with RT97, rhodamine-labelled goat anti-rabbit IgG to react with the polyclonal anti-Sp and anti-CGRP antibodies and FITC-conjugated goat anti-mouse IgM to react with 2C5.

In each series all neuronal sections with clear nuclei (most had nucleoli) were measured and their immunofluorescence was graded.

Combined with Electrophysiology

After a cell had been injected with dye the ganglion was fixed by immersion and processed as above. The labelled cell was found and immunocytochemistry carried out on the appropriate sections. Controls to examine whether the fluorescent dye interfered with the immunocytochemistry are reported by McCarthy and Lawson (this volume).

Results

Intracellular Recordings

All C cells (16/16), 60 % of the Aδ cells (25/41) and 23 % of the Aα/β cells (35/154) had APs with an inflection or hump on the falling phase (Table 1). These will be called C, AδI and Aα/βI neurones respectively. The remaining Aδ and Aα/β cells had no such inflection and will be called AδO and Aα/βO neurones or AO neurones collectively.

For the mean AP duration, statistically significant differences were seen between C cells and each of the groups of A cells. However, there were also significant differences between AI and AO cells. It can also be seen from Table 1 that the mean AP duration increases with decreasing CV for neurones with humps, that is AI and C cells. This may indicate that although C cells have much longer APs than A cells, the difference could be in the size of the inward Ca^{++} current rather than in the type of ion carrying the inward current in C cells.

Table 1. Conduction velocity (CV) range and action potential (AP) parameters for neurones with and without a hump

	CV range (m/s)	No. of cells	AP mean duration (ms)	AHP mean duration (ms)
C	0.3–1.3	16	3.84 ± 2.87	24.5 ± 9.7
AδI	1.5–12	25	1.41 ± 0.56	16.9 ± 13.5
Aα/βI	12–28	35	0.97 ± 0.16	15.6 ± 15.8
AδO	5.7–12	16	0.7 ± 0.18	5.7 ± 6.6
Aα/βO	12–50	119	0.57 ± 0.11	6.1 ± 6.6

Above: neurones with AP inflections (C, AδI, Aα/βI). Below: neurones without AP inflections (AδO, Aα/βO). AP mean duration was measured across the base of the AP. The after-hyperpolarisation (AHP) mean duration was measured to the time of 80 % recovery

The proportions of neurones with humps in each CV range increased with decreasing CV such that all C cells, but no neurones with CVs greater than 28 m/s, had humps.

The mean AHP duration was considerably longer in C cells than in A cells (see Table 1) and was also longer in all groups of neurones with humps than in those without.

Tetrodotoxin (TTX) caused a complete block of the intracellularly evoked AP in all neurones whose APs had no hump (13/13 including AδO and Aα/βO). In contrast, in 13/13 neurones whose APs displayed humps the APs were not abolished and were never reduced in height by more than a few mV, suggesting that both the Ca^{++} and the Na^{+} components were TTX-resistant. This group included C, AδI and Aα/βI neurones. In some of these neurones an increase in threshold was found.

Conduction Velocity and RT97 Immunocytochemistry

RT97 labelled all (20/20) of the neuronal somata whose peripheral nerve or dorsal root CV was in the A fiber range (Aα/β and Aδ). The sizes of these somata covered the entire size range in the DRG. None of those with peripheral C fibers were RT97-positive (0/7). These somata were all small, in the size range of the SD neurones.

Double-Labelling Immunofluorescence Study

It follows that double immunofluorescent labelling with RT97 can indicate for each antibody-labelled population the proportion of neurones which have CVs in the A fiber range, consistent with their fibers being myelinated.

Table 2. Percentages of immunocytochemically labelled neurones

Antibody	No. of rats	Mean % neurones	SD
RT97+	8	51 9	6.4
SPLI+	7	18.9	1.5
RT97+/SPLI+	7	4.1	2.8
2C5+	4	24.2	3.7
2C5+/RT97+	1	(3.85)	–
CGRPLI+	4	38.3	8.7
CGRPLI+/RT97+	3	8.5	1.4
CGRPLI+/2C5+	3	16.8	2.8

The means and standard deviations of the percentages of all measured neurones which were labelled by the antibody (ies) indicated. For example, 16.8/24.2 (69.4%) of the 2C5 neurones also showed CGRPLI. One L4 DRG was analysed from each rat. The mean number of neurones sampled for each series was 255, range 125–510

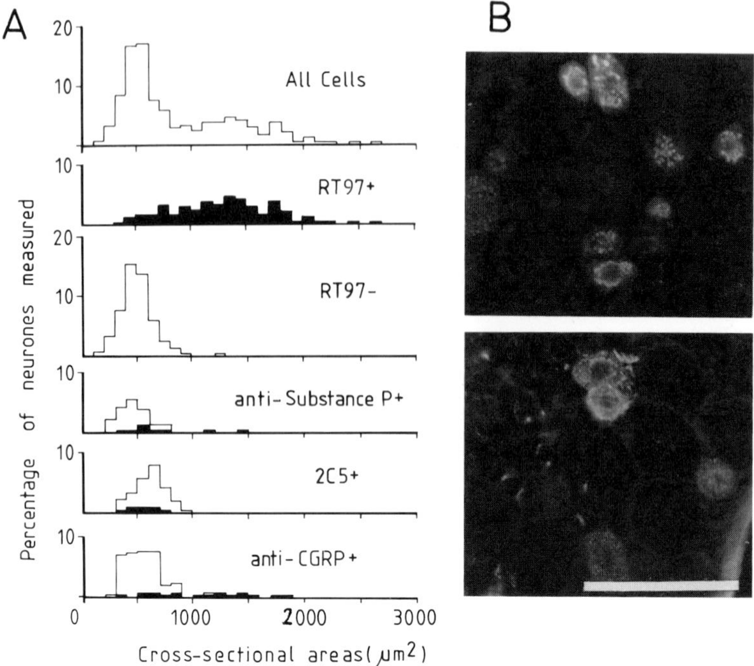

Fig. 1 A. The size distributions of antibody-labelled neurones from two series of sections from the same Zamboni-fixed L4 DRG from a 10-week-old female rat. Top four histograms from one series, lower two from another series of sections. The solid histograms indicate those neurones labelled by RT97 as well as by the antibody indicated. **B** Photomicrographs of a frozen section showing immunofluorescence with anti-CGRP (upper, rhodamine) and 2C5 (lower, FITC). Note that most 2C5-positive neurones also show CGRPLI. Bar = 100 μm

It was found (see Table 2, Fig. 1A) that about 50% of neurones were RT97-positive. About 19% of neurones showed SPLI, most of which fell in the size range of the SD (RT97-negative) population and were RT97-negative. One-fifth of the SPLI neurones were also RT97-positive. The values for overlap between SPLI and RT97 immunoreactivity were variable, perhaps indicating that these neurones are clustered within the DRG. Approximately 25% of all neurones were 2C5-positive; about one-sixth of these were also RT97-positive. About 38% of the neurones showed CGRPLI, of which about one-fifth were also RT97-positive. The CGRPLI/RT97-positive population covered the entire size range of L neurones, comprising about one-sixth of this population. The overlap between 2C5- and CGRP-positive neurones was very extensive (Table 2, Fig. 1B), about 70% of 2C5-positive neurones showing CGRPLI.

Electrophysiology Combined with Immunocytochemistry

Table 3 shows some preliminary results. Despite the small amount of data, there is remarkably good correlation between the population studies above and these results. That is, as we would predict from the overlap studies with RT97, 2C5-positive cells had C fibers, one-fourth of the neurones showing SPLI had A fibers (presumed to be myelinated) and neurones showing CGRPLI fell in all CV ranges.

Table 3. Immunoreactivity of neurones of known CV labelled intracellularly by Lucifer yellow or ethidium bromide

Antibody	C		Aδ		Aα/β	
	+ve	-ve	+ve	-ve	+ve	-ve
RT97	–	2	–	2	10	–
2C5	2	–	–	6	–	9
Anti-SP	3	1	1	6	–	10
Anti-CGRP	1	2	1	3	2	7

Discussion

From the analysis of AP duration it seems that there is no real evidence for fundamentally different AP mechanisms between A and C neurones, although detailed studies of the ionic mechanism are required to verify this. A real difference in mechanism does seem to exist between the neurones with and those without a hump, since not only is a substantial Ca^{++} inward current indicated but our results show that in rat DRGs a TTX-sensitive Na^{+} inward current was found only in neurones with no hump.

The mean duration of the AHP was much longer in C neurones than in A neurones. However, it was also generally longer in hump than no-hump neurones. Barrett and Barrett (1976) showed that some mammalian motoneurones have longer AHPs due to a Ca^{++}-dependent K^{+} current (IK Ca) while shorter duration AHPs were associated with voltage-dependent K^{+} currents (IK V). It was therefore suggested (Ransom and Holz 1977; Görke and Pierau 1980) that DRG neurones with humps have longer AHPs because of an IK Ca perhaps in conjunction with an IK V. Whatever the mechanism, it seems that taken as a whole group the C cells might differ from the A cells by displaying an extreme form of the behaviour intrinsic to DRG cells with Ca^{++} currents, rather than falling into a totally different group with respect to ionic mechanisms. However, further differences in ionic mechanisms may well emerge in subpopulations of DRG neurones divided according to sensory function.

RT97 antibody was found to label only the neurones whose CVs indicated that at least the peripheral process was myelinated. We have therefore used this antibody as a marker to distinguish between A and C neurones. We define C neurones as those which have C fiber CV (presumed to indicate no myelin) in both the central and peripheral processes and A neurones as those with any myelination (that is A-fiber CVs in either of these processes).

The proportions of DRG neurones labelled with the antibodies RT97, 2C5 and those against SP and CGRP were very close to those already reported in the literature (Lawson et al. 1984, 1985; Hökfelt et al. 1980; Dodd and Jessell 1985). The overlap studies showed that a part of each population was also labelled with RT97, indicating that one-fifth of the SPLI neurones, one-sixth of the 2C5 neurones and one-fifth of the CGRPLI neurones had A fibers. The RT97-positive parts of these populations had cell bodies of a size compatible with them having either Aδ or Aα/β fibers (see Harper and Lawson 1985a).

The immunocytochemistry showed a very good correlation between the results obtained from electrophysiologically identified neurones and the predicted results for each antibody on the basis of the overlap studies with RT97. This has increased our confidence in the use of RT97 as a marker for myelinated fiber cells in the rat. We are continuing this study seeking further correlations between the electrophysiological properties of neurones and their immunoreactivity to these and to other antibodies.

Acknowledgements. We are grateful to the MRC for supporting P.J. Waddell and P. McCarthy. We should also like to thank J. Wood, B.J. Randle, P. Keen and J. Polak for the gifts of antibodies RT97, 2C5, anti-SP and anti-CGRP respectively.

References

Andres KH (1961) Untersuchungen über den Feinbau von Spinalganglien. Z Zellforsch Mikrosk Anat 55 : 1–48

Barrett EF, Barrett JN (1976) Separation of voltage dependent potassium currents, and demonstration of a TTX-resistant calcium current in frog motoneurones. J Physiol (Lond) 255 : 737–774

Birren JE, Wall PD (1956) Age changes in conduction velocity, refractory period, number of fibers, connective tissue space and blood vessels in sciatic nerve of rats. J Comp Neurol 104 : 1–16

Dichter MA, Fischbach GD (1977) The action potential of chick dorsal root ganglion neurones maintained in cell culture. J Physiol (Lond) 267 : 281–298

Dodd J, Jessell TM (1985) Lactoseries carbohydrates specify subsets of dorsal root ganglion neurons projecting to the superficial dorsal horn of rat spinal cord. J Neurosci 5 : 3278–3294

GIBSON SJ, POLAK JM, BLOOM SR, SABATE IM, MULDERRY PM, GHATEI MA, McGREGOR GP, ET AL. (1984) Calcitonin gene-related peptide immunoreactivity in the spinal cord of man and of eight other species. J Neurosci 4 : 3101-3111

GÖRKE K, PIERAU F-K (1980) Spike potentials and membrane properties of dorsal root ganglion cells in pigeons. Pfluegers Arch 386 : 21–28

HARMER AJ, KEEN P (1986) Methods for the identification of neuropeptide processing products: somatostatin and the tachykinins. Methods Enzymol 124 : 335–348

HARPER AA, LAWSON SN (1985a) Conduction velocity is related to morphological cell type in rat dorsal root ganglion neurones. J Physiol (Lond) 359 : 31–46

HARPER AA, LAWSON SN (1985b) Electrical properties of rat dorsal root ganglion neurones with different peripheral nerve conduction velocities. J Physiol (Lond) 359 : 47–63

HEYER EJ, MACDONALD RL (1982) Calcium and sodium dependent action potentials of mouse spinal cord and dorsal root ganglion neurones in culture. J Neurophys 47 : 641–655

HÖKFELT T, JOHANNSSON O, LJUNGDAHL A, LUNDBERG JM, SCHULTZBERG H (1980) Peptidergic neurones. Nature 284 : 515–521

HOPKINS AP, LAMBERT EG (1973) Age changes in conduction velocity of unmyelinated fibers. J Comp Neurol 147 : 547–552

LAWSON SN, WADDELL PJ (1985) Intracellular recordings from rat primary afferent neurones with known peripheral and central conduction velocities. J Physiol (Lond) 364 : 13P

LAWSON SN, HARPER AA, HARPER EI, GARSON JA, ANDERTON BH (1984) A monoclonal antibody against neurofilament protein specifically labels a subpopulation of rat sensory neurones. J Comp Neurol 228 : 263–272

LAWSON SN, HARPER EI, HARPER AA, GARSON JA, COAKHAM HB, RANDLE BJ (1985) Monoclonal antibody 2C5: a marker for a subpopulation of small neurones in rat dorsal root ganglia. Neuroscience 16 : 365–374

LYNN B, CARPENTER SE (1982) Primary afferent units from the hairy skin of the rat hind limb. Brain Res 238 : 29–43

RANSOM BR, HOLTZ RW (1977) Ionic determinants of excitability in cultured mouse dorsal root ganglion and spinal cord cells. Brain Res 136 : 445–453

SKOFITSCH G, JACOBOWITZ DM (1985) Calcitonin gene-related peptide coexists with substance P in capsaicin sensitive neurons and sensory ganglia of the rat. Peptides 6 : 747-754

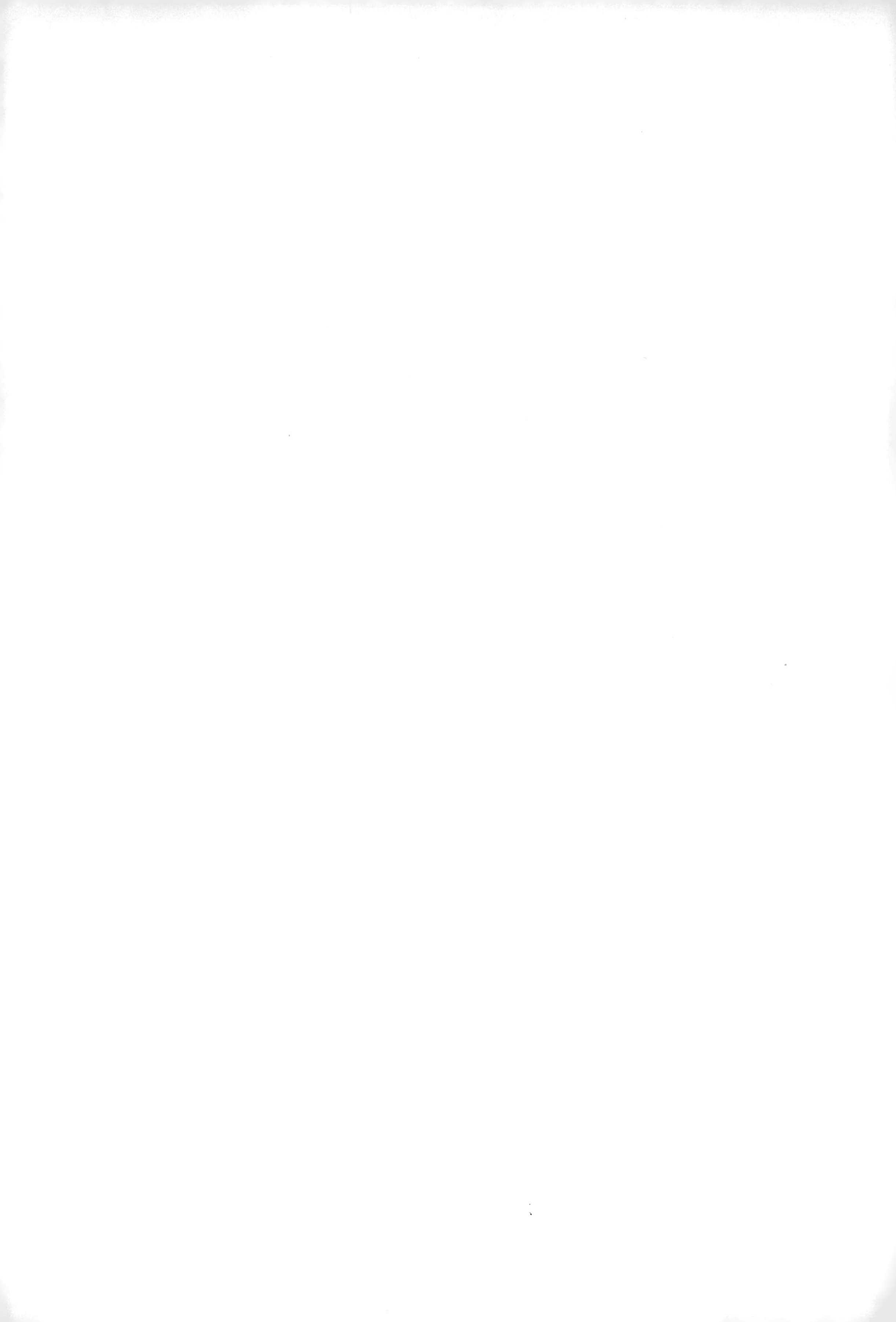

21 Intracellular Injection of Ethidium Bromide and Lucifer Yellow Allows the Positive Identification of Two Neurones in the Same Dorsal Root Ganglion

P. W. McCarthy and S. N. Lawson

Introduction

Intracellular injection of Lucifer yellow has been extensively used to label electrophysiologically identified neurones (Stewart 1981). The use of a second fluorescent dye would offer significant advantages, not least of which would be the ability to label and identify adjacent neurones in the same preparation. This would lead to a greatly increased number of neurones which could be studied in any preparation. Furthermore, such a technique would enable the direct comparison of the physical relationships between two adjacent cells.

To the authors' knowledge, the use of the fluorochrome, ethidium bromide, as an intracellular label has been reported only by Aghajanian and Vandermaelen (1982). Prompted by this report, we have compared ethidium bromide and Lucifer yellow as intracellular markers. These dyes have been used together in a study of the immunocytochemistry of electrophysiologically characterised rat dorsal root ganglion (DRG) neurones in vitro.

Methods

Preparation of the Dyes

Ethidium Bromide. Ethidium bromide (Sigma) was dissolved in distilled water (12 mM) and could be stored at 4 °C. This stock solution was mixed 1:1 with 2 M KCl and allowed to stand for 30 min before being used to fill microelectrodes. The resulting mixture could be stored for weeks in the dark at 4 °C.

Lucifer Yellow. We are grateful to W. Stewart for the gift of Lucifer yellow. This dye was dissolved as 5 % w/v in 0.1 M LiCl solution (ca. 110 mM). The final solution could be stored in the dark at 4 °C for months.

Preparation of the Electrodes

Intracellular recording microelectrodes were manufactured from 1.2 mm external diameter, thick-walled, filamented capillary glass (GC120-F15, Clark Electromedical). Microelectrode tips were filled with a small quantity of dye/electrolyte solution. The remainder of the microelectrode was filled with a pure electrolyte solution, either 2 M KCl (ethidium) or 1 M LiCl (Lucifer).

Electrophysiology

Recordings were made from rat DRG neurones in vitro (Lawson and Waddell 1985), using standard single-electrode intracellular voltage recording techniques. Dye (either ethidium or Lucifer) was injected after sufficient electrophysiological information had been obtained from the impaled neurone. Constant current pulses (±1 nA for 700 ms at 1 Hz) in a depolarising (ethidium) or hyperpolarising (Lucifer) direction were used for the purpose of dye injection. Approximate currents required to fill a 40 μm diameter neurone were 4 nA min for ethidium and -2.5 nA min for Lucifer.

Histology

The ganglia were lightly fixed (90 min) in Zamboni's fixative and left overnight in a 30 % sucrose 0.1 M phosphate buffer (pH 7.4) before frozen sectioning. Dye-filled cells were located using a Leitz Dialux 22 microscope with epifluorescence (filter details in Table 1 and Figs. 1,2) at a total magnification of x 160.

Table 1. Lists of the concentrations and properties of both ethidium and Lucifer as used in these experiments

	ethidium bromide	Lucifer yellow
Concentration in solution	6 mM	110 mM
Concentration of electrolyte	1 M KCl	0.1 M LiCl
Electrode resistance [MΩ]	60–90	150–200
Injection current	Positive	Negative
Colour of fluorescence	Orange/red	Yellow
Filter block	I_2/N_2	I_2
Excitation filters	N_2 [BP530–560]	I_2[BP450–490]
Suppression filters	N_2[LP580]	I_2(LP515]

The filter blocks listed are for use in the Leitz Dialux 22 microscope. The standard electrode resistance for 3 M KCl as the electrolyte was between 20 and 50 MΩ

Immunocytochemistry

The frozen sections were incubated for 24–48 h with the primary antibody (i.e. RT97, anti-substance P) and 30 min incubation with secondary (fluorescent labelled) antibody (see Lawson et al., this volume).

A series of controls have been performed to determine if the presence of dye interfered with the antibody reaction. In the controls, frozen sections of fixed rat DRGs were lightly stained with either Lucifer (50 μm) or ethidium (50 nM) in phosphate buffer (0.1 M, pH 7.4). These sections, and unstained controls, were then treated with antibodies as per normal.

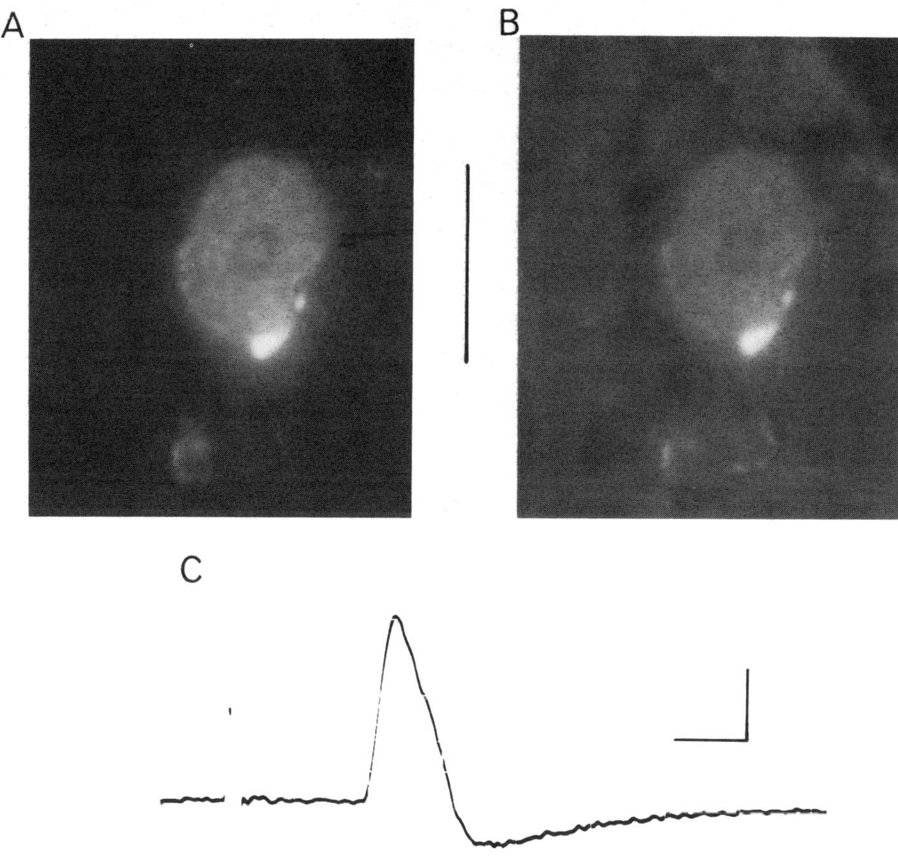

Fig. 1 A–C. The electrophysiology and histological appearance of an ethidium-filled neurone. **A, B** Two views of the same "dry" 7 μm frozen section of the neurone using N_2 and I_2 filter units respectively. Lucifer-filled neurones were only visible when using the I_2 unit. Note that the fluorescence of the neurone in **A** appears more intense, with respect to background, than that in **B**. The dye-filled neurone was just as obvious in **B**, however, owing to the difference in colour between the background (green) and the dye (orange). The scale bar represents 50 μm. **C** An intracellular voltage recording of an action potential. This was recorded in the soma and evoked by peripheral nerve stimulation; note the artefact. The resting membrane potential of this neurone was -58 mV. The scale bars indicate 25 mV (vertical) and 1 ms (horizontal)

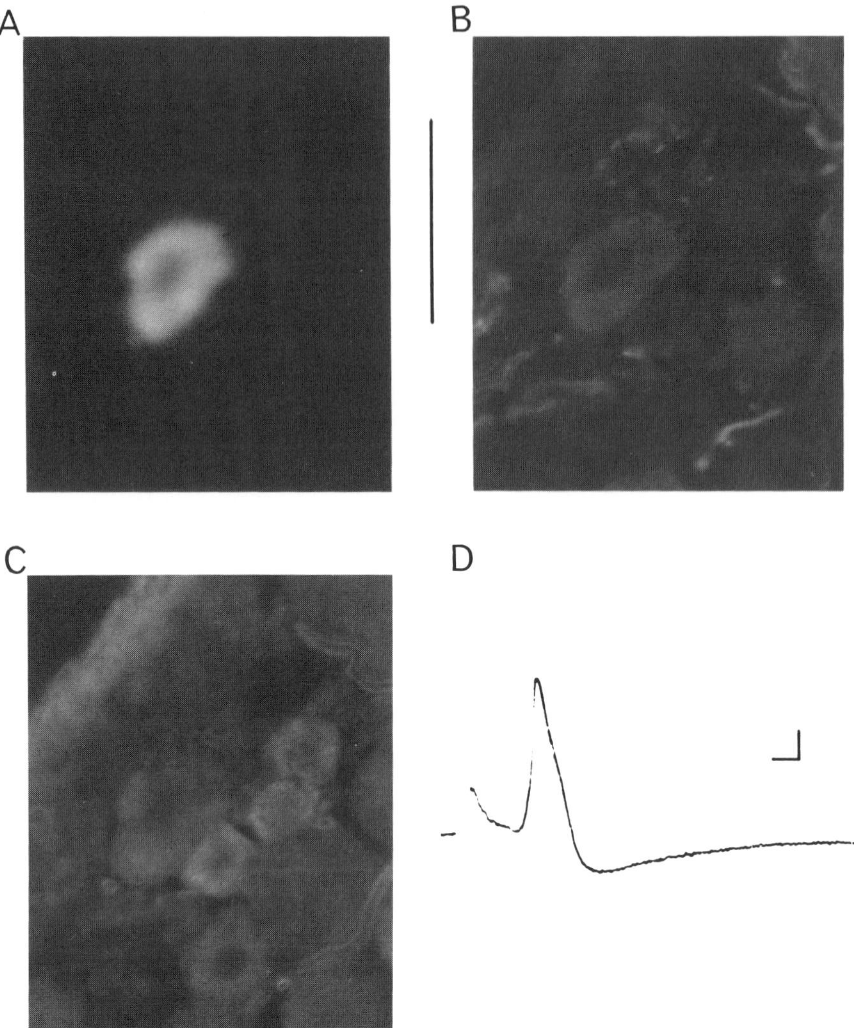

Fig. 2 A–D. The correlation of electrophysiology and immunocytochemistry. **A** A "dry" 7 μm frozen section through an ethidium-filled neurone. **B, C** The same section after treatment with RT97 and anti-substance P antibodies. The N_2 filter unit was used to view **A** and **C** and the I_2 in the case of **B**. This neurone was RT97-positive and substance P-negative. Note that the intensity of ethidium fluorescence was greatly reduced after the immunocytochemical processing (cf. **A** and **C**). The scale bar represents 50 μm. **D** The corresponding intracellular voltage recording of an action potential; details as in Fig. 1. The resting membrane potential of this neurone was -70 mV, the scale bars represent 20 mV (vertical) and 1 ms (horizontal)

Results

Electrophysiology

Dye-injection microelectrodes filled with ethidium had electrical resistances lower than those containing Lucifer (Table 1). Correspondingly, electrophysiological measurements made with microelectrodes used for ethidium dyeinjection were of a similar or higher quality than those made with Lucifer-filled microelectrodes. Although dye filling of neurones took slightly longer with ethidium, the lower microelectrode resistances and the use of positive injection current made the electrodes more stable and less prone to "blocking", a phenomenon seen occasionally with Lucifer-filled microelectrodes.

Histology

Both dyes could be located in fixed, frozen sections of tissue. No dye coupling was noticed between neurones; however, there was some evidence of dye coupling between the injected neurones and adjacent glial cells. One could select for ethidium over Lucifer by changing the excitation and suppression filters (Table 1, Fig. 1).

Immunocytochemistry

The area and antibody reactivity of a representative selection of neuronal sections were measured for a series of 7 μm sections of ganglion. Only neuronal sections with nuclei were measured and used in the assay. This method was used to ascertain whether the presence of either dye affected the percentage or actual population (based on size) of neurones reacting with antibody. So far RT97 and anti-substance P antibodies have been tested and appear to be unaffected by the presence of either dye. Further antibodies are in the process of being tested. The results so far have increased our confidence in this technique. Therefore, the dyes are still being used to correlate data obtained in electrophysiological experiments with the findings of immunocytochemical studies (Lawson et al., this volume).

Discussion

We have shown that ethidium bromide can be used alongside Lucifer yellow as an intracellular label. Using these two dyes it was found that adjacent cells could be labelled, relocated after histological processing and later studied immunocytochemically. Apparently, neither dye interferes with the immunocytochemical staining pattern of those antibodies we have tested. Further applications of this technique must include the direct morphological study of adjacent neurones, a field which has, as yet, been sadly neglected.

Summary

1. Ethidium bromide has been investigated as an intracellularly injected label for use in conjunction with Lucifer yellow.

2. Both dyes have been used histologically to identify rat DRG neurones which had been characterised electrophysiologically.

3. Ethidium bromide did not appear to alter the immunocytochemical properties of the injected rat DRG neurones.

Acknowledgements. We are grateful to the MRC for financial assistance. We would also like to thank J. Wood and P. Keen for the gifts of the antibodies RT97 and anti-substance P respectively.

References

Aghajanian GK, Vandermaelen CP (1982) Intracellular identification of central noradrenergic and serotonergic neurons by a new double labelling procedure. J Neurosci 2:1786–1792

Lawson SN, Waddell PJ (1985) Intracellular recordings from rat primary afferent neurones with known peripheral and central conduction velocities in vitro. J Physiol (Lond) 364:13P

Stewart WW (1981) Lucifer dyes – highly fluorescent dyes for biological tracing. Nature 292:17–21

22 Neuropeptides in Sensory Neurones of Pigeons and the Insensitivity of Avians to Capsaicin

Fr.-K. Pierau, H. Sann, G. Harti, and R. Gamse

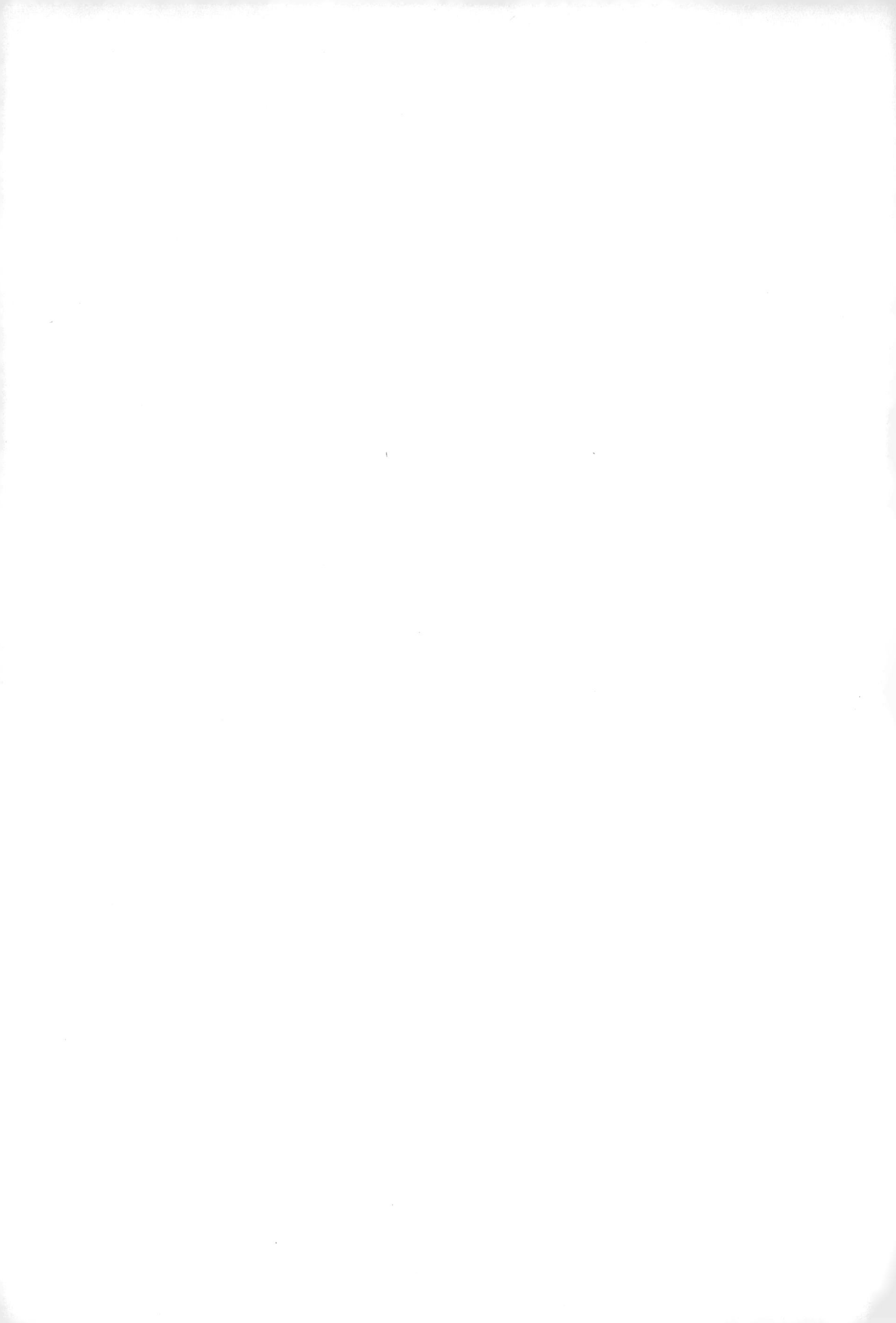

Introduction

Capsaicin, the hot principle of red pepper, is increasingly used as a tool to selectively excite and subsequently block peptidergic sensory neurones in mammals (Fitzgerald 1983; Szolcsányi 1984; Hori 1984). Avians appear to be profoundly insensitive to capsaicin. Pigeons do not react to instillation of 10^{-2} g/ml capsaicin into the eye (Pierau et al. 1986). The threshold for nociceptive responses to close arterial injection is 10 000 times higher than in guinea pigs (Szolcsányi et al. 1986).

One of the common characteristics of sensory neurones sensitive to capsaicin is that they contain a number of neuropeptides such as substance P (SP), neurokinin A, calcitonin gene-related peptide (CGRP), and somatostatin. Since the effect of capsaicin on peptidergic afferent neurones of different species has been most extensively studied in regard to SP (Fitzgerald 1983), we have compared the effect of capsaicin injected into the sciatic nerve upon the content and distribution of SP in dorsal root ganglia (DRG) and spinal cord of rats and pigeons. We also investigated the effect of locally applied capsaicin on SP release from the spinal cord (Gamse et al. 1979). The peripheral release of SP in response to antidromic stimulation or local application of capsaicin and other irritants was indirectly tested by Evans blue plasma extravasation (Jancsó et al. 1967).

Materials and Methods

Pigeons or rats of either sex were anesthetized with pentobarbital (Nembutal 45 mg/kg i.m.). In pigeons the trachea and the v. cutanea ulnaris were cannulated; ECG and body temperature were continously monitored.

Capsaicin Injection into the Sciatic Nerve

In anesthetized animals the sciatic nerve was carefully exposed in the middle of the thigh, leaving the perineural sheets intact. A total of 10 μl of a 1 % capsaicin solution (5 % Tween 80, 5 % alcohol) was injected into the two main branches of the nerve, the tibial and common peroneal nerves.

* This is part of Holger Sann's thesis, to be presented to the Fachbereich Biologie, Justus-Liebig-Universität Gießen

Immunohistochemistry

Anesthetized animals were perfused through the aorta with ice-cold Tyrode solution (pH 7.4) followed by 4% paraformaldehyde (pH 7.4) 14–16 days after capsaicin injection. Using the methods of Sharkey et al. (1983), cryostat sections (10 μm) of DRG and lumbar spinal cord were processed for indirect immunofluorescence (Coons and Kaplan 1950) and peroxidase-antiperoxidase (PAP) staining (Sternberger et al. 1970). DRG neurones were counted in alternate sections. Only cell profiles which demonstrated a nucleus were regarded. Although double counting of neurones is reduced by this procedure, the analysis is only semiquantitative. Relative numbers of labeled neurones were used in relation to the total number of counted cells. The amount of HRP reaction product in spinal cord sections was estimated by a computer-assisted intensity measurement program (field size 8 μm^2).

Measurement of SP Release from Spinal Cord Slices

Slices from the dorsal half of the spinal cord of six pigeons were prepared and treated according to Gamse et al. (1979). The SP content of the superfusate and the slice at the end of the experiment were determined by radioimmunoassay. To evoke SP release, either capsaicin dissolved in ethanol (3 μl/ml) or 60 mM KCl solution was added to the superfusion medium.

Topical Application of Irritants to the Skin

Ten minutes after i.v. injection of Evans blue (50 mg/kg), capsaicin, mustard oil, and xylene were painted twice with a 10-min interval on different skin areas in anesthetized pigeons with intact feathers. After transcardial perfusion the appropriate skin areas and conjunctiva were removed, weighed and extracted in formamide for Evans blue determination by spectrophotometry.

Antidromic Stimulation of the Brachial and Sciatic Nerve

In anesthetized pigeons pretreated with guanethidine (20 mg/kg s.c.), the brachial and sciatic nerves were exposed proximally, severed, and covered with paraffin oil. The distal part of each nerve was placed onto a pair of bipolar platinum electrodes for stimulation and recording of the compound action potential. Pulses of 2 Hz, 0.5 ms duration, and a voltage supramaximal for C fibers (10–20 V) were applied. Ten minutes later the birds were killed and the appropriate skin areas were removed and treated for the determination of Evans blue.

Subcutaneous Injection of Vasoactive Substances

SP, bradykinin, and histamine were injected subcutaneously into skin areas of anesthetized pigeons locally defeathered 1 day prior to the experiment. Ten minutes after the i.v. injection of Evans blue the test substances were injected in a constant volume of 0.05 ml into labeled skin areas. Treatment for Evans blue determination was as above.

Results

Capsaicin Effects on SP Content in DRG Neurones and the Spinal Cord

Immunohistochemistry for SP of sensory DRG neurones was performed with the immunofluorescence method. In both rat and pigeon about 10 % of the counted sensory neurones contained SP-like fluorescence. This percentage was surprisingly constant in all animals (Fig. 1). In agreement with the literature (Hökfelt et al. 1975; Price 1985), only small cells were labeled by SP immunofluorescence. Two weeks after the injection of capsaicin (100 μg) into the sciatic nerve, the number of neurones containing SP-like immunofluorescence was substantially reduced, by about 30 % - 40 %, in both species (exact numbers, Fig. 1). The different effect from ganglion to ganglion may be attributable to a different number of fibers ascending to each.

The reduction of SP neurones by capsaicin was not due to nonspecific fiber loss caused by the injection per se, since the absolute number of sensory neurones was similar on the treated and untreated sides (Fig. 1). Control injections of saline or the solvent into the sciatic nerve did not affect the number of immunofluorescent neurones in any of the DRG. In the spinal cord the PAP method was used for SP labeling, since the HRP reaction product was more suitable for the quantification of SP-like immunoreactivity. The distribution of SP-like reaction product in the spinal cord of rats was similar to that observed by other investigators (Hökfelt et al. 1975; Nagy and Hunt 1983). The highest density of SP labeling was seen in laminae I and II in the mediodorsal part of the dorsal horn. The superficial layer of lamina III was labeled to a lesser extent (Fig. 2B). Further labeling was seen in lamina V and the epithelial cells on the ventral side of the central canal (Cuello et al. 1981). Labeled nerve fibers were observed in the tract of Lissauer and in the lateral bundle projecting to lamina V.

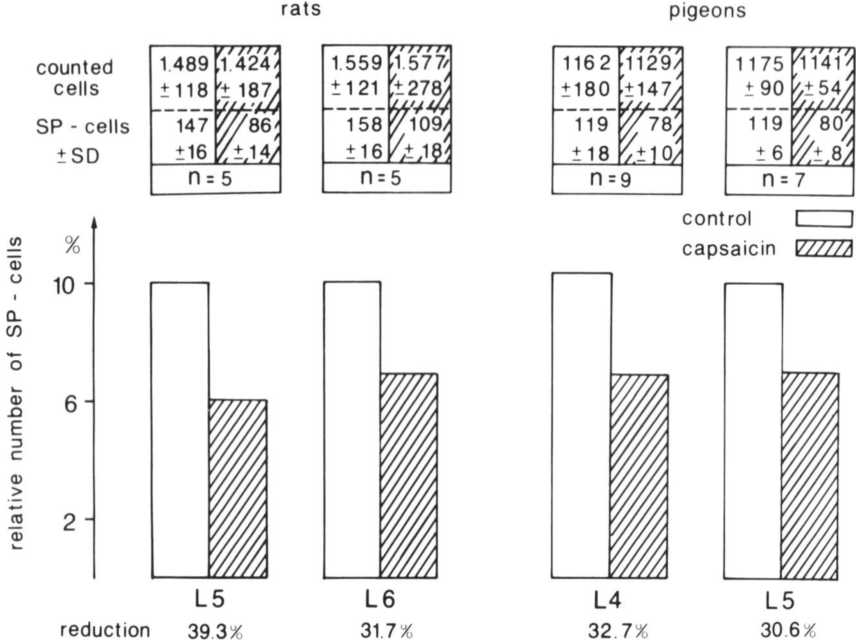

Fig. 1. Absolute and relative number of SP-containing neurones in lumbar DRG of rats and pigeons on the untreated control side (open columns) and the contralateral side where capsaicin was injected into the sciatic nerve (hatched columns). Reduction of SP neurones in percentage of the control side

The SP-like immunoreactivity in the spinal cord of pigeons displays distribution and density similar to that in rats (Figs. 2, 3). Since the dorsal horn of the spinal cord is ventrolaterally twisted in the lumbar region by the glycogen body, the greatest density of the reaction product was seen in the dorsolateral part of laminae I and II (Fig. 2A). Several nerve fibers which traversed the glycogen body also contained SP reaction products similar to those found in chickens (La Valley and Ho 1983). However, no SP-positive reaction was seen around the central canal in the pigeon, while it was quite dense in this area in the chicken.

Two weeks after treatment of the sciatic nerve with capsaicin, the SP-like immunoreaction product was highly reduced in the ipsilateral dorsal horn in rats. The depletion of SP reaction product was almost complete in the dorsomedial part of the dorsal horn, while the lateral dorsal horn was less affected (Figs. 2A, 3B, C). In contrast, no reduction of SP-like immunoreactivity was observed in the spinal cord of pigeons (Fig. 2C). It even appeared that the density of the reaction product was higher in the dorsolateral part of laminae I and II. Spectrophotometric measurements also indicated an increase in the density of reaction product on the treated site in pigeons by about 20 % (Fig. 3A). Similar results were obtained when SP immunohistochemistry was performed 28 days after the capsaicin injection.

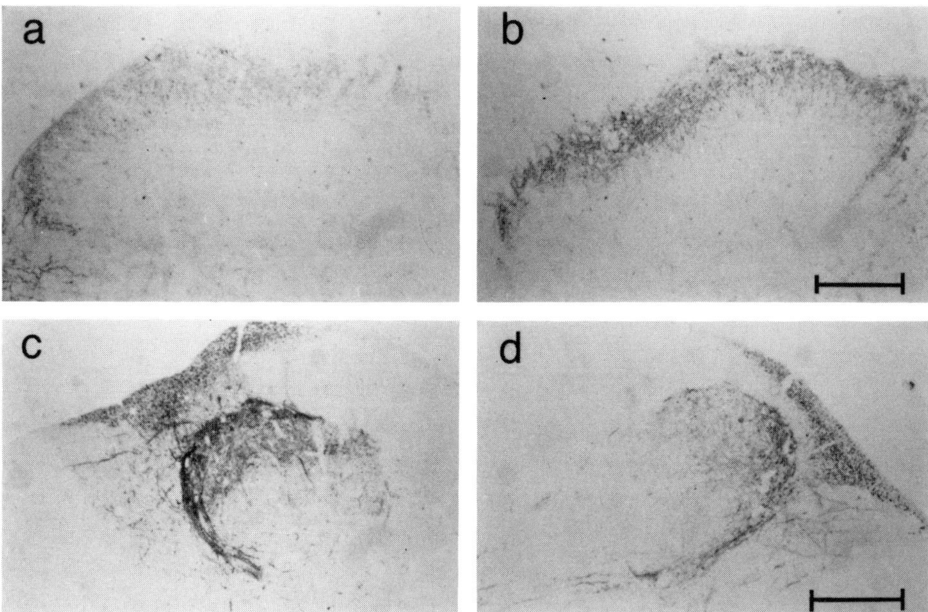

Fig. 2 A–D. Distribution of SP-like immunoreactivity (dark spots) in the lumbar spinal cord of rat (**A**, **B**) and pigeon (**C**, **D**) (PAP method). Transverse sections of the left dorsal horns after capsaicin injection into the sciatic nerve (**A**, **C**) and the untreated right dorsal horn (**B**, **D**). Cryostat section 10 μm, light field. Bars indicate 200 μm. Note: the lumbar dorsal horn of pigeons is lateroventrally twisted by the glycogen body

Capsaicin Effects on the Release of SP

The results appear to suggest that capsaicin does not cause a release of SP from afferent spinal terminals in pigeons. In rodents, the release of SP from the spinal cord has been demonstrated by superfusion of spinal cord slices with capsaicin (Gamse et al. 1979). In similar experiments with spinal cord slices of pigeons, superfusion with 10 μM capsaicin did not increase the spontaneous release of SP (Fig. 4). Superfusion of the same spinal cord slices with 60 mM potassium, however, induced a significant release of SP which was similar in concentration and kinetics to the release of SP by capsaicin and high potassium in spinal slices of rats (Gamse et al. 1979).

Local administration of capsaicin to the skin of mammals causes plasma extravasation, indicated by the appearance of Evans blue in the treated tissue (blueing reaction) (Jancsó et al. 1967; Szolcsányi 1984). This reaction is thought to be the consequence of SP release from peripheral afferent terminals and is therefore used as an indicator for peripheral SP release (Lembeck and Holzer 1979).

Painting the skin of pigeons with a solution of 1% capsaicin did not elicit Evans blue extravasation. Similarly, mustard oil (5%) in liquid paraffin applied to different skin areas

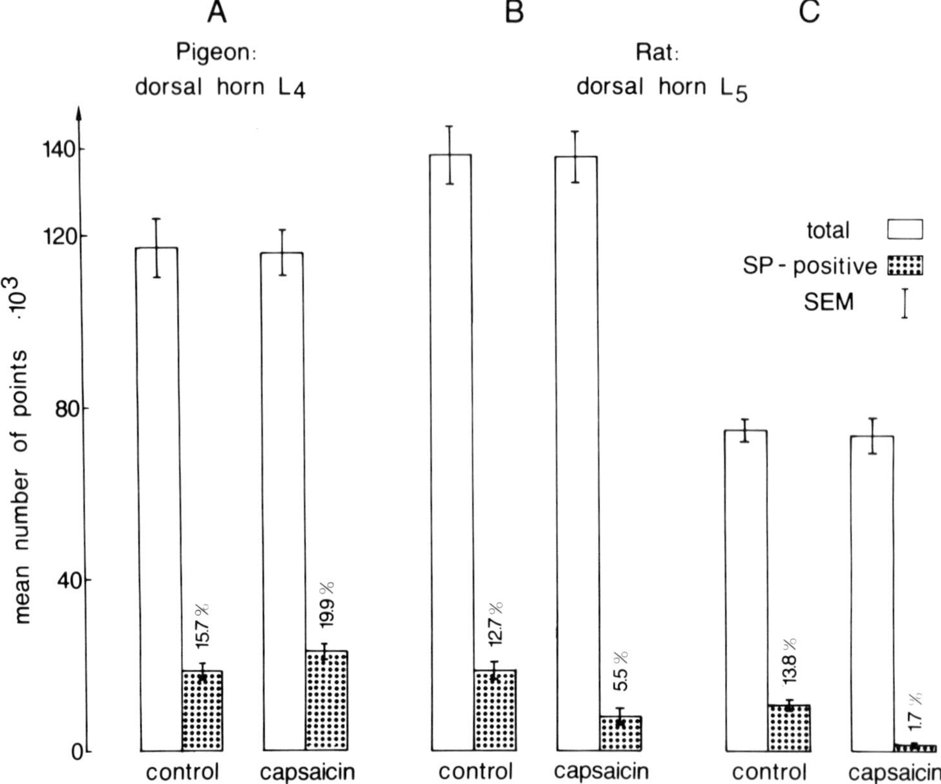

Fig. 3 A–C. Computer-assisted spectrophotometric determination of the density of immunoreactive SP-like reaction products of the lumbar spinal cord of pigeons and rats. **A, B** Total dorsal horn; **C** medio-dorsal part only. The total number of measured points (open columns) and the number of dark points (hatched columns) at the untreated side (control) is compared to the side in which capsaicin was injected into the sciatic nerve

did not induce plasma extravasation. Painting the skin with xylene always induced strong blueing reactions, but did not evoke nocifensive responses in conscious pigeons.

The hypothesis of a neurogenic mechanism for capsaicin-induced plasma extravasation has been supported by the observation that plasma extravasation produced by antidromic nerve stimulation is abolished by pretreatment with capsaicin (Szolcsányi 1984). Surprisingly, antidromic stimulation in pigeons (2 Hz, 0.5 ms, supramaximal for C fiber response, 10–15 min) did not induce any plasma extravasation. This might indicate that SP, although present in peripheral afferent nerve fibers (Harti et al., unpublished), is not released by electrical stimulation.

Alternatively, SP might be released from peripheral nerve terminals but the appropriate receptors might be lacking in the skin vessels. The effect of subcutaneous injection of SP into different areas of the pigeon's skin do not support this notion. As demonstrated in Fig. 5, subcutaneously injected SP produced plasma extravasation in a dose-dependent manner. Bradykinin as well as histamine induced plasma extravasation comparable to that induced in mammals (Arvier et al. 1977).

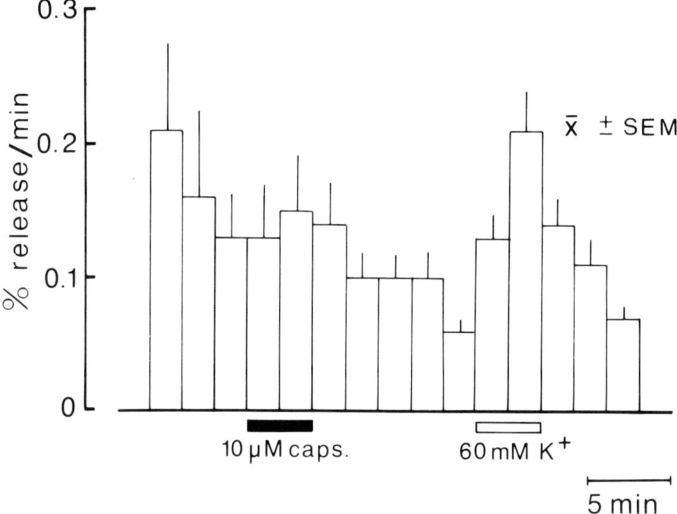

Fig. 4. Effect of capsaicin (caps.) and high potassium (K^+) on the release of SP from spinal cord slices of pigeons. SP efflux is expressed in terms of percent release per minute according to the equation of Gamse et al. (1979). n = 5

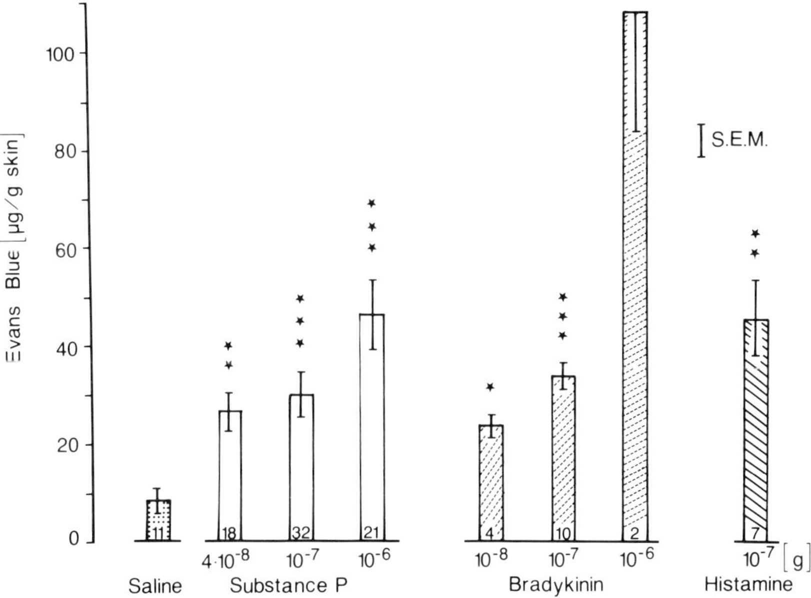

Fig. 5. Plasma extravasation expressed as Evans blue content of skin areas in which saline, SP, bradykinin, and histamine were injected subcutaneously. The number of injections for each concentration is given in the columns. T-test: *** $p < 0.001$; ** < 0.01; * < 0.05

Discussion

The immunohistochemical data presented here demonstrate that 10% of the sensory DRG neurones in the lumbosacral region of both pigeons and rats contain SP-like fluorescence. This is less than the 15%–20% SP neurones observed in the DRG of cats (Hökfelt et al. 1975). The distribution and density of SP reaction product in the lumbosacral spinal cord of pigeons is also similar to that in rats (Nagy and Hunt 1983) and in chickens (La Valley and Ho 1983), with the highest density of SP in laminae I and II and a lesser density in laminae III and V.

Injection of capsaicin into the sciatic nerve resulted in a similar reduction of SP-containing sensory neurones in the appropriate DRG in both species. On the other hand, depletion of SP in the dorsal horn was observed only in the spinal cord of rats, not in pigeons. One possible explanation for this discrepancy is that the axonal transport of the peripheral processes might be impaired wherever capsaicin has access to the axon. The depletion of SP from the afferent terminals of the spinal cord, however, would then be attributable to a different mechanism which might be in some way related to the excitatory effect of capsaicin. The present observation that capsaicin does not induce a release of SP from spinal cord slices of pigeons, together with the indirect evidence that SP is not released by capsaicin from peripheral C fiber endings of pigeons, would support the notion that central and peripheral nerve endings lack capsaicin "receptors."

It is intriguing, however, that antidromic stimulation of the brachial and sciatic nerves of pigeons did not produce plasma extravasation, although judging from the compound action potential, stimulation clearly excited C fibers (Szolcsányi 1984). This could mean that the inability of capsaicin to induce plasma extravasation is not due to a lack of the appropriate receptor sites, but is rather the consequence of an unknown mechanism which generally prevents the release of SP or other peptides upon electrical or chemical stimulation. The fact that even mustard oil does not elicit plasma extravasation in the skin of pigeons is consistent with this hypothesis. The plasma extravasation produced by xylene is probably not neurogenic in pigeons, but rather the result of direct drug action on vessels. In chicken, plasma extravasation in response to local xylene application was observed after chronic denervation (Sann et al., unpublished). The probably non-neurogenic nature of the mediation of xylene-induced plasma extravasation in pigeons might also be inferred from the observation that the substance does not evoke nociceptive responses when applied to the skin.

Endogenous mediators of vasoreaction and inflammation applied directly in the vicinity of the vessels by subcutaneous injection all produced a dose-dependent plasma extravasation. Consequently, the vessels of pigeons appear to be as sensitive to SP, histamine, and bradykinin as those of other species (Gamse and Saria 1985; Arvier et al. 1977). None of these mediators, however, seem to be released by electrical stimulation, capsaicin, and other irritants in pigeons.

References

ARVIER PT, CHAHL LA, LADD RJ (1977) Modification by capsaicin and compound 48/80 of dye leakage induced by irritants in the rat. Br J Pharmacol 59 : 61–68

COONS AH, KAPLAN MH (1950) Localization of antigen in tissue cells. II. Improvements in a method for detection of antigen by means of fluorescent antibody. J Exp Med 91 : 1–13

CUELLO CA, GAMSE R, HOLZER P, LEMBECK F (1981) Substance P immunoreactive neurons following neonatal administration of capsaicin. Naunyn Schmiedebergs Arch Pharmacol 315 : 185–194

FITZGERALD M (1983) Capsaicin and sensory neurones – a review. Pain 15 : 109–130

GAMSE R, SARIA A (1985) Potentiation of tachykinin induced plasma protein extravasation by calcitonin gene-related peptide. Eur J Pharmacol 114 : 61–66

GAMSE R, MOLNÁR A, LEMBECK F (1979) Substance P release from spinal cord slices by capsaicin. Life Sci 25 : 629–636

HÖKFELT T, KELLERTH JO, NILSSON G, PERNOW B (1975) Experimental immunohistochemical studies on the localization and distribution of substance P in cat primary sensory neurons. Brain Res 100 : 235–252

HORI T (1984) Capsaicin and central control of thermoregulation. Pharmacol Ther 26 : 389–416

JANCSÓ N, JANCSÓ-GABOR A, SZOLCSÁNYI J (1967) Direct evidence for neurogenic inflammation and its prevention by denervation and by pretreatment with capsaicin. Br J Pharmacol Chemother 31 : 138–151

LA VALLEY AL, HO RH (1983) Substance P, somatostatin, and methionine enkephalin immunoreactive elements in the spinal cord of the domestic fowl, *Gallus domesticus*. J Comp Neurol 213 : 406–413

LEMBECK F, HOLZER P (1979) Substance P as neurogenic mediator of antidromic vasodilation and neurogenic plasma extravasation. Naunyn Schmiedebergs Arch Pharmacol 310 : 175–183

NAGY JI, HUNT SP (1983) The termination of primary afferents within the rat dorsal horn: evidence for rearrangement following capsaicin treatment. J Comp Neurol 218 : 145–158

PIERAU FR.-K, SZOLCSÁNYI J, SANN H (1986) The effect of capsaicin on afferent nerves and temperature regulation of mammals and birds. J Therm Biol 11 : 95–100

PRICE J (1985) An immunohistochemical and quantitative examination of dorsal root ganglion neuronal subpopulations. J Neurosci 5 : 2051–2059

SHARKEY KA, WILLIAMS RG, SCHULTZBERG M, DOCKRAY GJ (1983) Sensory substance P innervation of the urinary bladder: possible site of action of capsaicin in causing urine retention in rats. Neuroscience 10 : 861–868

STERNBERGER LA, HARDY PH, CUCULIUS JJ, MEYER HG (1970) The unlabeled antibody enzyme method of immunohistochemistry – preparation and properties of soluble antigen-antibody complex (horseradish peroxidase–antihorseradish peroxidase) and its use in identification of spirochetes. J Histochem Cytochem 18 : 315–333

SZOLCSÁNYI J (1984) Capsaicin and neurogenic inflammation: history and early findings. In: CHAHL LA, SZOLCSÁNYI J, LEMBECK F (eds) Neurogenic inflammation and antidromic vasodilatation. Akadémiai Kiadó, Budapest, pp 7–25

SZOLCSÁNYI J, SANN H, PIERAU FR.-K (1986) Nociception in pigeons is not impaired by capsaicin. Pain 27 : 247–260

23 Opioid Receptor-Mediated Effects on Spinal Responses to Controlled Noxious Natural Peripheral Stimuli: Technical Considerations

P. M. Headley, C. G. Parsons, and D. C. West

Introduction

It has been clear for over a decade that there are opiate binding sites present in the spinal cord and that opiate analgesics have spinal actions which are increasingly being put to therapeutic use (for review see Cousins and Mather 1984). Nonetheless the physiological mechanisms which underlie such clinical applications are still only poorly understood. Amongst the questions which are still largely unanswered are those concerning (1) the range of spinal cells affected by activation of spinal opiate receptors and (2) the physiological consequences of selective activation of the various subclasses of opiate receptor.

We have begun to examine these questions in electrophysiological experiments and have become increasingly aware of differences in results obtained in these compared with behavioural tests using the productive technique of indwelling intrathecal catheters in freely moving animals (Yaksh and Rudy 1976). We shall describe here some of the problems which may arise in such experiments and some of the possible reasons for discrepancies.

Methods

Experiments are performed on decerebrate cats and on rats anaesthetised with alpha-chloralose, occasionally supplemented with halothane or pentobarbitone. Decerebrate but not anaesthetised animals are artificially respired. All animals are implanted with arterial, venous and tracheal cannulae. A laminectomy is performed so as to expose the lumbar spinal cord. All animals are spinalised so that any effects of intravenously administered opioid compounds on spinal neurones should be mediated within the spinal cord.

Recordings are made from neurones of laminae I and III–VIII using glass pipettes which are sometimes seven-barrelled so that microelectrophoretic tests can be performed. Recordings from single motoneurones are made from fine ventral root filaments. Cells are activated by peripheral stimuli which are designed to mimic natural conditions but which are nonetheless controlled electronically so as to ensure constancy of intensity, duration and repetition interval. The stimuli which we can control to this degree include noxious heat and pinch and non-noxious skin indentation and hair deflection. A regular cycle of one to three sensory and/or electrophoretic stimuli is established and this constant cycle is maintained throughout ensuing tests. Stimuli are adjusted so that the firing rates of the responses being evoked alternately are matched as closely as possible (see below). In establishing the interstimulus intervals a compromise has to be made between any tendency of responses to accommodate and the requirement to obtain as many data points as possible during individual drug tests; our usual cycle period is 3 min.

Neuronal responses are plotted on pen recorders and are also analysed on-line so that quantified data on stability of responses and on drug effects and recovery are always visible. Analysis is of the total number of spikes evoked by peripheral stimuli; alterations of responses are calculated from percentages of pre-test controls, where the control value is the mean of three to five successive responses.

In these experiments all opioid drugs have been tested by intravenous administration so that all regions of the cord should have been exposed to similar concentrations of the drugs. The receptor ligands were chosen so as (a) to be sufficiently selective for the receptor subtype, (b) to cross the blood-brain barrier readily and (c) to be sufficiently rapidly inactivated so that recovery could be observed and comparisons made of the actions of more than one drug on each cell. The drugs used were as follows: fentanyl for mu receptors (for selectivity in binding studies see Magnan et al. 1982); for kappa receptors, U-50,488 (Vonvoigtlander et al. 1983; gift of Dr P. Vonvoigtlander, Upjohn) and tifluadom (Römer et al. 1982; gift of Dr D. Römer, Sandoz); and as a sigma ligand, ketamine (see Sircar et al. 1986 for a discussion of the relation of ketamine to sigma receptors).

Results

The importance of the constancy of stimulus intensity and duration during tests involving repeated stimuli is self-evident; the importance of constant repetition interval is perhaps less so. Figure 1 illustrates a test in which peripheral noxious pinch and noxious contact heat were alternated. The 3-min repetition cycle was purposely interrupted after the first cycle of stimuli so as to examine possible variations of response with changing interval between responses. The response marked with the star was thus elicited after a longer interval than were the other responses to noxious pinch. In this trace of firing frequency the response appears not to be greatly different; however, in terms of the number of spikes elicited, it was 55 % larger than the mean of the preceding and succeeding responses, emphasising the importance of analysing spike count as well as firing frequency data. It should be clear that only rather limited qualitative analyses can be made unless stimuli are controlled for repetition interval as well as for intensity and duration.

The relative intensity of different modality stimuli is critical to the interpretation of modality selectivity. Figure 2 illustrates this important point. The left panel shows the effects of the kappa-specific opioid U-50,488 in a test on responses of a motoneurone to alternating noxious heat and pinch stimuli. In this test U-50,488 gives the appearance of having reduced the pinch responses to a considerably greater degree than the heat responses. However, when, on the same cell, the heat stimulus was moderated so that the evoked firing rate matched more closely that during the pinch stimulus, as shown on the right of Fig. 2, this apparent selectivity by U-50,488 was lost; both responses were similarly affected. This lack of selectivity by kappa agonists between thermal and mechanical nociceptive responses has been entirely consistent in our experiments. The result has direct implications for the interpretation of behavioural tests such as tail flick or writhing tests with opioid compounds, for in such experiments the different modality stimuli cannot be matched so as to elicit similar neuronal firing rates. Judging by the vigorousness of the motor responses, however, the intensity of the stimuli in the tail flick test results in considerably greater motoneuronal discharge rates than occur in other types of test such as the paw pressure or writhing tests. Reports of the ineffectiveness of kappa agonists against behavioural responses to thermal stimuli should therefore be treated with caution until further controls have been performed; it is quite clear from our results that spinal kappa receptors can and do mediate reduction of thermal nociceptive responses at the same doses as those affecting mechanical nociceptive responses.

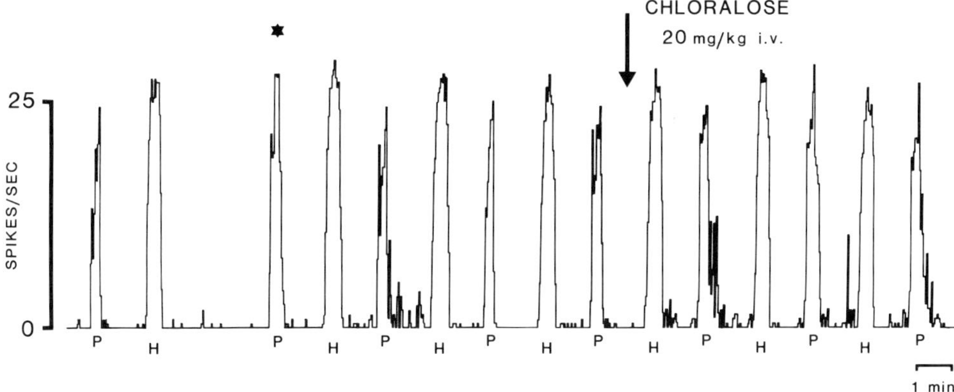

Fig. 1. Effects of varying the interstimulus intervals and of intravenously administered alpha-chloralose on the firing frequency of a motoneurone in L5 ventral root in response to alternating noxious pinch (P; fifth toe for 15 s) and contact heat (H; plantar foot, ramp from baseline 37.0 to 49.5 °C, total 30 s). Spinalised rat anaesthetised with alpha-chloralose

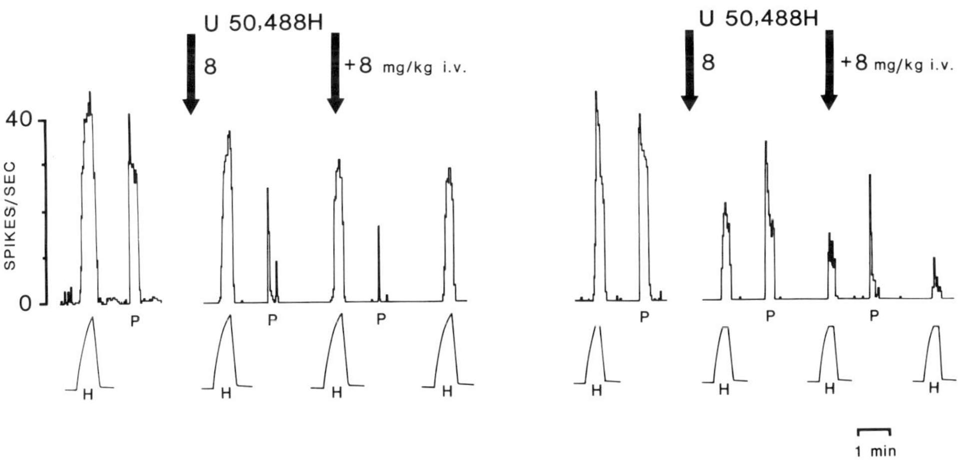

Fig. 2. Dependence of apparent modality selectivity by the kappa opioid U-50,488 (total 16 mg/kg in divided doses) on the relative intensity of alternating noxious heat and pinch stimuli. The pinch stimulus (P; fifth toe for 15 s) remained constant throughout, but the heat stimulus (H; plantar foot) was reduced between the periods shown in the sections of trace on the left (36.5–53 °C for 30 s) and on the right (37.0–47.5 °C for 25 s). The skin temperature profile is shown below the respective responses. Cycle period 3 min. Motoneurone in L4 ventral root of a spinalised rat anaesthetised with alpha-chloralose

The question of drug selectivity between different sensory responses has another aspect, namely the possibility that different modality responses have spike interval patterns which are differentially sensitive to compounds with central depressant actions. This possibility has been mooted many times but is still infrequently and insufficiently controlled for. Figure 3 illustrates one way of testing for such selectivity. With this dorsal horn neurone the mu agonist fentanyl left the responses to hair deflection virtually unaltered (counts of evoked spikes > 90% control). Responses to noxious pinch were however reduced, with the later phase (which presumably contains more nociceptive and less rapidly adapting mechanoreceptive information) being reduced to < 30% control. This result is what would be predicted from previous experiments with morphine (e.g. Duggan et al. 1977). To ascertain whether the lack of action of fentanyl on the non-nociceptive responses was related to a relative resistance of this response to depressant drugs in general, the short-acting barbiturate anaesthetic methohexitone was tested on the same cell. At half its anaesthetic induction dose, methohexitone caused a clear reduction of non-nociceptive as well as of nociceptive responses, thus giving weight to the selectivity displayed by the opiate.

The potency and non-selectivity with which this barbiturate anaesthetic reduced the synaptic responses underlines the significance of anaesthetic choice in electrophysiological investigations such as ours. In the absence of detailed information on the relative effects of different anaesthetics on spinal responses to adequately controlled peripheral stimuli, we use alpha-chloralose in nearly all experiments (unless the animals are decerebrated), although the chloralose "jerks" do sometimes need allaying with small doses of another anaesthetic. Figure 1 illustrates that, unlike the barbiturate illustrated in Fig. 3, alpha-chloralose at about 20% of the induction dose for rats had minimal effects on responses to noxious heat and pinch (this is the dose we regularly use for topping up anaesthetic levels).

There is a general assumption that opioid actions in the spinal cord are mediated in the dorsal horn. Such an assumption receives support from the findings that opiate binding

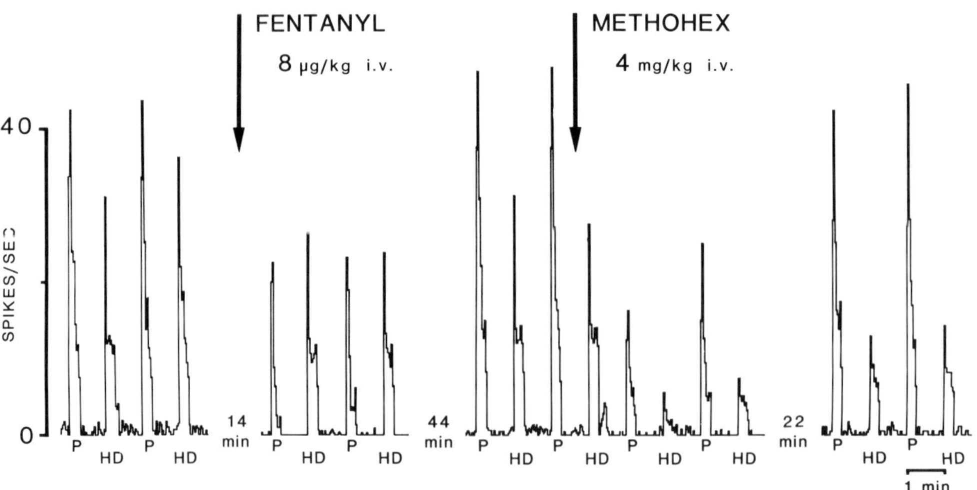

Fig. 3. Comparison of the effects of the opioid analgesic fentanyl and the barbiturate anaesthetic methohexitone on the responses of a spinal neurone to alternating noxious pinch (P; centre footpad for 15 s) and non-noxious hair deflection (HD; fourth toe for 15 s). Cycle period 2 min. Lamina V neurone in a decerebrate spinalised cat

sites and opioid immunoreactivity are concentrated in the dorsal horn and that opioids administered into the superficial dorsal horn do cause antinociception. However we find that mu, kappa and especially sigma agonists are effective at lower doses when tested on motoneuronal responses than when examined on responses of dorsal horn cells. For example, doses of $\leq$ 4mg/kg of the kappa agonist U-50,488 reduced motoneuronal nociceptive responses to noxious pinch to below 50% of control on 62% of cells tested ($n=69$), whereas the same dose was effective on only 21% of dorsal horn neurones ($n=37$). It thus seems likely that the greater sensitivity seen with motoneurones than with dorsal horn neurones is a reflection of some difference between our spinalised preparation and intact animals, since under most conditions opioids are thought to affect spinal sensory systems at

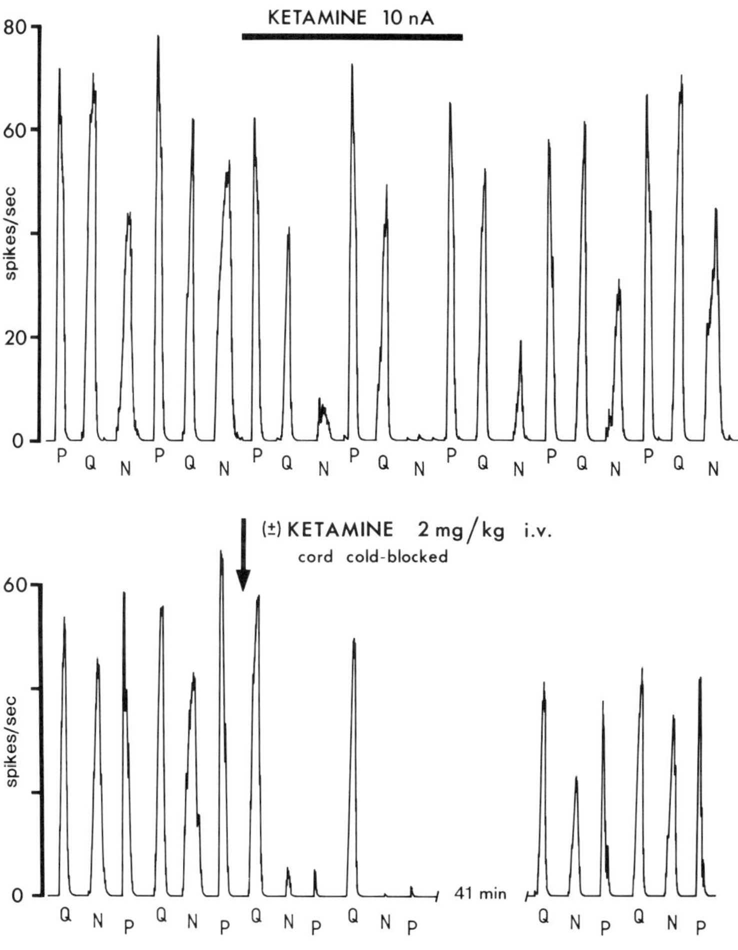

Fig. 4. Comparison of the effectiveness of microelectrophoretic (top) and intravenous (bottom) ketamine on the responses of a spinal neurone to noxious pinch (P; calcaneum for 15 s) and to microelectrophoretically administered excitatory amino acid analogues N-methyl-D-aspartate (N; 65 nA ejection current) and quisqualate (Q; 28 nA). Cycle period 2 min 30 s. Lamina VII–VIII border neurone in a decerebrate spinalised cat. (Lower trace reprinted, with permission, from Headley et al. 1985)

doses which do not cause overt signs of motor deficit. That there is a preferential ventral horn action under a variety of conditions is supported by preliminary clinical studies in which spinal spasticity can be relieved by locally administered opioids (Ochs 1983).

Figure 4 illustrates a problem familiar to any who use microelectrophoretic administrations of transmitter antagonists in attempts to identify the transmitters mediating synaptic responses. If in such tests the antagonist fails to affect the synaptic response it is impossible to know whether the lack of effect is disproof of a role for the putative transmitter or whether it results simply from the failure of the antagonist to reach the appropriate synaptic sites. We have run into this problem in our studies with ketamine, which is not only a dissociative anaesthetic and a sigma agonist but also, as illustrated in Fig. 4, a selective antagonist of actions mediated by the N-methylaspartate (NMA) class of excitatory amino acid receptor (Anis et al. 1983). The figure shows cycles of responses of a ventral horn interneurone to excitatory amino acid analogues and to noxious pinch. When administered microelectrophoretically, as shown in the top panel, ketamine was without effect on the synaptic responses at ejection currents sufficient to block responses to NMA. The uncertainty of the interpretation of such a result can be resolved if the antagonist can also be administered systemically. For most antagonists of excitatory amino acid transmitters this is not practicable, but ketamine can readily be given systemically. The lower panel shows, on the same cell, that intravenous ketamine, at a sub-anaesthetic yet NMA-blocking dose, did block responses to NMA and to noxious pinch in parallel whilst leaving virtually unaffected the responses to quisqualate, an amino acid selective for a different receptor. The result with electrophoretic administration would therefore seem to have been a false negative. This kind of test thus highlights the problems of access of locally administered drugs to synaptic sites.

The importance of bearing in mind the dose of drug which is effective systemically is illustrated by the grossly different potency ratios of the mu agonists morphine and fentanyl depending on the route of administration. In our experiments in spinalised animals, intravenous fentanyl has clear antinociceptive actions at doses in the low microgram per kilogram range, agreeing with results of behavioural tests with systemic administration (Janssen et al. 1963). This result is illustrated in Fig. 5, in which fentanyl was active at 1 μg/kg. On the same cell the dose of morphine required to cause a similar degree of reduction was 4 mg/kg, indicating a potency ratio of the order of 1000 : 1. In behavioural tests with intrathecal or epidural administration, in contrast, the relative potencies of fentanyl and morphine are less than 10 : 1 and the absolute dose of fentanyl given intrathecally may exceed the systemically effective dose. This point has been discussed elsewhere (Durant and Yaksh 1986; Yaksh et al. 1986), and there are ready explanations in terms of the different physicochemical properties of these two opioids resulting in very different distributions of the drugs through nervous tissue. Nonetheless, important conclusions are drawn from the relative potencies of drugs administered by local spinal administration despite inadequate information on drug distribution from the site of local administration. One such conclusion is that kappa agonists are ineffective against thermally induced responses in tests such as the tail flick and hot plate (see Yaksh and Noueihed 1985). Quite apart from considerations of relative stimulus intensities (see above and Fig. 2), the degree of drug access needs to be clearly established. It is our contention that conclusions based on local drug administration should be treated with caution unless there is corroborative evidence from systemic administration of the same drugs.

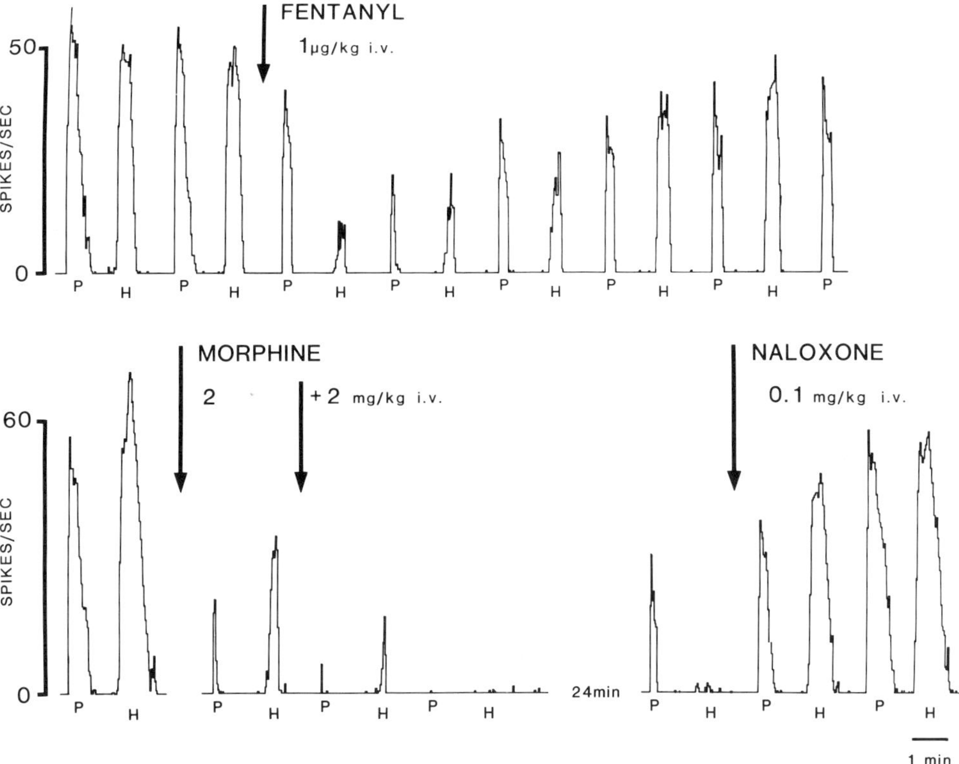

Fig. 5. Comparison of the effect of the mu receptor-selective opioid analgesics fentanyl (top trace) and morphine (4 mg/kg in divided doses; bottom trace) on responses to noxious pinch (P; toe 5 for 15 s) and noxious heat (H; plantar foot, 37.0 °C to 48.0 °C for 30 s). Cycle period 3 min. Reversal of the morphine effect by naloxone is shown. Motoneurone in L5 ventral root of a spinalised rat anaesthetised with alpha-chloralose supplemented with 0.5 % halothane in oxygen

Discussion

The results presented above have been selected to illustrate some of the many difficulties encountered in studies designed to elucidate the physiological and antinociceptive effects of activating the various opioid receptor subtypes in the spinal cord. Some of these technical points have been raised frequently over the years but are apparently still not fully appreciated. The importance of the constancy, regularity and relative intensities of peripheral stimuli cannot be overemphasized.

Behavioural testing with local spinal administration of opiate and other agents is a relatively new technique, and the possible causes of disparities between the results in these highly productive experiments and the results using other techniques have not often been discussed (but see e.g. Yaksh et al. 1986). We wish to emphasise that in some cases there is a gross mismatch between the relative potencies of analgesic agents in these behavioural tests and the relative effectiveness observed in experiments which utilise systemic administration of drugs. In many of the latter experiments the cellular site of action of the systemically administered agents cannot be known. In our type of electrophysiological experiment, however, the drugs must have been having their principal action in the spinal cord, since the animals were spinally sectioned; moreover, we can define the approximate laminar effectiveness of drug action. Our results match those of behavioural tests using systemic administration better than those of local spinal administration, indicating that the distribution of drug through the spinal cord must be taken into account when interpreting the results of tests with localised drug administration. Despite the undoubted problems in acute electrophysiological experiments of anaesthetic and surgical interference with nociceptive processing mechanisms, the type of electrophysiological result described above does have considerable credence.

Acknowledgements. We thank the Medical Research Council, The Wellcome Trust and the University of London C.R.F. for financial support.

References

Anis NA, Berry SC, Burton NR, Lodge D (1983) The dissociative anaesthetics, ketamine and phencyclidine, selectively reduce excitation of central mammalian neurones by N-methyl-aspartate. Br J Pharmacol 79 : 565–575

Cousins MJ, Mather LE (1984) Intrathecal and epidural administration of opioids. Anesthesiology 61 : 276–310

Duggan AW, Hall JG, Headley PM (1977) Suppression of transmission of nociceptive impulses by morphine: selective effects of morphine administered in the region of the substantia gelatinosa. Br J Pharmacol 61 : 65–76

Durant PAC, Yaksh TL (1986) Epidural injections of bupivacaine, morphine, fentanyl, lofentanyl, and DADL in chronically implanted rats: a pharmacologic and pathologic study. Anesthesiology 64 : 43–53

Headley PM, West DC, Roe CA (1985) Actions of ketamine and the role of N-methyl-aspartate receptors in the spinal cord: studies on nociceptive and other neuronal responses. Neurol Neurobiol 14 : 325–331

Janssen PAJ, Niemegeer CJE, Dony JGH (1963) The inhibitory effect of fentanyl and other morphine-like analgesics on the warm water induced withdrawal reflex in rats. Arzneimittelforsch 13 : 502–507

Magnan J, Paterson SJ, Tavani A, Kosterlitz HW (1982) The binding spectrum of narcotic analgesic drugs with different agonist and antagonist properties. Naunyn Schmiedebergs Arch Pharmacol 319 : 197–205

Ochs G (1983) The effect of epidural application of opioids on spasticity of spinal origin. Life Sci 33 : 607–610

Römer D, Büscher HH, Hill RC, Maurer R, Petcher TJ, Zeugner H, Benson W, Finner E, Milkowski W, Thies PW (1982) An opioid benzodiazepine. Nature 298 : 759–760

Sircar R, Nichtenhauser R, Ieni JR, Zukin SR (1986) Characterization and autoradiographic visualization of (+)-(^{3}H) SKF10.047 binding in rat and mouse brain: further evidence for phencyclidine/"sigma opiate" receptor commonality. J Pharmacol Exp Ther 237 : 681–688

VonVoigtlander PF, Lahti RA, Ludens JH (1983) U-50,488: a selective and structurally novel non-mu (kappa) opioid agonist. J Pharmacol Exp Ther 224 : 7–12

White PF, Way WL, Trevor AJ (1982) Ketamine – its pharmacology and therapeutic uses. Anesthesiology 56 : 119–136

Yaksh TL, Noueihed R (1985) The physiology and pharmacology of spinal opiates. Ann Rev Pharmacol Toxicol 25 : 433–462

Yaksh TL, Rudy TA (1976) Analgesia mediated by a direct spinal action of narcotis. Science 192 : 1357–1358

Yaksh TL, Noueihed RY, Durant PAC (1986) Studies of the pharmacology and pathology of intrathecally administered 4-anilinopiperidine analogues and morphine in the rat and cat. Anesthesiology 64 : 54–66

24 The Roles of Tachykinin and Opioid Receptor Types in Nociceptive and Non-Nociceptive Processing in Superficial Dorsal Horn

S. M. Fleetwood-Walker, R. Mitchell, P. J. Hope, N. El-Yassir, and V. Molony

Tachykinins in Dorsal Horn

A number of biochemical markers including neuropeptide transmitters have been found in dorsal root ganglion neurons with small-diameter fibres. Amongst these, the tachykinin substance P (SP) has been the prominent candidate for the transmitter of nociceptive afferents. Intrathecally administered tachykinins are either pro-algesic or elicit behaviour similar to that induced by peripheral irritation (e.g. Moochhala and Sawynok 1984; Post and Folkers 1985), whilst antagonists or capsaicin produce analgesia in some tests. Substance P in dorsal horn is derived from sensory ganglia, local interneurons and perhaps also descending systems (Hökfelt et al. 1980) Immunoreactive SP is released from spinal cord (although not necessarily originating from afferents) by high-intensity electrical stimulation of peripheral afferents (Yaksh et al. 1980) or by noxious mechanical, but not thermal, stimuli to the skin (Kuraishi et al. 1985). Ionophoretic application of SP in the vicinity of dorsal horn neurons elicits excitatory effects (Henry 1976; Randic and Miletic 1977; Zieglgänsberger and Tulloch 1979; Willcockson et al. 1984; our unpublished results on identified spinocervical tract neurons). In some cases, inhibitory components have also been observed, suggesting multiple sites of action. In no case, however, has the effect of SP been rigorously compared on cell responses to different modalities of peripheral input.

In addition to SP, two novel tachykinin peptides, neurokinins A and B (NKA, NKB) have recently been isolated from spinal cord (Kimura et al. 1983) (Fig. 1). One of the two SP precursor peptides sequenced from bovine brain also codes for NKA, and there is some evidence for the coexistence of immunoreactive SP and NKA in primary afferents (Sundler et al. 1985). Whilst NKA, and to a lesser extent SP, in the dorsal horn appear to be provided by afferent fibres, NKB seems to be associated with segmental or ascending spinal neurons (Ogawa et al. 1985).

Substance P	Arg - Pro - Lys - Pro - Gln - Gln - Phe - Phe - Gly - Leu - MetNH_2
Neurokinin A	His - Lys - Thr - Asp - Ser - Phe - Val - Gly - Leu - MetNH_2
Neurokinin B	Asp - Met - His - Asp - Phe - Phe - Val - Gly - Leu - MetNH_2

Fig. 1. The mammalian tachykinins

There is evidence that tachykinins and their analogues show selectivity for different receptor subtypes, which have been designated SP-P, SP-E and SP-N (Iversen et al. 1986). [Met-OMe^{11}]-SP is a highly selective agonist at SP-P sites, whilst NKA and NKB may show selectivity for SP-E and SP-N sites respectively.

Neuropeptides and Somatosensory Processing at the Single Neuron Level

Our approach to investigating the roles of tachykinins in somatosensory processing has been to use a dual electrode protocol, administering drugs into the region of the substantia gelatinosa whilst recording responses of lamina IV/V spinocervical tract (SCT) neurons that transmit both nociceptive and non-nociceptive information to supraspinal levels. As fine nociceptor afferents predominantly terminate in the region of the substantia gelatinosa (Perl 1984) and the greatest concentrations of tachykinin-like immunoreactive terminals are also seen here (Sundler et al. 1985), this seems the most appropriate location to administer tachykinin receptor agonists in these experiments. Concomitant recording of the responses of identified ascending transmission neurons, however, displays the integration of processing events that has occurred in the more superficial dorsal horn prior to the information being relayed to these SCT cells. In view of the abundant evidence for specific antinociceptive actions of opioids (Duggan and North 1984; Schmauss and Yaksh 1984) and the long-postulated association of opioid receptors with SP afferents, we have also investigated the effects of a series of receptor-selective opioids on nociceptive and non-nociceptive responses of these cells.

Extracellular recordings were made from antidromically-identified SCT neurons in lumbar segments L6–7 of cats, using methods described in detail previously (Fleetwood-Walker et al. 1985a,b, 1986). After multireceptive neurons had been identified, a multibarrelled glass electrode was advanced into the region of the substantia gelatinosa, directly dorsal to the recording site. Electrode positions were marked by dye spots. Drugs were prepared freshly, usually in distilled water at a concentration of 5 or 10 mM and pH 4.5–5.0 or 8.0–8.5 and ejected using a Neurophore BH2 unit. Current compensation and independent ejection of NaCl were used to discount the possibility of current artefacts in any of the drug effects (see Fig. 4). In some cases, both recording and ionophoresis were carried out using a single multibarrelled electrode, close to SCT cell bodies.

Controlled noxious and innocuous cutaneous stimuli were provided by thermistor-controlled radiant heat or calibrated pinch and by a motorised rotating brush respectively. Stimuli were generally applied for 10 s. In the case of the heat stimulus, the skin temperature was held at 48 °C for this time after a 5-s rising ramp. Regular cycles of these stimuli were applied every 3 min (together with direct excitation by D,L-homocysteic acid in the case of cell body experiments). Drugs were usually applied for 1 min before each test cycle and ionophoretic currents were increased stepwise. Changing the stimulus order did not affect the results. Increases in cell firing rate elicited by each stimulus were integrated from the computer record and normalised. Responses to the mechanical stimuli were integrated from the 10-s span over which the stimuli were presented. Responses to noxious thermal stimuli were integrated over 25-30 s from the start of the 48 °C plateau, to include the long-latency activity evoked by this type of stimulus. Results were expressed graphically on a continuous time scale, plotting responses during consecutive cycles of stimuli in which ionophoretic currents were progressively increased. These cumulative "current-response curves" allow comparison of drug potency on the different types of activity.

Tachykinins and Sensory Processing: Results

Our results with [Met-OMe[11]]-SP, NKB and NKA in spinal cord support the concept of heterogeneity of tachykinin receptors. When [Met-OMe[11]]-SP was ejected into superficial laminae, it caused a clear selective reduction in activity evoked by low-threshold mechanical stimuli, in six of nine SCT neurons tested (Fig. 2). The ineffectiveness of [Met-OMe[11]] SP in altering nociceptive responses or spontaneous activity suggests that it is acting at SP-P receptor sites restricted to the non-nociceptive input pathway, either on an interneuron or afferent terminal. Action at some distance from the ionophoretic electrode may explain the high currents required. This SP-P receptor-mediated effect in the region of substantia gelatinosa is quite distinct from that in laminae IV/V, where a general excitation of cells (not spe-

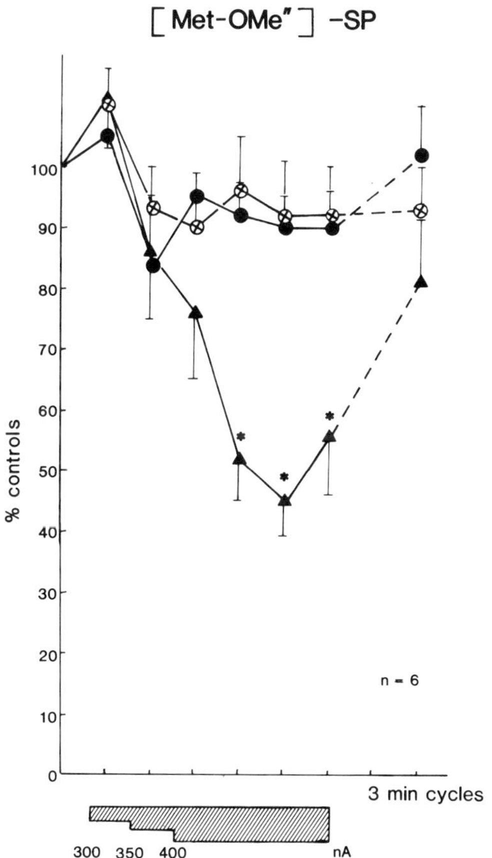

Fig. 2. Effects of [Met-OMe[11]]-SP administration into substantia gelatinosa on nociceptive and non-nociceptive responses of SCT neurons (mean ± S.E.M. of results from six neurons). ●, noxious heat; ▲, innocuous brush; ⊗, spontaneous activity. * $p < 0.05$ compared with pre-drug control (by matched t-test on raw data)

cifically related to nociceptive inputs) is produced by [Met-OMe[11]]-SP (our unpublished data) or the marginally-selective SP-P agonist physalaemin (Salter and Henry 1985).

Neurokinin B, ejected into the region of the substantia gelatinosa, selectively inhibited non-nociceptive responses, thereby displaying a functionally similar profile to [Met-OMe[11]]-SP, in five of six neurons tested (Fig. 3). However, during NKB (but not [Met-OMe[11]]-SP) ejection, the low-threshold mechanical receptive field expanded to adjacent regions, a phenomenon never normally seen in these SCT neurons, whose field boundaries otherwise remain quite constant.

In contrast, NKA caused a potent and selective facilitation of responses to noxious heat, without altering brush-evoked or spontaneous activity, in all seven neurons tested (Fig. 4). A maximal effect could be observed even at the lowest currents tested. In view of the prominent effect of NKA on thermal nociception, responses of these cells were also tested to noxious pinch. These responses, however,were unaffected (five of seven neurons) or only slightly facilitated. Such facilitation appeared only on the very long latency components of

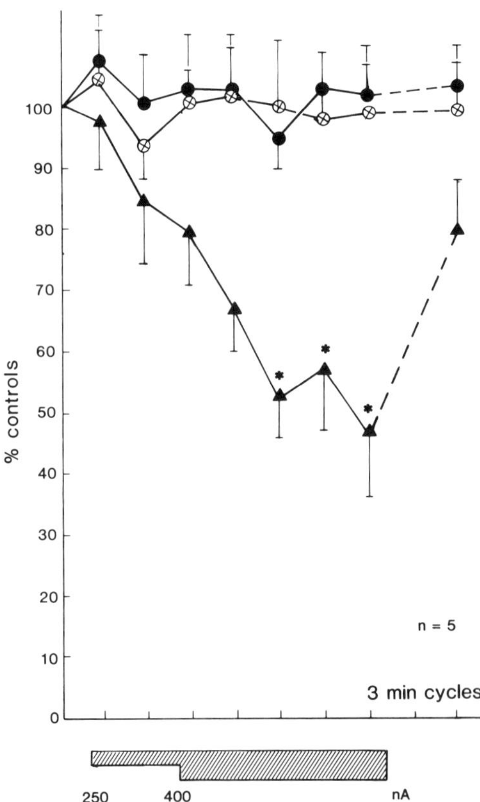

Fig. 3. Effects of NKB administration into substantia gelatinosa on sensory responses of SCT neurons (mean ± S.E.M. of results from five neurons). ●, noxious heat; ▲, innocuous brush; ⊗, spontaneous activity. *$p < 0.05$ compared with pre-drug control (by matched t-test on raw data)

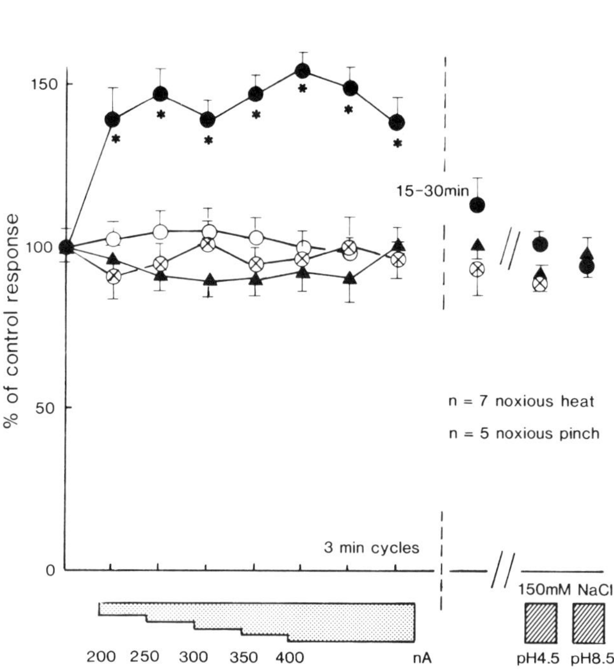

Fig. 4. Effects of NKA administration into substantia gelatinosa on sensory responses of SCT neurons (mean ± S.E.M. of results from seven neurons; five neurons for noxious pinch: see text). ●, noxious heat; ○, noxious pinch; ▲, innocuous brush; ⊗, spontaneous activity. * **p** < 0.05 compared with pre-drug control (by matched t-test on raw data)

the pinch responses and made only a minor contribution to the overall response. The pinch responses here are likely to involve a contribution from mechanoreceptors with fine myelinated (Aδ) afferents as well as unmyelinated (C) afferents. The predominant population of C fibre nociceptors (polymodal nociceptors) respond regularly to thermal as well as mechanical stimuli, although solely mechanical C nociceptors have been described (Iggo 1974). In contrast, the majority of Aδ mechanical nociceptors either require repeated sensitisation in order to respond to thermal stimuli or fail entirely to respond (Perl 1984). It may be, therefore, that the noxious thermal responses here (and the selective facilitatory effects of NKA thereon) are predominantly associated with impulses in polymodal C nociceptor afferents. The lack of marked effect of NKA on the pinch responses might thus be consistent with a greater contribution to them of nociceptors other than those of the polymodal C group. Responses to noxious heat and their facilitation by NKA could be reduced by the tachykinin receptor antagonist [D-Arg^{1}, D-Trp^{7,9}]-SP in preliminary experiments, suggesting that NKA may also exert such effects endogenously.

These results are consistent with NKA being a neurotransmitter of nociceptive primary afferents. The selective facilitation of thermal nociceptive responses may represent an action additive to that of endogenously released NKA. Alternatively, as NKA did not cause general excitation of SCT neurons, it may be that a synergistic action of NKA with other substances is required to fully activate the nociceptive pathway.

[Met-OMe[11]]-SP and NKB both act in superficial dorsal horn to reduce responses to non-nociceptive inputs relative to nociceptive inputs. If the ratio of activity evoked in ascending neurons by noxious vs innocuous stimuli can be interpreted at supraspinal levels,then both SP and NKB may also contribute in a pro-nociceptive fashion to the processing of nociceptive information. SP-P receptors appear generally to excite neurons in lamina IV/V as well, but this effect would not act to reverse the prior shift towards nociceptive responsiveness dictated by effects of tachykinins in the region of the substantia gelatinosa.

Opioid Receptors and Nociceptive Processing

Several classes of receptor may be important in mediating the spinal analgesic actions of opioids reported in behavioural studies. Mu and perhaps δ opioid agonists appear to be effective against a wide variety of noxious stimuli (Schmauss and Yaksh 1984). Kappa agonists are also effective, but some workers report greatly reduced potency against thermal nociception (Schmauss and Yaksh 1984). Other groups, however, have provided evidence for the potent effectiveness of κ agonists in analgesia with respect to thermal stimuli (Piercey et al. 1982; Han and Xie 1982).

In studies carried out at the single neuron level, administration of opioids near neuron somata in laminae IV/V has shown little evidence of selective influence on nociceptive inputs (Duggan and North 1984). Morphine or enkephalins appear to exert a partially selective antinociceptive effect if ejected in the region of the substantia gelatinosa whilst recording responses of laminae IV/V neurons (Duggan and North 1984). Apart from the μ-selective alkaloid morphine, no drugs capable of discriminating receptor types have been used, so at the single neuron level, no antinociceptive actions could up till now be specifically attributed to δ or κ receptors. Table 1 summarises our observations on a uniform identified population of neurons in laminae IV/V, using for the first time, selective receptor agonists applied into either lamina II or laminae IV/V. The κ agonists dynorphin A_{1-13} and U50488H (trans-3,4-dichloro-N-methyl-N-(2(pyrroylidinyl) cyclohexyl) -benzeneacetamide) produced a selective (naloxone-reversible) antinociceptive effect when applied close to SCT neurons. Responses to noxious stimuli, but not innocuous stimuli or D,L-homocysteic acid, were reduced. As spontaneous activity too was unaltered, it seems likely that the κ agonist antinociception is exerted at an indirect site. This effect, (observed using either noxious thermal or mechanical stimuli and also seen on unidentified laminae IV/V neurons in the rat), may represent the basis for spinal analgesic actions of κ agonists. Dynorphin A_{2-13} (lacking the 1-position tyrosyl, essential for interaction with opioid receptors) failed to reproduce this effect, in contrast to reports of depressant effects of dynorphins on motor function where such specificity is not apparent. Neither the highly selective μ receptor agonist DAGO ([D-Ala^2, MePhe^4, Gly-ol^5] enkephalin) nor the partially selective δ receptor agonist DADL ([D-Ala^2, D-Leu^5] enkephalin) had any marked effect on the responses of SCT neurons when applied nearby. Some non-selective depression was seen on occasions at very high currents, but no evidence of any discrete antinociceptive action. In contrast, when

Table 1. Effects of receptor-selective opioids administered into lamina II or laminae IV/V on sensory responses of SCT neurons

Peptide (preferred receptor type)	Ionophoresis in lamina II Selective antinociceptive effect	Marginal selectivity	No effect	Ionophoresis in lamina IV/V Selective antinociceptive effect	Marginal selectivity	No effect
DAGO (μ)	17/18	-	1/18	-	-	5/5
DYNO (ϰ)	-	-	7/7	14/16	-	2/16
U50488H (ϰ)	-	-	-	4/5	1/5	-
DADL (δ)	-	4/5	1/5	-	1/7	6/7
DSLET (δ)	-	2/3	1/3	-	-	-
DLPEN (δ)	-	2/3	1/3	-	-	-

The fractions indicated show the number of neurons affected in a particular manner compared with the total population of neurons tested. The compounds employed all show at least eight-to tenfold greater potency at the receptor subtype indicated than at other subtypes. In the cases of DAGO (μ), U50488H (ϰ) and DLPEN (δ) a much higher degree of selectivity is present, and these compounds are therefore rather unlikely to cause significant activation of receptor subtypes other than those indicated. The nociceptive responses of SCT neurons in laminae IV/V were selectively inhibited by μ receptor agonist administered in the region of lamina II or by ϰ receptor agonists applied close to their somata in laminae IV/V. In no other case was a selective antinociceptive effect observed in these experiments.

applied into superficial laminae, DAGO exerted a powerful and selective antinociceptive influence over SCT neurons. Neither the ϰ receptor agonists nor the δ receptor agonist DADL showed any evidence of similar prominent antinociceptive effects. As two rather more selective δ receptor agonists became available (DSLET: [D-Ser^2, L-Leu^5] enkephalyl-Thr, and DLPEN: [D-Pen^2, L-Pen^5] enkephalin), we investigated the effects of their administration into the region of the substantia gelatinosa. Again no clear-cut antinociceptive effects were apparent, even with DLPEN, which shows a many-fold selectivity for δ against μ or ϰ receptors (Corbett et al. 1984). These results therefore demonstrate that there are two distinct sites at which μ and ϰ agonists can exert an antinociceptive influence over dorsal horn neurons. The relevant μ and ϰ receptors appear to be located in superficial and deeper dorsal horn respectively.

Acknowledgements. This work was supported by the Wellcome Trust.

References

Corbett AD, Gillan MGC, Kosterlitz HW, McKnight AT, Paterson SJ, Robson LE (1984) Selectivities of opioid peptide analogues as agonists and antagonists at the δ-receptor. Br J Pharmacol 83 : 271–279

Duggan AW, North RA (1984) Electrophysiology of opioids. Pharmacol Rev 35 : 219–281

Fleetwood-Walker SM, Mitchell R, Hope PJ, Molony V, Iggo A (1985a) An α_2 receptor mediates the selective inhibition by noradrenaline of nociceptive responses of identified dorsal horn neurons. Brain Res 334 : 243–254

Fleetwood-Walker SM, Mitchell R, Hope PJ, Molony V (1985b) Effects of opioid peptide agonists selective for μ, δ and ϰ receptors on identified dorsal horn neurons. Philos Trans R Soc Lond [Biol] 308 : 427

Fleedwood-Walker SM, Hope PJ, Mitchell R, Molony V (1986) Effects of receptor-selective opioid peptides in superficial dorsal horn of the cat. J Physiol (Lond) 373 : 72P

Han JS, Xie CW (1982) Dynorphin: potent analgesic effect in spinal cord of the rat. Life Sci 31 : 1781–1783

Henry JL (1976) Effects of substance P on functionally identified units in cat spinal cord. Brain Res 114 : 439–451

Hökfelt T, Johansson O, Ljungdahl A, Lundberg JM, Schultzberg M (1980) Peptidergic neurons. Nature 284 : 515–521

Iggo A (1974) Activation of cutaneous nociceptors and their actions on dorsal horn neurons. Adv Neurol 4 : 1–9

Iversen LL, Foster AC, Watling KJ, McKnight AT, Williams BJ, Lee CM (1986) Multiple receptors and binding sites for tachykinins. Eur J Pharmacol (in press)

Kimura S, Okada M, Sugita Y, Kanazawa I, Munekata E (1983) Novel neuropeptides, neurokinin α and β, isolated from porcine spinal cord. Proc Jpn Acad 59 (B) : 101–104

Kuraishi Y, Hirota N, Sato Y, Hino Y, Satoh M, Takagi H (1985) Evidence that substance P and somatostatin transmit separate information related to pain in the spinal dorsal horn. Brain Res 325 : 294–298

Moochhala SM, Sawynok J (1984) Hyperalgesia produced by intrathecal substance P and related peptides: desensitisation and cross desensitisation. Br J Pharmacol 82 : 381–388

Ogawa T, Kanazawa I, Kimura S (1985) Regional distribution of substance P, neurokinin α and neurokinin β in rat spinal cord, nerve roots and dorsal root ganglia, and the effects of dorsal root section or spinal transection. Brain Res 359 : 152–157

Perl ER (1984) Characterisation of nociceptors and their activation of neurons in the superficial dorsal horn: first steps for the sensation of pain. Adv Pain Res Ther 6 : 23-51

Piercey MF, Lahti RA, Schroeder LA, Einspahr FJ, Barsahn C (1982) U-50488H, a pure kappa receptor agonist with spinal analgesic loci in the mouse. Life Sci 27 : 971–978

Post J, Folkers K (1985) Behavioural and anti-nociceptive effects of intrathecally injected substance P analogues in mice. Eur J Pharmacol 113(3) : 335–342

Randic M, Miletic V (1977) Effect of substance P on cat dorsal horn neurons activated by noxious stimuli. Brain Res 128 : 164–169

SALTER MW, HENRY JL (1985) Effects of physalaemin on functionally identified spinal dorsal horn neurons in the cat. Neurosci Abstr 11:966
SCHMAUSS C, YAKSH TL (1984) In vivo studies on spinal opiate receptor systems mediating antinociception. II. Pharmacological profiles suggesting a differential association of Mu, Delta and Kappa receptors with visceral, chemical and cutaneous thermal stimuli in the rat. J Pharmacol Exp Ther 228:1–12
SUNDLER F, BRODIN E, EKBLAD E, HAKANSON R, UDDMAN R (1985) Sensory nerve fibres: distribution of substance P, neurokinin A and calcitonin gene-related peptide. In: HAKANSON R, SUNDLER F (eds) Tachykinin antagonists. Elsevier, Amsterdam, pp 3–14
WILLCOCKSON WS, CHUNG JM, HORI V, LEE KH, WILLIS WD (1984) Effects of iontophoretically released peptides on primate spinothalamic tract cells. J Neurosci 4:741-750
YAKSH TL, JESSELL TM, GAMSE R, MUDGE AW, LEEMAN SE (1980) Intrathecal morphine inhibits substance P release from mammalian spinal cord in vivo. Nature 286:155–157
ZIEGLGÄNSBERGER W, TULLOCH IF (1979) Effects of substance P on neurons in the dorsal horn of the spinal cord of the cat. Brain Res 166:273–282

25 Peptidergic Neurotransmission in the Dorsal Horn of the Rat Spinal Cord

C. Mayer and W. Zieglgänsberger

Introduction

The characterization of neuropeptides as potential intercellular messengers has opened up new vistas for the signaling capacity of the nervous system (see: Bloom 1983, 1984). Unfortunately, for most of the hitherto known neuropeptides a role in any type of behavioral effect still awaits detection (Krieger et al. 1983; Luttinger 1984). Current research suggests that neuropeptides which have been characterized in primary afferent and descending nerve fibers, as well as axons and terminals of spinofugally projecting or intrinsic neurons, play key roles in the integration of somatosensory afferent information in the dorsal horn of the spinal cord, including signals from nociceptors (Siggins and Gruol 1986; Zieglgänsberger 1984, 1986). Specific binding sites have already been identified for most of these neuropeptides (Krieger et al. 1983; Björklund and Hökfelt 1985).

The principal aim of this study was the electrophysiological characterization of synaptic mechanisms at sites within the dorsal horn of the spinal cord thought to be peptidergic in nature. The present results have been obtained from multireceptive neurons (MRNs) in laminae I and IV-V of the rat dorsal horn. The dendrites of these neurons become intermingled with peptidergic primary afferents, terminals of descending fibers, and also with axons and dendrites of peptide-containing neurons in the substantia gelatinosa (Cervero 1980; Hunt et al. 1982; Hökfelt et al. 1983; Dodd et al. 1984).

Methods

A laminectomy was performed on male Wistar rats (body weight 150–250 g) in order to expose the lower thoracic and upper lumbar regions of the spinal cord. The animals were spontaneously breathing a mixture of normal air and halothane (0.5 %–0.8 %) from a reservoir. Extracellular recordings of spinal neurons were made in the most superficial layers, probably mainly lamina I, and deeper layers, probably mainly laminae IV-V, with four- or five-barrelled pipettes which had an overall tip diameter of 4–6 μm (resistance 5–80 MΩ). The compounds were applied either by microiontophoresis or pneumatically from multibarrelled micropipettes, in conjunction with extracellular recording techniques. In experiments where pneumatic ejection was used, electrode assemblies with the recording electrode protruding 100–150 μm were employed (for technical details see Zieglgänsberger and Tulloch 1979). By the use of such pneumatic ejections of diluted solutions from micropipettes, the major disadvantage of the microiontophoretic administration method, i.e., the unknown concentration of the substance applied in the region of the neuron being studied, can be at least partially overcome (Fig. 1). This technique allows the effective concentration of neuroactive substances to be established and can be combined with extra- and intracellular recording techniques (Stanzione and Zieglgänsberger 1983; Zieglgänsberger et al. 1986). Since diluted solutions are used the ejected volume need not be controlled. Prior to

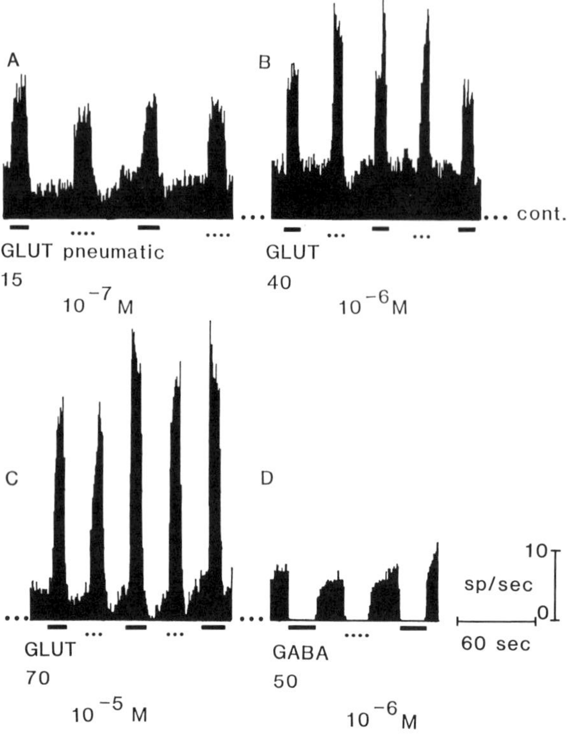

Fig. 1 A–D. Microiontophoretic (bars) and pneumatic (dots) application of GLUT and GABA on a spontaneously discharging MRN in lamina V. **A–C** GLUT was applied with increasing phoretic currents (15, 40, 70 nA) and from three barrels containing different concentrations of GLUT (10^{-7}, 10^{-6}, 10^{-5} M) in ACSF. **D** The effect of pneumatically applied GABA was compared to phoretic administration. The ejecting pressure was between 10 and 20 kPa; the intervals between **A, B, C,** and **D** were 20–60 s. Phoretic currents (nA) are indexed. Sp/sec, neuronal discharge activity in spikes per second

the experiment the necessary pneumatic pressure (5–20 kPa) was adjusted in order to increase the bulk flow from the pipette, as visualized under the microscope. Automatic current balancing was used during phoretic applications. Vehicle ejections were employed to check for mechanical artifacts during pneumatic administration. Few mechanical artifacts were observed, and those which were seen were abrupt in onset. Consequently, the recorded unit usually had to be abandoned. Substances used for iontophoretic or pneumatic application were as follows: D-ala^2, D-Leu^5-enkephalin: (phoretic) 5 x 10^{-3}M, pH 5.0; (pneumatic) 10^{-5}–10^{-8}M, in $Na_2HPO_4/Na_2H_2PO_4$, pH 6.0, 50 mM (Bachem). Morphine-HCl: (phoretic) 5 x 10^{-3}M, in Na-acetate buffer (NAB), pH 5.0, 20 mM (Merck); (pneumatic) 10^{-5}–10^{-8}M, in artificial cerebrospinal fluid (ACSF; Zieglgänsberger and Sutor 1983), pH 7.0. U 50 488H: 5 x 10^{-3}M, in NAB, pH 5.0, 20 mM (Upjohn). Naloxone: (phoretic) 10^{-3} and 10^{-2}M, pH 5.5; (pneumatic) 10^{-4}–10^{-7}M, in ACSF, pH 7.0 (Endo). Substance P: (phoretic) 2 x 10^{-3}M, in NAB, pH 5.0; (pneumatic) 10^{-4}–10^{-7}M, in ACSF, pH 7.0 (Sigma). (D-Pro^2, D-Trp^{7,9})-substance P: 2 x 10^{-3}M, in NAB, pH 5.0, 20 mM (Peninsula). Neurotensin: (phoretic) 10^{-5} – 5 x 10^{-5}M, in 165 mM NaCl, pH 7.0; (pneumatic) 10^{-5}–10^{-7}M, in ACSF, pH 7.0

(Peninsula). Somatostatin: 10^{-5}M, in 165 mM NaCl, pH 7.0 (Peninsula). L-Glutamate: (phoretic) 0.5 M, pH 8.0; (pneumatic) 10^{-5}–10^{-8}M, in ACSF, pH 7.0. Gamma-amino-butyric acid: (phoretic) 0.5 M, pH 5.0; (pneumatic) 10^{-5}–10^{-7}M, in ACSF, pH 7.0. Baclofen D,L: 10^{-2}M, in NAB, pH 4.5, 150 mM (Ciba-Geigy).

Only those units which responded to phoretically applied L-glutamate (GLUT) were included in this study. The phoretic currents were all cationic in polarity, except for GLUT.

Results

Extracellular recordings (n = 250) were obtained from dorsal horn neurons of 85 rats. The neurons were classified by their responses to physiological stimuli, such as hair movement, light touch, pinch, joint movement, and deep pressure (noxious). Only recordings from MRNs were included in this sample. About 50 % of them were spontaneously active and could be activated by light touch and pressure to the center of the receptive field on the hind limb. They responded with an increase in firing when the mechanical pressure was increased. Neurons not spontaneously discharging were activated by repetitively applied short phoretic pulses of GLUT (5–10 nA/2–20 s; intervals 30–60 s). Pneumatically ejected GLUT excited these neurons at concentrations in the range of 10^{-5}–10^{-7}M to a similar extent as phoretic currents of 15–70 nA (Fig. 1 A–C).

In order to analyze potential interactions between GABAergic and peptidergic synaptic processes, both gamma-amino butyric acid (GABA) (Fig. 1D) and the prototypic $GABA_B$ receptor agonist baclofen were applied iontophoretically (5–80 nA/5–30 s) and pneumatically (10^{-5}–10^{-7} M). Both GABA and baclofen inhibited all neurons tested. The therapeutically used racemic mixture of D- and L-baclofen (Lioresal) was administered with phoretic currents of 50–100 nA and dose-dependently inhibited (more than 50 % reduction of control discharge activity) spontaneous activity and synaptically, GLUT- and substance P-induced (see below) activity within 5-30 s (12 of 14 neurons). The L-enantiomer was clearly more effective than the D-enantiomer at comparable phoretic currents (compared in nine neurons). The L-enantiomer did not antagonize the depressant actions of D-baclofen (tested in 12 neurons).

Application of substance P (SP), either from pressurized micropipettes or by iontophoresis, dose-dependently excited most neurons (25 of 35). Five neurons were consistently inhibited (repeated applications). In the majority of tests the phoretic application of SP, with currents ranging from 50–130 nA, evoked an increase in excitability after 20–120 s, which outlasted the termination of application by some 2–3 min. Pneumatic administration of SP at concentrations of 10^{-4}–10^{-7}M resulted in excitatory effects over a similar time course. The phoretic application of the SP analogue (D-Pro^2, D-$Trp^{7,9}$)-SP, (50–120 nA) antagonized this action in four of 25 cells tested. The antagonistic action appeared within 20–150 s and outlasted the application by 50–120 s. In 16 cells the analogue evoked excitatory responses similar to these evoked by SP itself. The excitatory effect of SP on spontaneous activity was much less than on GLUT-induced activity. In 12 neurons the excitatory action of GLUT was markedly enhanced by SP without any detectable effect on spontaneous activity (Fig. 2).

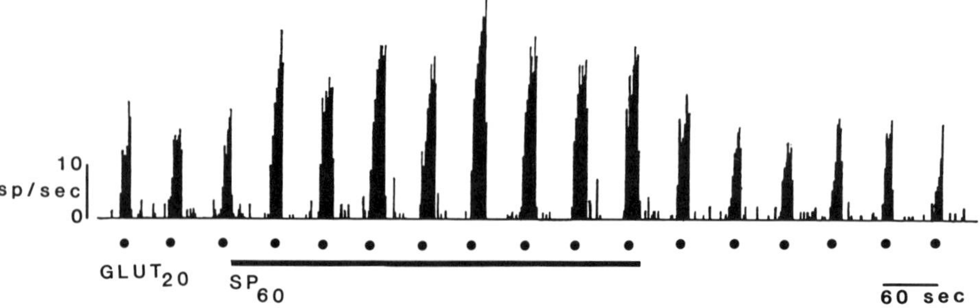

Fig. 2. SP enhances GLUT-induced (dots, 20 nA/15 s) excitation in an MRN. The spontaneous activity is not affected by this administration (bar). Phoretic current (nA) is indexed. sp/sec, neuronal discharge activity in spikes per second

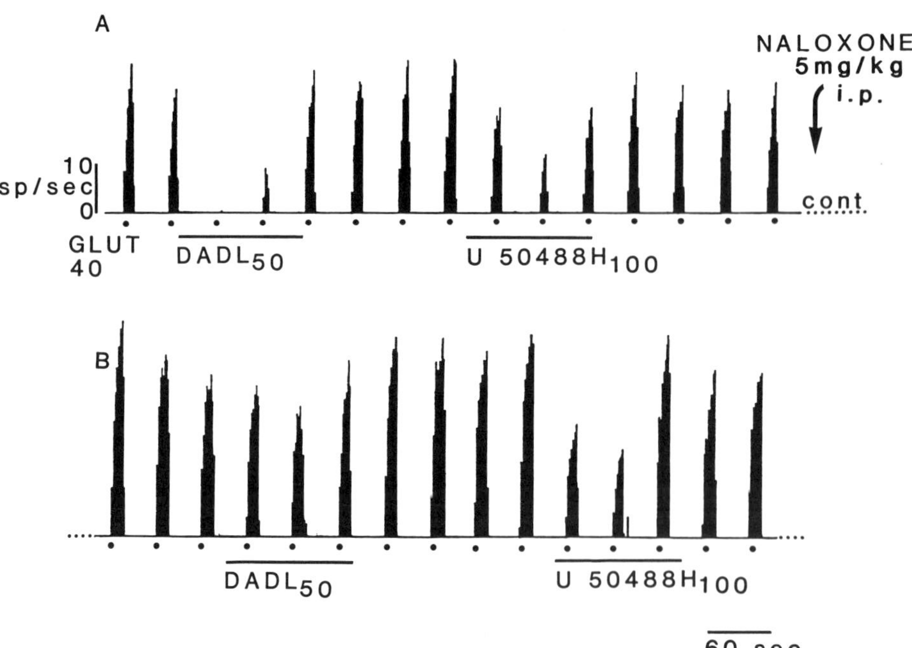

Fig. 3 A, B. Effect of systemically applied NAL on delta- and kappa-preferring agonists. The intraperitoneal administration of NAL (5 mg/kg, in 165 mM NaCl) antagonized the depressant effect of phoretically administered D-ala^2, D-leu^5-enkephalin (DADL, 50 nA) on GLUT-evoked activity (dots, 40 nA/20 s) without affecting the depressant effect of the phoretically applied kappa-preferring agonist U 50488H (100 nA). **A** Control; **B** 35 min after i.p. injection of NAL. Applications of DADL and U 50488H are indicated by bars. Phoretic currents (nA) are indexed. sp/sec, neuronal discharge activity in spikes per second

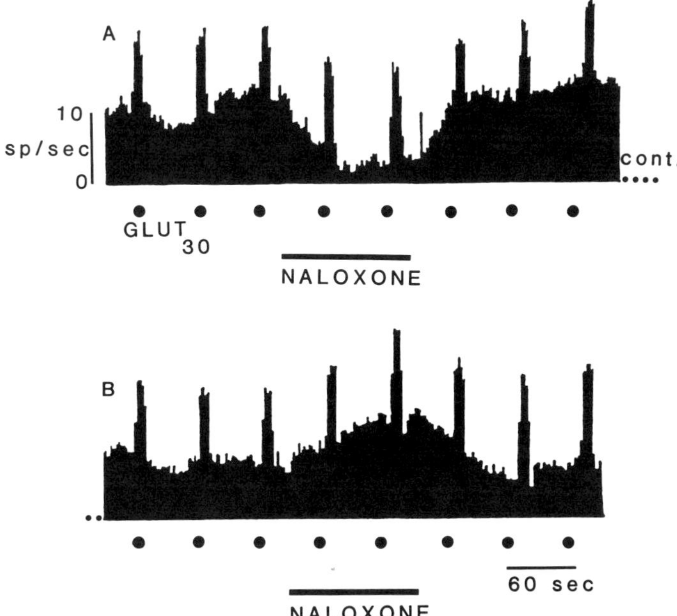

Fig. 4 A, B. Effect of NAL on GLUT-induced discharge activity of an MRN. NAL was iontophoretically applied (80 nA) from barrels filled with different concentrations. **A** 1 mM; **B** 10 mM. Note: With identical phoretic currents the release of NAL from more concentrated solutions is higher. sp/sec, neuronal discharge activity in spikes per second

All opioid agonists tested depressed spontaneous activity and both chemically and synaptically induced activity (45 of 50 neurons tested). The mu-preferring agonist, morphine, depressed neuronal firing (more than 75 % of control value) at phoretic currents in the range of 20–120 nA within 20–40 s. The depressant effect outlasted the application by 50–120 s. Pneumatic administration of the delta-preferring agonist, D-ala^2, D-leu^5-enkephalin, and morphine in concentrations of 10^{-6}–10^{-8} M resulted in a similar depression of neuronal excitability. The neuronal excitability was affected to a comparable extent by the kappa-preferring agonist, U 50 488H (Lahti et al. 1982), when phoretic currents in the same range as that for the mu- and kappa-agonists were employed. However, intraperitoneal administration of naloxone (NAL; 5 mg/kg) antagonized the actions of the mu- and delta-preferring agonists more readily than those of the kappa-preferring agonist (tested in 10 neurons). In eight neurons the effects of the enkephalin analogue and morphine were either completely antagonized or markedly reduced without an obvious effect on the depressant action of U 50488H (Fig. 3). The antagonistic action of NAL appeared some 10 min after injection and lasted some 60 min.

Phoretic (50–120 nA) and pneumatic (10^{-6}M) administration of NAL to cells which had not previously been exposed to an opioid agonist frequently evoked a moderate increase (20 %–50 % of control activity) in neuronal discharge rate (10 of 15 neurons). Unexpectedly, the increase in firing rate was often preceeded by a transient decrease. In the majority of cases (12 of 15 neurons), where increasing doses of NAL were applied, the lowest doses employed induced a decrease in firing rate (Fig. 4).

Twenty-five of 28 neurons which had been continuously exposed to opioids by phoretic application for 20–30 min and had become tolerant to this dosage showed a consistent increase (up to 300 %) in discharge rate in response to phoretically or pneumatically administered NAL. None of the actions of NAL on neuronal excitability described above were associated with a detectable change in spike shape.

Iontophoretically administered neurotensin (NT; 20–150 nA) evoked, in all 12 cells tested, a dose-dependent excitation. The delay between application and onset of action was clearly shorter (15–60 s) than that for SP, and the recovery of the firing rate to control levels was faster (10–30 s). Application of NT (10^{-5}–10^{-7} M) from pressurized micropipettes produced, after a delay of 2–20 s, an excitatory response in 10 of 16 neurons. The remainder were unaffected by NT. No depressant actions of NT were observed. In the same sample of neurons, phoretically applied somatostatin (SOM) evoked a decrease in neuronal excitability in all 12 cells tested. Spontaneous discharge activity was decreased (more than 75 %) by phoretic currents in the range of 50–120 nA more readily than the synaptically or chemically evoked neuronal activity of non-spontaneously firing neurons. The inhibitory effect became apparent after a delay of 15–45 s and reached control levels 50–150 s after termination of application.

Discussion

Substance P was the first neuropeptide considered to have a function in synaptic transmission within the CNS (Henry 1982a; Jessel 1983; Dun 1985). The present data, obtained using pneumatic application of SP, indicates that the slow "turning on" of excitatory effects (Randić and Miletic 1977) in MRNs in the dorsal horn can be elicited by concentrations in the micro- to nanomolar range. The ionic mechanism underlying this excitatory action remains to be established. Previous intracellular studies, performed in various types of spinal neurons, reported increases (Otsuka et al. 1975; Otsuka and Konishi 1977; Nicoll 1978), decreases, or no effect (Krnjevic 1977; Sastry 1979; Zieglgänsberger and Tulloch 1979) on ionic conductances accompanying the excitatory action of SP. Studies performed on cultured spinal neurons of the mouse (Nowak and Macdonald 1982) suggest that SP probably depolarizes these cells by blocking a voltage-dependent potassium conductance (resembling the M-current). There is evidence from studies performed on isolated spinal cord preparations of the neonatal rat that bath-applied SP reduces the duration of a tetrodotoxin-resistant (Ca) spike and may evoke indirect effects (Murase et al. 1982; Murase and Randić 1984).

Interestingly, SP seems to enhance GLUT-induced activity more than the spontaneous discharge of dorsal horn neurons. An increase in input resistance of the neuron which is associated with the depolarizing action of SP could explain the increase in GLUT responses. In addition, a voltage-dependent potassium conductance resembling the M-current, which is inactive at resting membrane levels, is probably switched on during GLUT-induced depolarizations. Since GLUT and SP have recently been shown to co-localize in primary afferent terminals (Battaglia et al., this volume) SP might function as a neuromodulator in this case, enhancing the excitatory actions of GLUT, e.g., after repetitive stimulation (wind-up), as suggested by earlier in vivo and in vitro electrophysiological investigations (Zieglgänsberger and Tulloch 1979; Zieglgänsberger and Sutor 1983). Recent patch-clamp studies performed on isolated bovine chromaffin cells showed that SP antagonizes the acetylcholine-induced inward current without evoking an ionic current itself (Clapman and Neher 1984), thus strengthening the concept that SP is a modulatory neuropeptide.

A multiplicity of actions seem to exist for SP in different spinal cord neurons. In cultured spinal neurons of the rat it has been reported that SP blocks the excitatory actions of GLUT (Vincent and Barker 1979), wheras in Renshaw cells SP preferentially reduces the nicotinic excitatory action of acetylcholine without affecting responses to GLUT (Belcher and Ryall 1977).

Unfortunately, the presently available SP analogues retain much of their agonist activity and are more selective for SP effects in peripheral organs than for synaptic processes in the CNS. However, the present results show that SP analogues are able to antagonize the excitatory action of SP in the spinal cord, although in most cases, clear agonistic properties were found, thus precluding any further analysis. As in previous investigations (Phillis 1976), the present study does not provide any evidence in favor of a selective antagonistic action of baclofen against SP.

The most extensive studies regarding peptidergic mechanisms in the dorsal horn have been carried out on the actions of opioid peptides (Zieglgänsberger 1986). The inhibitory action of the enkephalins on spontaneous activity and both chemically and synaptically induced neuronal activity of spinal neurons provides a clear example of a differing receptor/ionophore coupling in different neurons. As in numerous other structures within the CNS, opioid peptides transiently alter the responsiveness of various spinal neurons to excitatory amino acid neurotransmitters, without directly influencing membrane potential or conductance (Zieglgänsberger 1984). Using an in vitro preparation of the rat lumbar spinal cord it was found, in a significant number of neurons in the substantia gelatinosa, that opioid peptides caused hyperpolarization due to an increase in potassium conductance (Yoshimura and North 1983; Duggan and North 1983).

Within the spinal enkephalinergic circuit, interneurons probably exert their inhibitory action on spinofugally projecting neurons preferentially via postsynaptically located receptors (Ruda 1982; Bennett et al. 1982; Basbaum and Fields 1984; Dubner et al. 1984; Willis 1985; Zieglgänsberger 1986). Mixed inputs (e.g., low-threshold stimuli excite, high-threshold stimuli inhibit; Iggo 1980) from low-threshold afferents as well as from nociceptors, converging mainly on spontaneously active interneurons in the substantia gelatinosa, are most likely a prerequisite for the modulation of primary nociceptive information by afferent, segmental, and descending pathways in this spinal enkephalinergic circuit.

There is, at present, only circumstantial evidence that a certain opioid receptor subtype (mu, delta, kappa) is specifically related to a particular opioid peptide action. The enzymatically stable enkephalin analogue used in the present study shows mainly delta-receptor activity, U 50488H shows kappa preference (Lahti et al. 1982), whereas morphine is the prototypic agonist for the mu-receptor (Akil et al. 1984; Höllt 1983). Multiple, postsynaptic, non-cross-tolerant subclasses of opioid receptors, which might even be part of the same supramolecular entity, have been suggested to exist on the same neuron in the spinal cord, as in various other sites within the CNS (Zieglgänsberger 1984, 1986). In addition, for various agonists evidence for presynaptic actions through separate mechanisms has been reported. The finding that systemically applied NAL preferentially antagonizes the actions of the mu- and delta-preferring agonists is in keeping with current research on opioid receptor kinetics, which suggests a lower potency of NAL on kappa-mediated effects (Siggins and Gruol 1986). Unexpectedly, the lowest doses of the opioid antagonist NAL employed in this study often reduced the firing rate of MRNs. Such an inhibitory effect of NAL on neuronal discharge activity could explain the findings reported in arthritic rats that systemic NAL at low doses decreased the responses of ventrobasal thalamic neurons, which is a major target area of spinofugally projecting MRNs (Guilbaud et al. 1982). The increase in discharge activity often evoked by NAL in opioid-naive neurons indicates the existence of an opiopidergic tonus upon MRNs. A reduction of such a tonus may be the explanation for the hyperalgesia reported to follow NAL administration (Zieglgänsberger 1984; Zieglgänsberger et al. 1986).

The discovery of an NAL-reversible analgesia following intrathecal application of NT suggests that NT-containing neurons may activate opioid peptide-containing spinal interneurons (Luttinger 1984). Interneurons, axon terminals, and varicosities containing NT-reactive material and interneurons containing enkephalin are located in close proximity within lamina II (Seybold and Elde 1982; Seybold and Maley 1984). NT excited most cells and increased their response to GLUT without obvious selectivity for a particular type of spinal neuron (Miletic and Randić 1979; Henry 1982b; Stanzione and Zieglgänsberger 1983). It is conceivable that the increase in the input resistance observed in spinal cord neurons of the rat would also facilitate other synaptic inputs (Stanzione and Zieglgänsberger 1983).

As in previous studies on dorsal horn neurons of the cat responding to noxious stimuli (Randić and Miletic 1978), SOM had, preferentially, an inhibitory action on spontaneous, synaptically, or GLUT-evoked neuronal activity in MRNs. In the present study the C-terminal 14-amino-acid molecule was used. The presence of SOM in small primary afferent fibers suggests the possibility of inhibitory processes which may be initiated by primary afferent stimulation of high-threshold fibers. Electropohysiological studies have provided evidence that SOM has both pre- and postsynaptic actions on central neurons, triggering inhibitory as well as excitatory events, possibly via different receptors. An inverted U-shaped dose-response relationship has been postulated from such studies (Delfs and Dichter 1985). When added to the perfusing medium of a spinal cord slice preparation, SOM caused a hyperpolarization and increased membrane conductance in the majority of dorsal horn neurons (Murase et al. 1982). From intracellular recordings of mouse cultured spinal cord neurons, mostly excitatory actions of SOM were reported. The depolarizing actions were associated, in some cases, with a fall in input resistance due to a decrease in conductance for potassium or chloride (Macdonald and Nowak 1981; Delfs and Dichter 1985).

Electrophysiological studies suggest that some of the effects of neuropeptides on synaptic transmission resemble those of the more classical neurotransmitters, whereas others seem to be involved in nonconventional modes of information transfer, where neuropeptides are either co-released from the same terminal or released from adjacent terminals (Chan-Palay and Palay 1984). Since the dorsal horn of the spinal cord is a structure in which more experimental controls can be satisfied than in most other sites within the CNS, this area might prove to be a good model from which to study and establish the physiological significance of peptide action on neurohumoral transmission. Neuropeptides like vasoactive intestinal polypeptide, cholecystokinin, angiotensin II, and other peptides known for their role in endocrine function, e.g., thyrotropin-releasing hormone, lutein-hormone-releasing hormone, vasopressin, and oxytocin, are present in the dorsal horn of the spinal cord (Sofroniew 1983) and may have effects on neuronal excitability. The introduction of peptide analogues (Rosell and Folkers 1982) or compounds with selective antagonistic actions (Chiodo and Bunney 1983) will help to elucidate the function of neuropeptides in the CNS, where a peptidergic synaptic link has yet to be shown.

Summary

Multireceptive neurons (MRN) in the dorsal horn of the rat spinal cord were recorded extracellularly and amino acid neurotransmitters and neuropeptides were applied iontophoretically or pneumatically from multibarrelled micropipettes. Pneumatically applied L-glutamate markedly excited these neurons at concentrations of 10^{-6}–10^{-7} M; gamma-aminobutyric acid (GABA) inhibited all neurons tested within a similar dose range.

Substance P (SP) excited most neurons at concentrations between 10^{-5} and 10^{-7} M. The analogue D-Pro^2, D-Trp^{7,9}-SP antagonized the excitatory action in several neurons but usually showed strong agonistic actions. The $GABA_B$ receptor agonist, baclofen, which inhibited the spontaneous or induced discharge activity in all neurons tested, had no specific antagonistic action against SP-induced excitations.

The iontophoretically and pneumatically applied opioid agonists (morphine-HCl, D-ala^2, D-leu^5-enkephalin, U 50488H) suppressed spontaneous activity and both chemically and synaptically induced activity. Intraperitoneal administration of 5 mg/kg naloxone (NAL) could only antagonize the effects of the mu- and delta-preferring agonists morphine and D-ala^2, D-leu^5-enkephalin respectively. Pneumatically applied NAL (10^{-4}–10^{-7} M) antagonized the actions of D-ala^2, D-leu^5-enkephalin and morphine. In the majority of cases NAL itself slightly excited the neuron. Unexpectedly, inhibition of discharge was the predominant effect at low doses of NAL.

Phoretically and pneumatically administered neurotensin (10^{-5}–10^{-7} M) excited most neurons, whereas somatostatin caused a strong suppression of discharge activity.

The present study shows that neuropeptides exert distinct actions on MRNs in the dorsal horn of the rat spinal cord; however, the elucidation of the ionic mechanisms involved in the excitatory and inhibitory peptidergic synaptic links awaits more intracellular studies and the development of more selective antagonists.

Acknowledgements. This work was supported by a grant from the Stiftung Volkswagenwerk and by the Deutsche Forschungsgemeinschaft SPP Neuropeptide (ZI 222/3-1) and SPP Nociception und Schmerz (ZI 222/2-3).

References

Akil H, Watson SJ, Young E, Lewis EL, Khachaturian H, Walker JM (1984) Endogenous opioids: Biology and function. Annu Rev Neurosci 7:223–255

Basbaum AI, Fields HL (1984) Endogenous pain control systems: brainstem spinal pathways and endorphin circuitry. Annu Rev Neurosci 7:309–338

Belcher G, Ryall RW (1977) Substance P and Renshaw cells: a new concept of inhibitory synaptic transmission. J Physiol (Lond) 272:105–119

Bennett GJ, Ruda MA, Gobel S, Dubner R (1982) Enkephalin immunoreactive stalked cells and lamina IIb islet cells in cat substantia gelatinosa. Brain Res 240:162–166

Björklund A, Hökfelt T (eds) (1985) GABA and neuropeptides in the CNS, vol 4. Elsevier, Amsterdam

Bloom FE (1983) The endorphins: A growing family of pharmacologically pertinent peptides. Annu Rev Pharmacol Toxicol 23:151–170

Bloom FE (1984) The functional significance of neurotransmitter diversity. Am J Physiol 246:184–194

Cervero F, Iggo A (1980) The substantia gelatinosa of the spinal cord. A critical review. Brain 102:717–772

Chan-Palay V, Palay SL (1984) Coexistence of neuroactive substances in neurons. Wiley, New York

Chiodo LA, Bunney BS (1983) Proglumide: selective antagonism of excitatory effects of cholecystokinin in central nervous system. Science 219:1449–1451

Clapham DE, Neher E (1984) Substance P reduces acetylcholine-induced currents in isolated bovine chromaffin cells. J Physiol (Lond) 347:255–277

Delfs JR, Dichter MA (1985) Somatostatin. In: Rogawski MA, Barker JL (eds) Neurotransmitter actions in the vertebrate nervous system. Plenum, New York, pp 411–437

Dodd J, Jahr CE, Jessell TM (1984) Neurotransmitters and neuronal markers at sensory synapses in the dorsal horn. In: Kruger L, Liebeskind JC (eds) Neural mechanisms of pain. Raven, New York, pp 105–121 (Advances in pain research and therapy, vol 6)

Dubner R, Ruda MA, Miletic V, Hoffert MJ, Bennett GJ, Nishikawa N, Coffield J (1984) Neural circuitry mediating nociception in the medullary and spinal dorsal horns. In: Kruger L, Liebeskind JC (eds) Neural mechanisms of pain. Raven, New York, pp 151–166 (Advances in pain research and therapy, vol 6)

Duggan AW, North RA (1983) Electrophysiology of opioids. Pharmacol Rev 35:219–281

Dun NJ (1985) Substance P. In: Rogawski MA, Barker JL (eds) Neurotransmitter actions in the vertebrate nervous system. Plenum, New York, pp 385–410

Guilbaud G, Benoist JM, Gautron M, Kayser V (1982) Effects of systemic naloxone upon ventrobasal thalamus neuronal responses in arthritic rats. Brain Res 243:59–66

Henry JL (1982a) Relation of substance P to pain transmission: neurophysiological evidence. In: Porter R, O'Connor M (eds) Substance P in the nervous system. Pitman, Bath, pp 206–224

Henry JL (1982b) Electrophysiological studies on the neuroactive properties of neurotensin. In: Nemeroff CB, Prange AJ Jr (eds) Neurotensin, a brain and gastrointestinal peptide. The New York Academy of Sciences, New York, pp 216–227

Hökfelt T, Skirboll L, Lundberg JM, Dalsgaard CJ, Johansson O, Pernow B, Jancso G (1983) Neuropeptides and pain pathways. In: Bonica JJ, Lindblom U, Iggo A (eds) Advances in pain research and therapy, vol 5. Raven, New York, pp 227–246

Höllt V (1983) Multiple endogenous opioid peptides. Trends Neurosci 6 : 24–26

Hunt SP, Nagy JI, Ninkovic M (1982) Peptides and the organization of the dorsal horn. In: Sjölund BH, Björklund A (eds) Brain stem control of spinal mechanisms. Elsevier, Amsterdam, pp 159–178

Iggo A (1980) Segmental neurophysiology of pain control. In: Kosterlitz HW, Terenius LY (eds) Pain and society. Verlag Chemie, Weinheim, pp 123–140

Jessell TM (1983) Substance P in the nervous system. In: Iversen L, Iversen SD, Snyder SH (eds) Handbook of Psychopharmacology. Plenum, New York, pp 1–105

Krieger DT, Brownstein MJ, Martin JB (eds) (1983) Brain peptides. Wiley, New York

Krnjevic K (1977) Effects of substance P on central neurons in cats. In: von Euler US, Pernow B (eds) Substance P. Raven, New York, pp 217–230

Lathi RA, von Voigtlander PF, Barsun C (1982) Properties of a selective kappa-agonist U 50 488 H. Life Sci 31 : 2237–2260

Luttinger D (1984) Peptides and nociception. Int Rev Neurobiol 25 : 185–241

Macdonald R, Nowak L (1981) Somatostatin has excitatory actions on murine spinal cord neurons in primary dissociated cell culture. Soc Neurosci Abstr 7 : 429

Miletic V, Randić M (1979) Neurotensin excites cat spinal neurons located in laminae I-III. Brain Res 169 : 600–604

Murase K, Randić M (1984) The actions of substance P on rat spinal dorsal horn neurones. J Physiol (Lond) 346 : 203–217

Murase K, Nedeljkov V, Randić M (1982) The actions of neuropeptides on dorsal horn neurons in the rat spinal cord slice preparation: an intracellular study. Brain Res 234 : 170–176

Nicoll RA (1978) Peptide receptors in the CNS: neurophysiologic studies in neurobiology of peptides. Neurosci Res Prog Bull 16 : 272–285

Nowak LM, Macdonald RL (1982) Substance P: ionic basis for depolarizing responses of mouse spinal cord neurons in cell cultures. J Neurosci 2 : 1119–1128

Otsuka M, Konishi S (1977) Electrophysiological and neurochemical evidence for substance P as a transmitter of primary sensory neurons. In: von Euler US, Pernow B (eds) Substance P. Raven, New York, pp 207–214

Otsuka M, Konishi S, Takahashi T (1975) Hypothalamic substance P as a candidate for transmitter of primary neurons. Fed Proc 34 : 1922–1928

Phillis JW (1976) Is β-(4-chlorophenyl)-GABA a specific antagonist of substance P on cerebral neurons? Experientia 32 : 593–594

Randić M, Miletic V (1977) Effect of substance P on cat dorsal horn neurons activated by noxious stimuli. Brain Res 128 : 164–169

Randić M, Miletic V (1978) Depressant actions of methionine-enkephalin and somatostatin in cat dorsal horn neurones activated by noxious stimuli. Brain Res 152 : 196–202

Rosell S, Folkers K (1982) Substance P antagonists: a new type of pharmacological tool. Trends Pharmacol Sci 3 : 211–212

Ruda MA (1982) Opiates and pain pathways: demonstration of enkephalin synapses and dorsal horn projection neurons. Science 215 : 1523–1525

Saito KS, Konishi S, Otsuka M (1975) Antagonism between lioresal and substance P in the rat spinal cord. Brain Res 97 : 177–180

Sastry BR (1979) Substance P effects on spinal nociceptive neurones. Life Sci 24 : 2169–2178

Seybold V, Elde RP (1982) Neurotensin immunoreactivity in the superficial laminae of the dorsal horn of the rat. I. Light microscopic studies of cell bodies and proximal dendrites. J Comp Neurol 205 : 89–100

Seybold V, Maley B (1984) Ultrastructural study of neurotensin immunoreactivity in the superficial laminae of the dorsal horn of the rat. Peptides 5 : 1179–1189

Siggins GR, Gruol DL (1986) Mechanisms of transmitter action in the vertebrate central nervous system. In: The nervous system IV. Williams & Wilkins, Baltimore, pp 1–114 (Handbook of physiology)

Sofroniew MV (1983) Morphology of vasopressin and oxytocin neurons and their central and vascular projections. Prog Brain Res 60 : 101–114

Stanzione P, Zieglgänsberger W (1983) Action of neurotensin on spinal cord neurons in the rat. Brain Res 268 : 111–118

Vincent JD, Barker JL (1979) Substance P: evidence for diverse roles in neuronal function from cultured mouse spinal neurons. Science 205 : 1409–1412

Yoshimura M, North RA (1983) Substantia gelatinosa neurones hyperpolarized in vitro by enkephalin. Nature 305 : 529–530

Willis WD (1985) The pain system. The neuronal basis of nociceptive transmission in the mammalian nervous system. In: Gildenberg PL (ed) Pain and headache, Karger, Basel

Zieglgänsberger W (1984) Opioid actions on mammalian spinal neurons. Int Rev Neurobiol 25 : 243–275

Zieglgänsberger W (1986) Central control of nociception. In: The nervous system IV. Williams & Wilkins, Baltimore, pp 581–645 (Handbook of physiology)

Zieglgänsberger W, Sutor B (1983) Responses of gelatinosa neurons to putative neurotransmitters in an in vitro preparation of the adult spinal cord. Brain Res 279 : 316–320

Zieglgänsberger W, Tulloch IF (1979) Effects of substance P on neurones in the dorsal horn of the spinal cord of the cat. Brain Res 166 : 273–282

Zieglgänsberger W, Mercuri N, Stanzione P, Sutor B (1986) Neurophysiological characterization of opioid peptide actions on neurohumoral transmission in the mammalian central nervous system. In: Stefanos GB (ed) Handbook of comparative opioid and related neuropeptide mechanisms, vol 2. CRC, Boca Raton, pp 41–48

26 Substance P and Cholecystokinin Octapeptide Modify a Slow Inward Calcium-Sensitive Current Relaxation in Rat Spinal Dorsal Horn Neurons

K. Murase, M. Randić, P. D. Ryu, and S. Usui

Introduction

Experimental evidence supports the concept that substance P (SP) may function as a neurotransmitter and/or neuromodulator in synaptic transmission between primary afferent fibers and neurons within the spinal cord (Nicoll et al. 1980). SP produces a slow neuronal depolarization accompanied by an increase (Krnjević 1977; Murase et al. 1982; Murase and Randić 1984), decrease (Murase et al. 1982, Murase and Randić 1984), or no change in input resistance (Sastry 1979; Zieglgänsberger and Tulloch 1979). The ionic mechanisms of the SP depolarization or increase in neuronal membrane excitability are, however, presently unresolved. Data obtained in cultured mouse and rat spinal neurons (Hösli et al. 1981; Nowak and MacDonald 1982) and bullfrog sympathetic neurons (Adams et al. 1983) suggested that SP inhibits the M current (I_M), a species of voltage-dependent K current (Brown and Adams 1980; Nowak and MacDonald 1981, 1983), and that the I_M inhibition is the primary cause of the membrane depolarization. It was reported, furthermore, that SP raises neuronal membrane excitability by reducing inward rectification in cultured rat globus pallidus neurons and that modulation of the inward rectification by SP implies a self-enforcing element to the depolarization caused by the peptide (Stanfield et al. 1985). As it will be shown in this presentation, we have recently demonstrated that SP induces an inward current at the holding potential close to the original resting level and augments a slow time- and voltage-dependent inward calcium (Ca)-sensitive current relaxation and inward current tails in immature rat spinal dorsal horn neurons in vitro. We have suggested that this effect may be instrumental in generating the slow membrane depolarization, increase in excitability, and "bursting" behavior in the immature rat dorsal horn neurons (Murase et al. 1985, 1986a).

Possible involvement of cholecystokinin octapeptide (CCK-8) in the sensory transmission in the spinal dorsal horn has also been suggested, although its role in the spinal cord is presently not understood (see Willetts et al. 1985 for review). Using the current-clamp technique we have investigated membrane actions of CCK-8 on dorsal horn neurons in the immature rat spinal cord slice preparation, and suggested that CCK-8 and SP might share a common neuronal mechanism although they do not act at the same receptor site (Willetts et al. 1985). We have therefore undertaken a further series of experiments on the membrane effects produced by CCK-8 in voltage-clamped immature rat spinal dorsal horn neurons. Similarly to SP, CCK-8 induces an inward current at the holding potential close to the resting level and augments time- and voltage-dependent Ca-sensitive inward current relaxations and inward current tails. These results suggest that induction of a slow inward current shift and augmentation of Ca-sensitive slow inward current relaxations and inward current tails may account, in part, for the CCK-8-induced slow depolarization and increase in excitability of the immature rat spinal dorsal horn neurons.

Preliminary results of our finding have already been communicated (Murase et al. 1985, 1986a,b,c).

Methods

Experiments were performed on 10- to 26-day-old Sprague-Dawley rats. The procedures with respect to the spinal cord slice technique were similar to those reported previously (Murase and Randić 1983; Murase et al. 1986a). The slices were cut transversally, and under visual control neurons in laminae III, IV, and V of the spinal dorsal horn were impaled (several neurons in lamina II were also examined for comparison) with a single microelectrode filled with 3 M potassium acetate (pH 7.2) having a resistance of 70–110 Mohm. Cells were voltage-clamped using a sample-and-hold amplifier (Dagan 8100) set at 3 kHz switching frequency and 25 % duty cycle. Responses were filtered with a low-pass filter (cut-off frequency 100 Hz, 12 dB/oct.) and recorded on a Gould-Brush 2200S pen recorder and a Nicolet 4094 digital oscilloscope. Tetrodotoxin (TTX, $0.5\text{–}1 \times 10^{-6}$ M) was regularly added in the Krebs solution to block the fast sodium inward current. The NaCl concentration was adjusted to maintain the osmolarity when tetraethyl-ammonium chloride (TEA, $1\text{–}2 \times 10^{-2}$ M, Kodak, Aldrich) or $MgCl_2$ (1×10^{-2} M) was added to the Krebs solution to reduce the fast potassium outward current and the Ca-activated outward current, and also, when external Ca^{2+} ions were removed. In the latter experiments the Mg^{2+} concentration of the Krebs solution was raised to 10 mM to offset the effect of changes in the total divalent cation concentration. SP and CCK-8 (Cambridge Research Biochemicals, Sigma) were dissolved in the perfusate and in known concentrations applied to the bath.

Since in the voltage-clamped dorsal horn neurons, complex time- and voltage-dependent current relaxations and tails were observed at membrane potentials close to the resting level, the "leak" component in the current responses was not subtracted in the illustrations shown in this presentation. In 20 mM TEA-containing solution, an inward current of more than -1 nA was regularly recorded during 1 s depolarizing voltage commands to membrane potentials to between −40 and −30 mV. This voltage-dependent Ca-sensitive current, which presumably supports a regenerative high-threshold Ca spike, was not possible to clamp satisfactorily with relatively high resistance electrodes used (Murase et al. 1986a,b). We present here, therefore, the current records obtained at membrane potentials below the threshold for the Ca-spike current generation or in the condition when the TEA concentration was reduced to 5–10 mM so that the total current could be clamped.

Results

A total of 39 dorsal horn neurons in laminae II–V perfused with the Krebs solution containing TTX (5×10^{-7} M) or TTX and TEA ($1\text{–}2 \times 10^{-2}$ M) were successfully voltage-clamped, and each result described below was observed in at least three neurons.

In about 75 % of examined neurons clamped at a holding potential close to the resting level and perfused with a TTX-containing solution (Fig. 1A), a slow inward current relaxa-

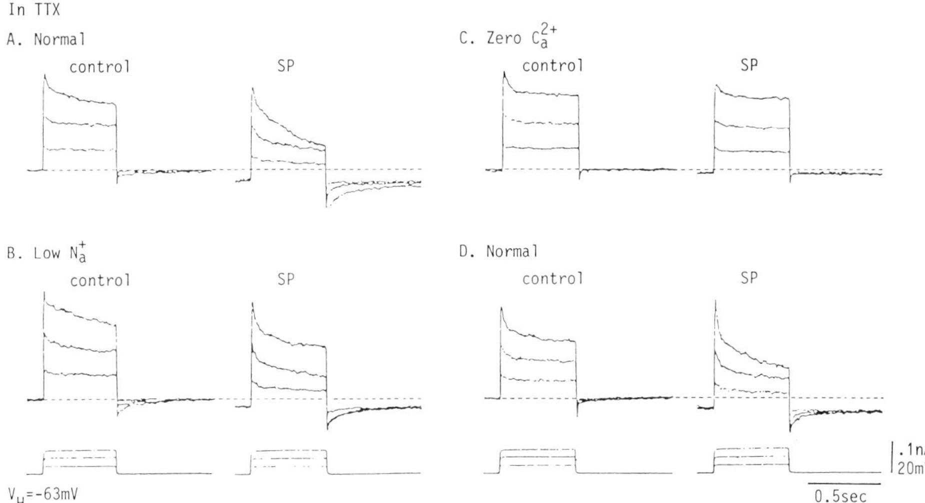

Fig. 1 A–D. Ionic dependence of the slow inward current relaxations and inward current tails, and the actions of SP on a dorsal horn neuron of a 15-day-old rat in TTX solution (5×10^{-7} M). Upper records are sampled current, lower records are membrane voltage. **A** Before SP (2×10^{-6} M), small slow inward relaxations and inward tails were seen. After the application of SP, an inward current developed at the holding potential, and in addition SP, augmented the slow time- and voltage-dependent inward relaxations as well as the inward current tails. **B** When external Na^+ was reduced from 127 to 36 mM by replacing Na^+ with Tris, the actions of SP on the holding current, the slow inward current relaxations, and inward current tails remained, although the effects were somewhat reduced. **C** However, the slow inward current relaxations and tails, and the effects of SP on the holding current, the relaxations, and the tails were reversibly depressed by removing external Ca^{2+} ions. **D** The SP effects were restored on replacing the 2.4 mM Ca^{2+}

tion could be recorded during depolarizing voltage commands to membrane potentials positive to about –40 mV. When external Na^+ ion concentration was reduced to 36 mM, by replacing Na^+ with Tris, the inward current relaxation persisted (Fig. 1B). The inward current relaxation was markedly depressed by removing external Ca^{2+} (Fig. 1C), or by adding 0.1–0.2 mM Cd, 5 mM Co, or 0.1 mM verapamil, and was increased by adding Ba or Bay K 8644 (Murase, et al. 1986a). In TEA-containing solution (with TTX present), the slow inward current relaxations and inward current tails were significantly augmented. The inward relaxation frequently persisted for more than 5 s. In respect to the activation and deactivation kinetics it appears that this Ca-sensitive inward relaxation and underlying conductance is distinct from the one supporting the high-threshold Ca spike (Murase et al. 1986a).

Under current-clamp conditions, SP produced a reversible dose-dependent slow depolarization in a majority of tested neurons. Bath application of SP (3×10^{-7} to 1×10^{-5} M for 1 min) induced an inward current in 30 out of 39 cells voltage-clamped at a holding potential close to the original resting level. Four neurons examined in the substantia gelatinosa region developed an outward current. The rest of the cells were unresponsive to 10^{-5} M SP. In 22 neurons SP augmented the slow time- and voltage-dependent inward relaxations, as

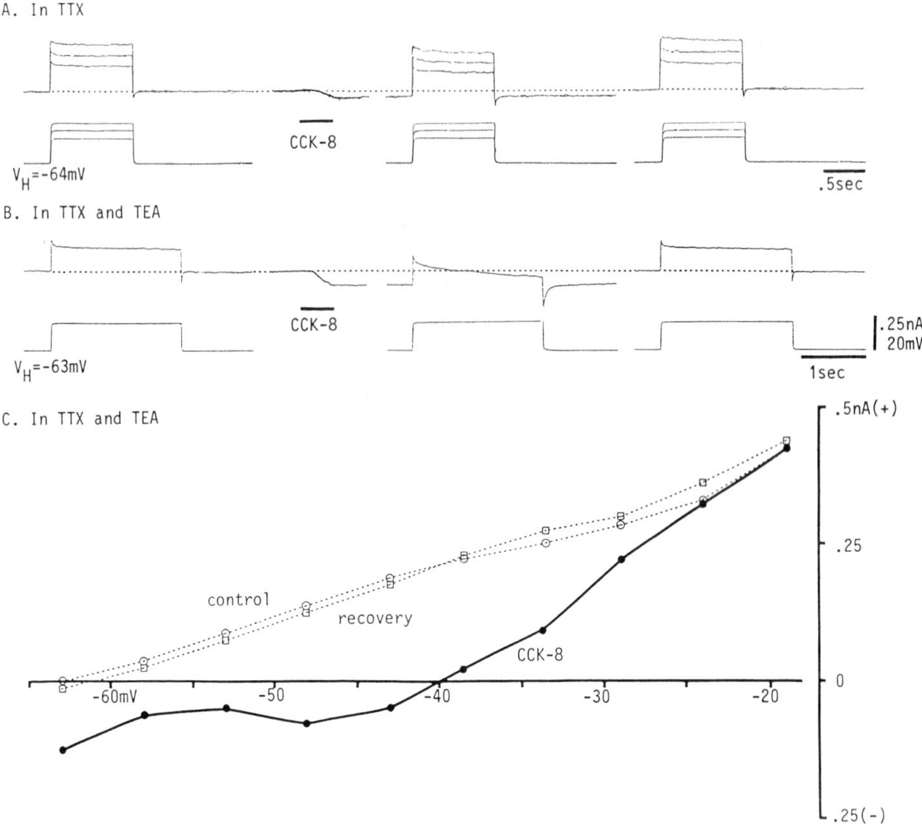

Fig. 2 A–C. Effects of CCK-8 on the inward current relaxations and inward current tails of a dorsal horn neuron of a 19-day-old rat in TTX (5×10^{-7} M) solution **(A)**, and TTX and TEA (1×10^{-2} M)-containing solution **(B,C)**. **A** The cell in TTX solution was clamped at a holding potential of –64 mV and subjected to a series of 1 s depolarizing voltage commands (lower records) before, during, and after the bath application of CCK-8 (1.5×10^{-6} M for 1 min). After CCK-8, an inward current developed at the holding potential, and the peptide, in addition, augmented the slow time- and voltage-dependent relaxations, as well as inward current tails. **B** The effects of CCK-8 were significantly augmented in TTX- and TEA-containing solution. **C** The current-voltage relationships were constructed from the current excursions measured at the end of 2 s voltage commands before (○), during (●), and after (□) application of CCK-8

well as inward current tails recorded in response to 1 s depolarizing command pulses to approximately –40 mV. Furthermore, in 10 neurons, an increase in the outward current, which may or may not be associated with the augmentation of the inward relaxations, was also observed. Some of the described actions of SP are illustrated in Fig. 1.

After the bath application of SP (2×10^{-6} M) in a control Krebs solution, an inward current developed at the holding potential, and in addition SP augmented the slow time- and voltage-dependent inward relaxations as well as inward current tails (Fig. 1A). In a low-Na^+ solution, the actions of SP on the holding current, the inward current relaxation, and the inward current tail remained, although the effects were somewhat reduced (Fig. 1B). However, the effects of SP on the holding current, the inward current relaxations, and the inward current tails were reversibly depressed by removing external Ca^{2+} ions (Fig. 1C). The inward current and the effects of SP were rapidly restored on replacing the 2.4 mM Ca^{2+} (Fig. 1D). In TEA-containing solution, the actions of SP were markedly enhanced (not illustrated).

In about half of the tested neurons perfused with the Krebs solution containing TTX or TTX + TEA and voltage-clamped at a holding potential close to the original resting level, bath application of CCK-8 (0.5–3 x 10^{-6} M) also induced an inward current and augmented the slow time- and voltage-dependent current relaxations and inward current tails (Fig. 2A,B). Similarly to the actions of SP described above, the actions of CCK-8 were reversibly depressed by removing external Ca^{2+}, remained in a low-Na^{+} solution, and were augmented in the TEA-containing solution (Fig. 2B). The voltage dependency of the CCK-8 actions was illustrated with current-voltage relationships constructed from current excursions measured at the end of the 2 s voltage commands before, during, and after the application of the peptide (Fig. 2C). The inward current induced by CCK-8, as well as one induced by SP, is more pronounced at membrane potentials positive to the rest.

Discussion

Our experiments indicate that in the immature rat spinal dorsal horn neurons SP and CCK-8 can induce an inward shift in the holding current when voltage-clamped at a holding potential close to the original resting level, and in response to depolarizing command steps can in addition augment a slow time- and voltage-dependent Ca-sensitive inward relaxation as well as inward current tails. This Ca-sensitive inward current relaxation seems to be present at around the resting level, and SP and CCK-8 seem to modify the kinetics. Since I_M inhibition by the peptides alone appears not to be sufficient to account for the inward current produced (Murase et al. 1986a), and the anomalous rectifier (Murase and Randić 1985) appears not to be significantly modified by the peptides (Randić, unpublished observation), the augmentation of the slow inward relaxations might be an important neuronal mechanism that leads the cells to depolarize in response to the application of the peptides. Since the actions of SP and CCK-8 on the slow inward current and the slow inward relaxation were more pronounced at membrane potentials positive to the rest, these effects might be instrumental in generating the peptide-induced slow depolarization, increase in the neuronal excitability, and burst discharges in the immature rat spinal dorsal horn neurons.

Reduction of the effects of SP and CCK-8 in low-Ca^{2+} solution is consistent with our previous findings that the peptide-induced slow membrane depolarizations were significantly reduced in the absence of external Ca^{2+} ions (Murase and Randić 1984; Willetts et al. 1985). However, an important question remaining to be resolved in a future work is to find out whether the induction of the slow inward current and the augmentation of the slow inward relaxation occur as a result of a direct effect of the peptides on receptor-coupled slow Ca^{2+}-sensitive current channels or secondarily via a mechanism such as a reduction of a Ca^{2+}-sensitive outward current(s). Appropriate ion-substitution experiments should provide necessary information about possible modification by SP and CCK-8 of either Ca^{2+}-dependent chloride conductance (Owen et al. 1986), or existence and/or change of a nonspecific inward cation conductance similar to one described in bursting pacemaker neurons of *Aplysia* (Kramer and Zucker 1985) and *Helix pomatia* (Hofmeier and Lux 1981; Swandulla and Lux 1985), and also in cardiac cells (Colquhoun et al. 1981).

Acknowledgements. The authors thank Drs. N. Akaike, D.A. Brown, and M. Sugimori for helpful comments on this work. This research was supported in part by grants from the National Science Foundation (BNS 8418042) and the United States Department of Agriculture to M.R., and from the Japanese Ministry of Education (61750357) to K.M.

References

Adams PR, Brown DA, Jones SW (1983) Substance P inhibits the M-current in bullfrog sympathetic neurones. Br J Pharmacol 79 : 330–333

Brown DA, Adams PR (1980) Muscarinic suppression of a novel voltage sensitive K^+ current in a vertebrate neurone. Nature 283 : 673–676

Colquhoun D, Neher E, Reuter H, Stevens CF (1981) Inward current channels activated by intracellular Ca in cultured cardiac cells. Nature 294 : 752–754

Hösli L, Hösli E, Zehntner C, Landolt H (1981) Effects of substance P on neurones and glial cells in cultured rat spinal cord. Neurosci Lett 24 : 165–168

Hofmeier G, Lux HD (1981) The time courses of intracellular free calcium and related electrical effects after injection of $CaCl_2$ into neurons of the snail, *Helix pomatia*. Pflugers Arch 391 : 242–251

Kramer RH, Zucker RS (1985) Calcium dependent inward current in *Aplysia* bursting pacemaker neurones. J Physiol (Lond) 362 : 107–130

Krnjević K (1977) Effects of substance P on central neurones in cats. In: von Euler US, Pernow B (eds) Substance P. Raven, New York, pp 217–230

Murase K, Randić M (1983) Electrophysiological properties of rat spinal dorsal horn neurones in vitro: calcium-dependent action potentials. J Physiol (Lond) 334 : 141–153

Murase K, Randić M (1984) Actions of substance P on the rat spinal dorsal horn neurones. J Physiol (Lond) 346 : 203–217

Murase K, Nedeljkov V, Randić M (1982) The actions of neuropeptides on dorsal horn neurons in the rat spinal cord slice preparation: an intracellular study. Brain Res 234 : 170–176

Murase K, Ryu PD, Randić M (1985) Voltage dependent slow membrane currents in rat spinal dorsal horn neurons and the actions of substance P. Soc Neurosci Abstr 11 : 842

Murase K, Ryu PD, Randić M (1986a) Substance P augments a persistent slow inward calcium-sensitive current in voltage-clamped spinal dorsal horn neurons of the rat. Brain Res 365 : 369–376

MURASE K, RYU PD, RANDIĆ M (1986b) Substance P augments a persistent slow inward calcium-sensitive current in voltage-clamped spinal dorsal horn neurons of the rat. Nippon Seirigaku Zasshi 48 : 210

MURASE K, RYU PD, RANDIĆ M (1986c) Neuropeptides modify a persistent slow inward calcium-sensitive current in rat spinal dorsal horn neurons (Abstr). 30th International Congress of Physiological Sciences, p 437

NICOLL RA, SCHENKER C, LEEMAN SE (1980) Substance P as a transmitter candidate. Annu Rev Neurosci 3 : 227–268

NOWAK LM, MACDONALD RL (1981) DL-muscarine decreases a potassium conductance to depolarize mammalian spinal cord neurons in cell culture. Soc Neurosci Abstr 7 : 725

NOWAK LM, MACDONALD RL (1982) Substance P: ionic basis for depolarizing responses of mouse spinal cord neurons in cell culture. J Neurosci 2 : 1119–1128

NOWAK LM, MACDONALD RL (1983) Muscarine-sensitive voltage-dependent potassium current in cultured murine spinal cord neurons. Neurosci Lett 35 : 85–91

OWEN DG, SEGAL M, BARKER JL (1986) Voltage-clamp analysis of a Ca^{2+}- and voltage-dependent chloride conductance in cultured mouse spinal neurons. J Neurophysiol 55 : 1115–1135

SASTRY BR (1979) Substance P effects on spinal nociceptive neurons. Life Sci 24 : 2169–2178

STANFIELD PR, NAKAJIMA Y, YAMAGUCHI K (1985) Substance P raises neuronal membrane excitability by reducing inward rectification. Nature 315 : 498–501

SWANDULLA D, LUX HD (1985) Activation of a nonspecific cation conductance by intracellular Ca^{2+} elevation in bursting pacemaker neurons of *Helix pomatia*. J Neurophysiol 54 : 1430–1433

WILLETTS J, URBÁN L, MURASE K, RANDIĆ M (1985) Actions of cholecystokinin octapeptide on rat spinal dorsal horn neurons. Ann NY Acad Sci 448 : 385–402

ZIEGLGÄNSBERGER W, TULLOCH IF (1979) Effects of substance P on neurones in the dorsal horn of the spinal cord of the cat. Brain Res 166 : 273–282

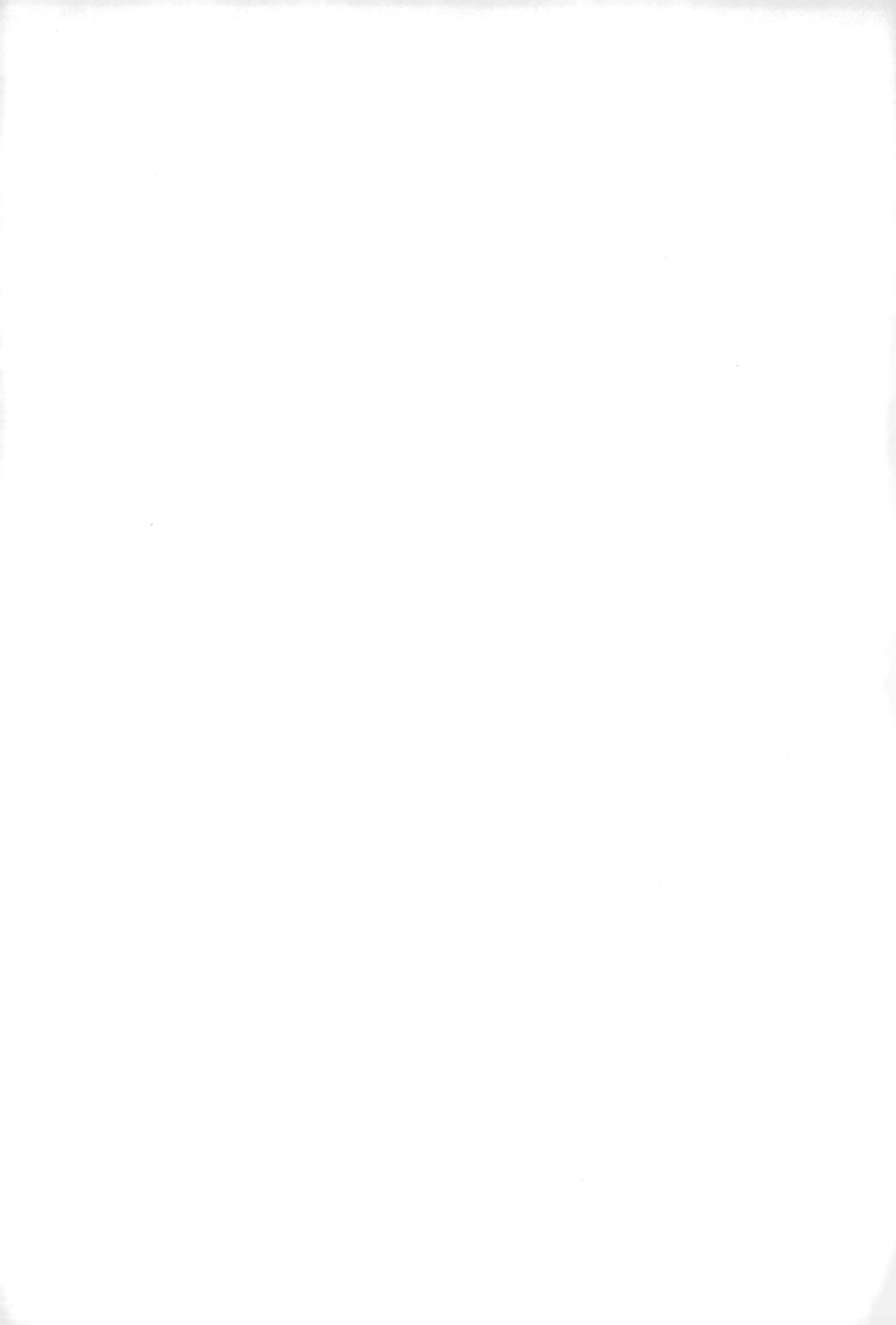

27 Slow Potentials in Rat Spinal Dorsal Horn Neurons Studied In Vitro

S. Jeftinija, L. Urban, I. Kangrga, P-D. Ryu, and M. Randić

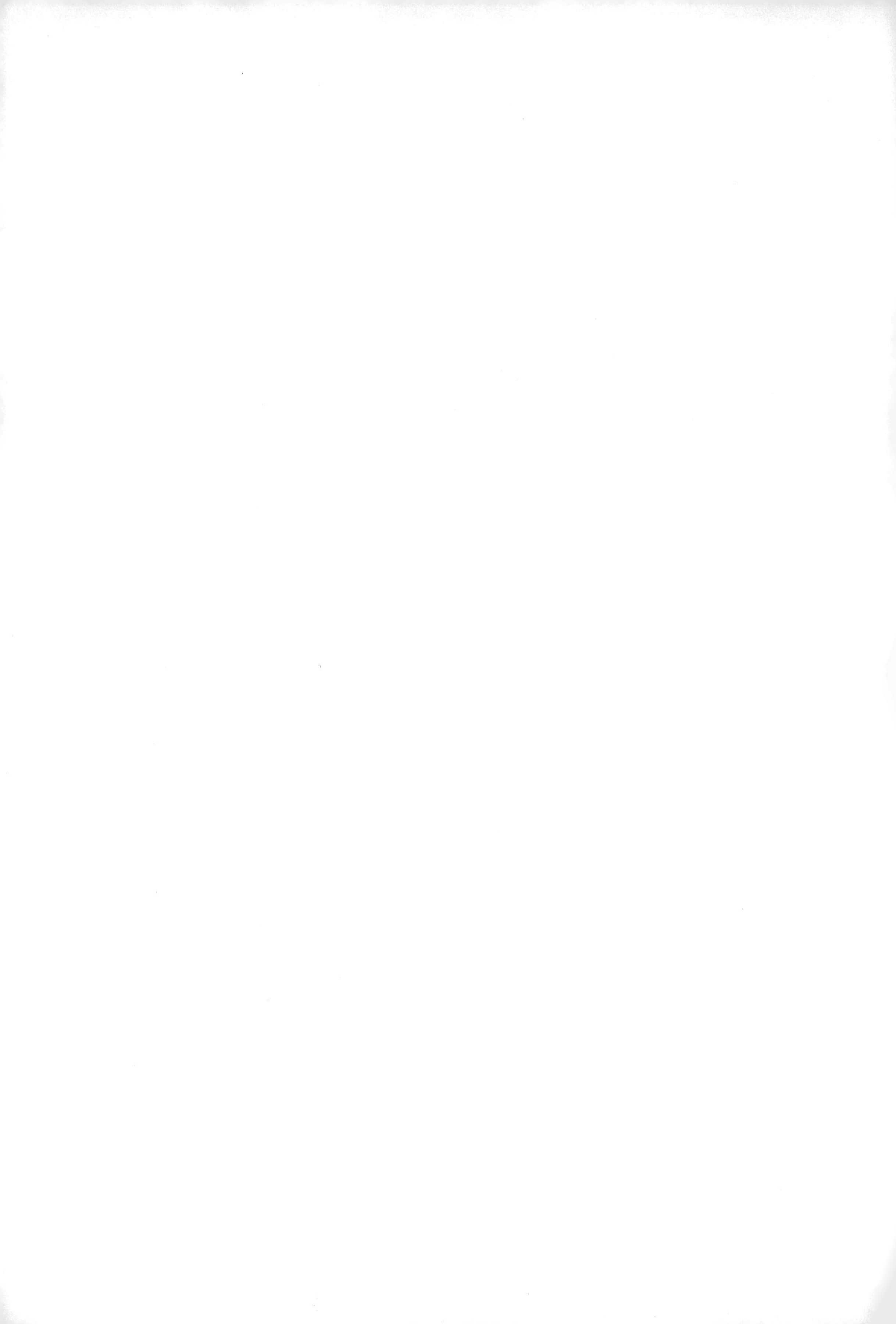

Introduction

We have recently demonstrated that repetitive stimulation of a dorsal root elicits a slow depolarization in more than half of the rat spinal dorsal horn neurons located in laminae I-V. In a smaller proportion of dorsal horn neurons a slow hyperpolarization was observed (Jeftinija et al. 1985). The slow depolarization was markedly depressed or abolished in the presence of substance P (SP), SP antagonists, monoclonal and polyclonal SP antisera, and capsaicin (Urban and Randić 1984; Urban et al. 1985; Randić et al. 1986). These results led us to suggest that SP, or SP-like peptide, may be an agonist that mimics in several important aspects the action of the natural transmitter for the slow depolarizing potential.

Norepinephrine, enkephalins, somatostatin and (-)-baclofen were considered as inhibitory neurotransmitter candidates since they hyperpolarize rat spinal dorsal horn neurons (Randić and Miletić 1978, Murase et al. 1982, North and Yoshimura 1984).

Methods

Experiments were performed on 10- to 30-day-old Sprague-Dawley rats. The procedures with respect to the spinal cord slice technique were similar to those reported previously (Murase and Randić 1983; Urban and Randić 1984; Jeftinija et al. 1985). Intracellular recordings from dorsal horn neurons were performed with micropipettes filled with 3 M potassium acetate (pH 7.2) having DC resistances of 90–120 MΩ. Synaptic activation of the dorsal horn neurons was obtained with a coaxial stainless steel stimulating electrode (outer diameter of inner and outer electrodes 25 and 200 μm respectively) or a bipolar platinum electrode positioned on the dorsal roots. Substance P (Cambridge Research Biochemicals, CRB, England), (D Pro^2, D-Trp^{7,9})-SP or (D-Arg^1, D-Pro^2, D-Trp^{7,9}, Leu^{11})-SP (Peninsula Labs, CRB), vasoactive intestinal polypeptide (Peninsula Labs, Beckman), cholecystokinin octapeptide (CCK-8; Bachem), (D-Ala^2, Met^5)- or (D-Ala^2, Leu^5)-enkephalinamide (CRB), somatostatin (SS; CRB), norepinephrine (NE; Regis), (-)-baclofen (Ciba-Geigy), polyclonal SP antisera (17H12T, Immuno Nuclear; AMSP-2 kindly supplied by Dr. T. M. Jessell, Harvard Medical School), and monoclonal SP antiserum 11E6 (supplied by Dr. T. M. Jessell) were applied by bath perfusion in known concentrations or dilutions. The chemicals were, as routine, applied for a minute, while the application time for antiserum varied between 30 and 90 min. Twenty-three rats of both sexes taken from two different litters were injected subcutaneously with 50 mg/kg of capsaicin in vehicle [10 % ethanol, 10 % Tween (v/v) in 0.9 % (w/v) saline] 48 h after birth. Six control litter mates received equal volumes of vehicle alone. After a survival time of 9-14 days the animals were subjected to the experimental procedure described above. Data were recorded on a Gould-Brush pen recorder (model 2200S) or stored in the disks of a Nicolet digital oscilloscope (model 4094) until processed and printed out on a digital plotter.

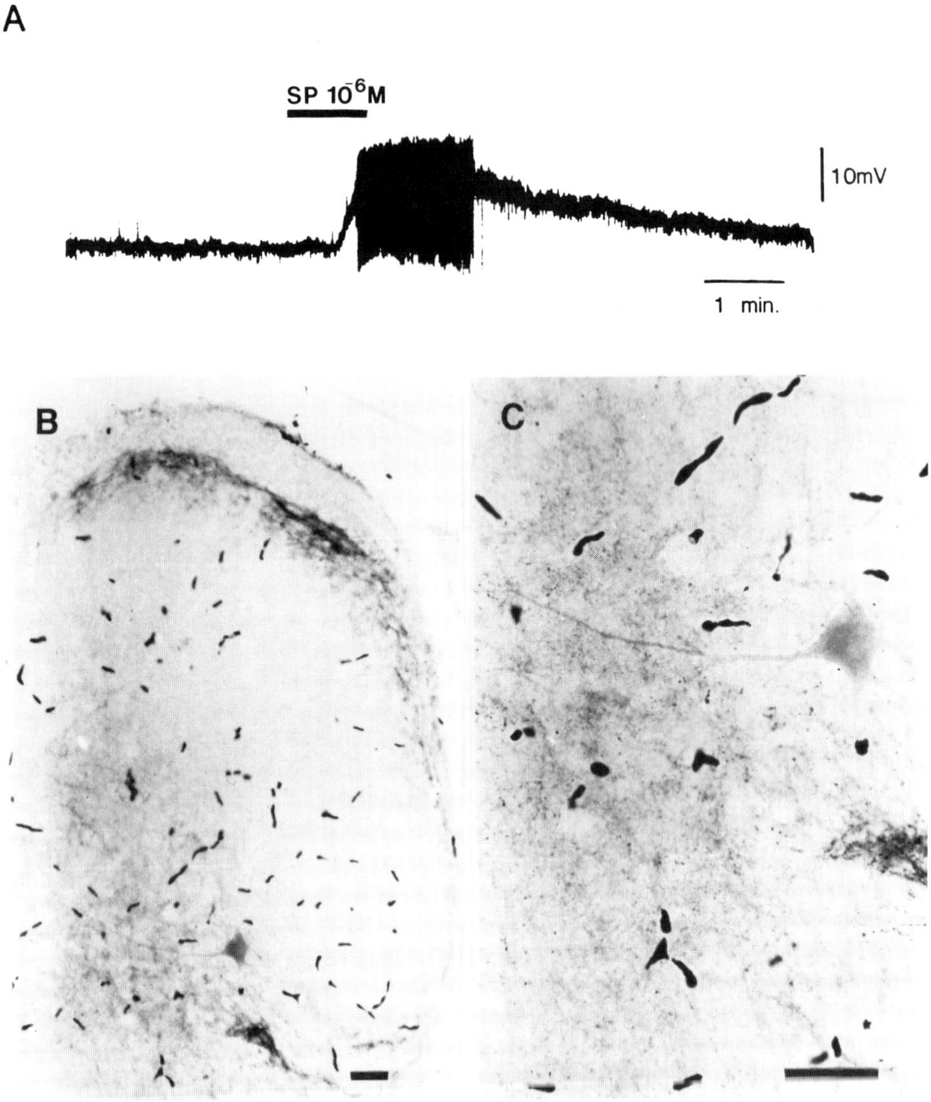

Fig. 1 A-C. SP-induced depolarization **(A)** is present in a horseradish peroxidase-labeled dorsal horn neuron possibly receiving inputs from SP-containing fibers **(B, C)**. Scale bar 50 μm, 14-day-old rat. (Reprinted from Randić and Urban, in press)

Results

Electrophysiological Properties of a Dorsal Root-Evoked Slow Depolarization

We recorded intracellularly from about 200 dorsal horn neurons located in laminae I-V, and in order to initiate responses the lumbar dorsal roots were electrically stimulated. In more than half of the cells examined, repetitive stimulation of the dorsal root (5- to 20-V pulses of 0.2- to 0.5-ms duration applied at 1-20 Hz for 3-5 s) elicited, in addition to the monosynaptic and polysynaptic excitatory synaptic potentials, a slow depolarization which reached a peak in 28 ± 10 s (mean $\pm$ S.D., $n = 46$) and lasted 103 ± 53 s. The mean amplitude of 7 ± 5 mV was recorded at resting membrane potentials between -60 and -75 mV. A low Ca^{2+} (0–0.6 mM), high Mg^{2+} (10–12 mM) solution or tetrodotoxin (10^{-6} M) reversibly abolished the slow depolarization, suggesting the presynaptic origin for this response (Urban and Randić 1984).

Intracellular recordings demonstrated that substance P produces slow depolarization of dorsal horn neurons (Sastry 1979; Zieglgänsberger and Tulloch 1979; Murase et al. 1982; Murase and Randić 1984), the characteristics of the response being in some aspects similar to those of the dorsal root-elicited slow depolarization. Therefore, we have analyzed conductance changes, voltage dependence and effects of SP antagonists and SP antisera on both types of depolarizations. Furthermore, using a combined method of horseradish peroxidase (HRP) staining of dorsal horn neurons and SP immunohistochemistry, we have observed that the cells responding to SP receive inputs from SP-containing fibers (Fig. 1).

Voltage Dependence and Membrane Input Resistance Changes During Dorsal Root-Elicited Slow Depolarization and SP Depolarization

When the membrane potential was manually clamped at the resting level, we found that the neuronal input resistance during the slow depolarization and SP-induced depolarization, as determined from the change in the amplitude of superimposed hyperpolarizing electrotonic potentials, appeared to increase in some cells, but decreased in other cells. The average values of the resistance decrease and increase were 18 % and 7 % respectively. These values were not statistically significant. In a similar fashion to the SP-induced depolarization, a decrease in amplitude of the dorsal root-induced slow depolarizing response could be effected by soma hyperpolarization (Fig. 2), but inversion of the response to a hyperpolarizing one could not be achieved even at a membrane potential of –106 mV. These results suggested that both depolarizations may be due to a decrease in a voltage-dependent G_K (potassium conductance). As shown in Fig. 3, we found that the dorsal root-induced slow depolarization and the SP depolarization were dependent upon extracellular potassium concentration. At higher external K^+ concentration (11.2 mM) both depolarizing responses were reduced.

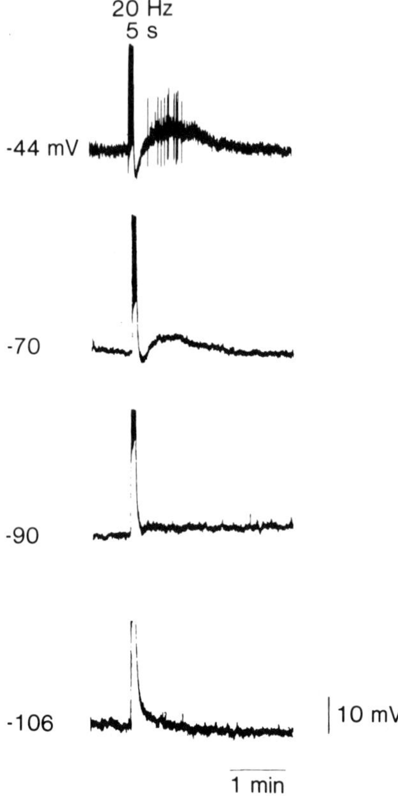

Fig. 2. The effects of soma depolarization and hyperpolarization with a DC current on the amplitude of dorsal root-evoked slow depolarization in a dorsal horn neuron. Soma depolarization from −70 to −44 mV increased the size of the slow depolarization and elicited synaptic and action potentials. Soma hyperpolarization from −70 to −106 mV abolished the slow depolarization. (Reprinted from Urban and Randić 1984)

Effects of Putative SP Antagonists on the Dorsal Root-Induced Slow Depolarization and SP Depolarization

Since synthetic analogues of SP with antagonist properties have recently been developed (Rosell et al. 1983), we examined the possible interaction between the two SP analogues (D-Pro^2, D-Trp^{7,9})-SP and (D-Arg^1, D-Pro^2, D-Trp^{7,9}, Leu^{11})-SP and SP-induced depolarization and dorsal root-elicited slow depolarization of the dorsal horn neurons. We found that bath application of these two SP analogues in concentrations of 1–2 x 10^{-5} M for 2–4 min markedly reduced or abolished both the SP depolarization and the dorsal root-evoked slow depolarization in 70% of examined cells (n = 25). (D-Pro^2, D-Trp^{7,9})-SP exhibited more frequent SP-agonist activity and weaker SP-antagonist properties than (D-Arg^1, D-Pro^2, D-Trp^{7,9}, Leu^{11})-SP. An example of the depressant effect of (D-Arg^1, D-Pro^2, D-Trp^{7,9}, Leu^{11})-SP is illustrated in Fig. 4.

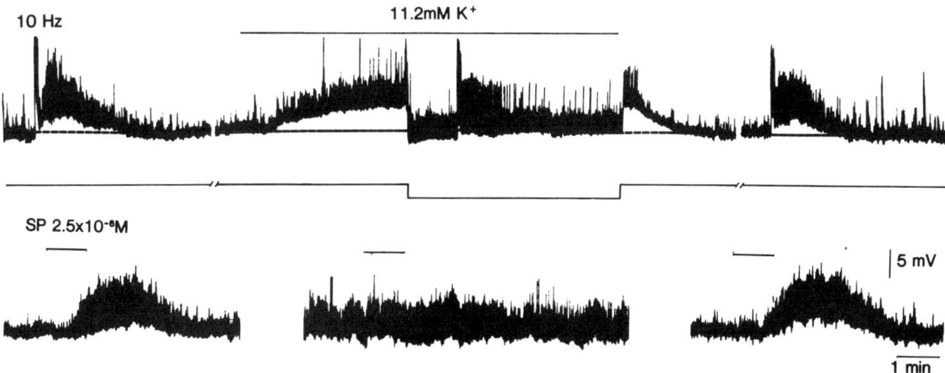

Fig. 3. Dorsal root-evoked slow depolarization and SP depolarization are potassium-dependent. Records from a 13-day-old rat, resting membrane potential = –62 mV. Top record: Dorsal root-elicited slow depolarization before, during, and after perfusion with a high K^+ medium (11.2 mM). At the peak of K^+-induced depolarization membrane potential was restored to the resting level by passage of a hyperpolarizing current (as indicated by the continuous line below the record). There is a clear decrease in the amplitude of slow depolarization. Bottom record: K^+ dependency of the SP depolarization is shown. (Reprinted from Randić and Urban, in press)

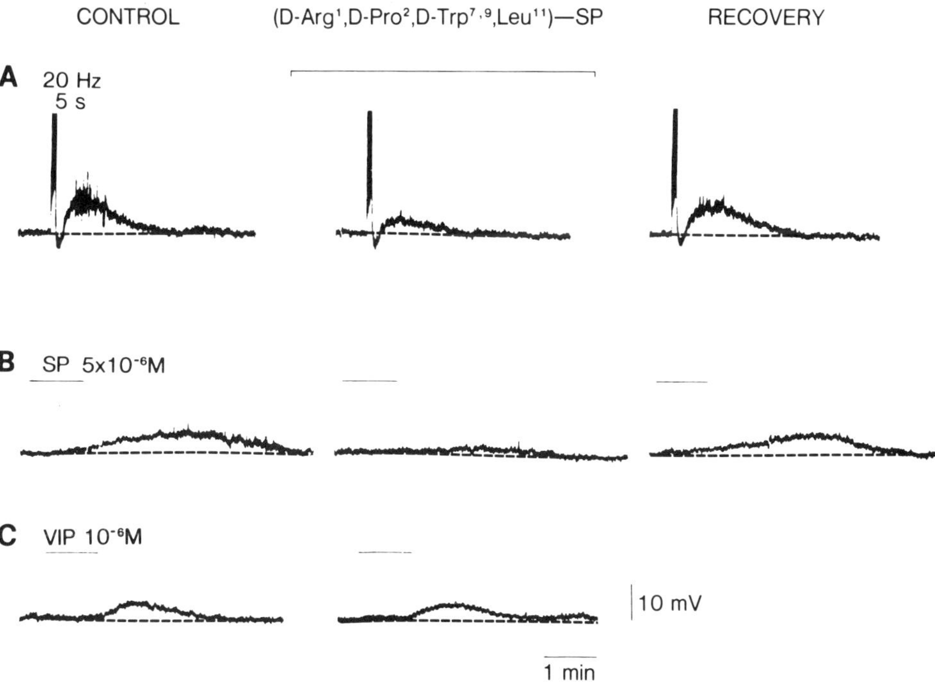

Fig. 4 A-C. Effects of (D-Arg[1], D-Pro[2], D-Trp[7,9], Leu[11])-SP on the responses of a dorsal horn neuron to dorsal root stimulation **(A)**, SP **(B)**, and vasoactive intestinal polypeptide **(C)**. In each record, the left trace represents control response, the middle trace shows response obtained 1 min after stopping the perfusion with (D-Arg[1], D-Pro[2], D-Trp[7,9], Leu[11])-SP, and the right trace represents response obtained 9 min after the removal of the SP antagonist. A 14-day-old rat, resting membrane potential = –64 mV. (Reprinted from Randić and Urban, in press)

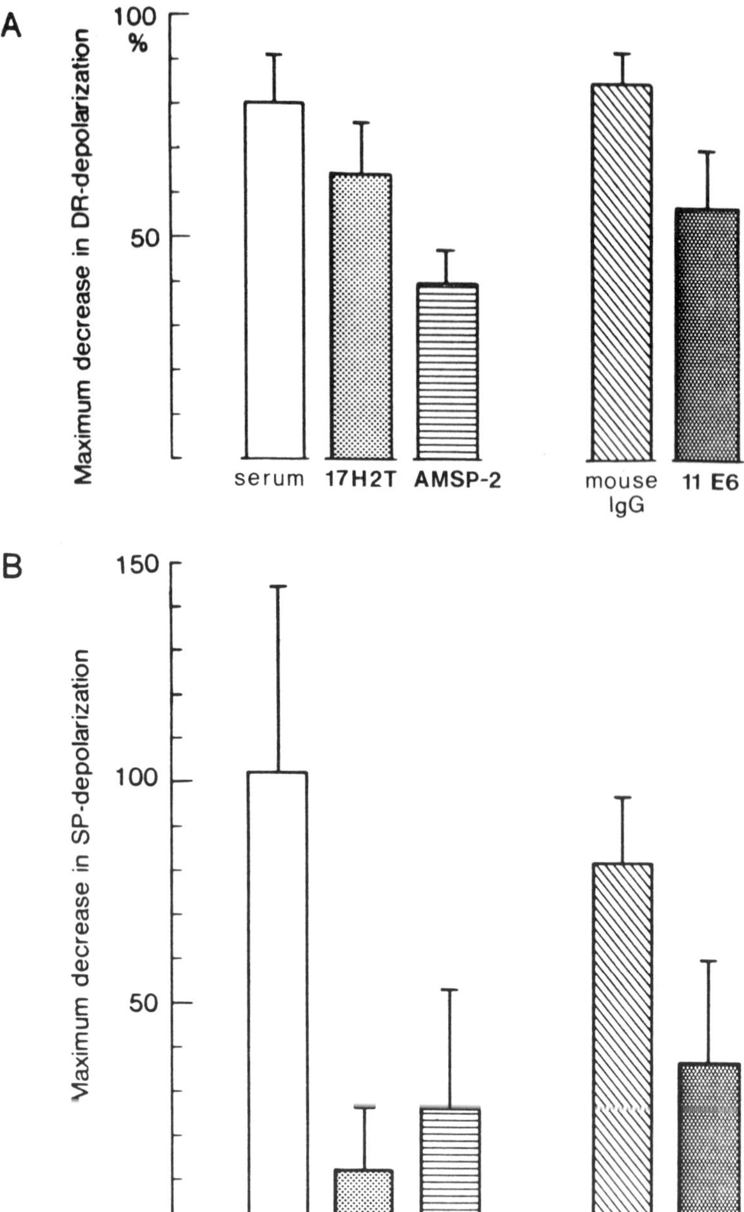

Fig. 5 A, B. Effects of immune and nonimmune sera on the slow depolarization evoked by dorsal root stimulation **(A)** and exogenous SP application **(B).** Note that both polyclonal, antibodies to SP (AMSP-2, n = 4 ⊟; 17H2T, n = 3, ▨) and also the monoclonal antibody to SP (11E6, n = 3, ▩) significantly reduced the dorsal root-elicited slow depolarization, P values being: AMSP-2 <0.005; 17H2T <0.05; 11E6 <0.025. P values for the SP depolarization were: AMSP-2 <0.05; 17H2T <0.05; 11E6 <0.10. Perfusion with normal rabbit serum (□, n = 4) or nonspecific mouse IgG (⧅) resulted in no significant change in the size of the slow depolarization. Histograms show mean values and standard deviations. (Reprinted from Randić et al. 1986)

Effects of SP Antisera on Slow Excitatory Transmission in Spinal Dorsal Horn Neurons

Because of mixed agonist-antagonist properties of the SP analogues, and in an attempt to provide a further support for the neurotransmitter role of SP, the effects of bath perfusion of polyclonal and monoclonal antibodies to SP on slow excitatory transmission in rat dorsal horn neurons have been investigated. As shown in Fig. 5, both polyclonal and monoclonal SP antisera produced a significant decrease in the amplitude and the duration of the slow depolarization generated in dorsal horn neurons by dorsal root stimulation or exogenous SP application. An effect of endogenous SP, or a SP-related peptide, released during dorsal root stimulation appears likely, since bath perfusion of a slice with a normal rabbit serum, affinity chromatography-preadsorbed SP antiserum, polyclonal 5-hydroxytryptamine antiserum, or nonspecific IgG had no similar depressant effect (Fig. 5).

Effects of Chronic Administration of Capsaicin on Slow Excitatory Transmission

Attempts were also made to determine the origin of the fibers generating slow depolarization of dorsal horn neurons during stimulation of dorsal roots by administering capsaicin to neonatal rats. It is known that neonatal capsaicin treatment results in a destruction of small B type sensory ganglion cells (Jancso et al. 1977), significant loss in the number of C fibers and their terminals in the dorsal horn, and depletion of several neuropeptides, including SP, from the small primary sensory neurons and the dorsal horn (Fitzgerald 1983).

As shown in Table 1, about 67 % of dorsal horn neurons in a control group responded with a characteristic slow depolarization to both repetitive stimulation of a dorsal root and administration of SP. The residual 33 % of the cells did not show any sign of the slow excitatory transmission and had no or very low sensitivity to SP. After neonatal capsaicin treatment, the proportion of dorsal horn neurons responding to dorsal root stimulation was very much reduced (17 %). Instead, there appeared to exist a dominant group of cells (83 % of all tested cells) in which a prolonged repetitive stimulation of dorsal roots failed to evoke a slow excitatory transmission, while the fast EPSPs remained unchanged.

Electrophysiological Properties of a Dorsal Root-Evoked Slow Hyperpolarization

High-intensity repetitive stimulation of lumbosacral dorsal roots (10- to 25-V pulses of 0.2- to 0.5-ms duration applied at 10–20 Hz for 2–5 s) elicited a slow hyperpolarizing potential in less than half of the dorsal horn neurons examined in the rat spinal cord slice preparation (Fig. 6). Slow hyperpolarizing potential was reversibly abolished in a low Ca^{2+}, high

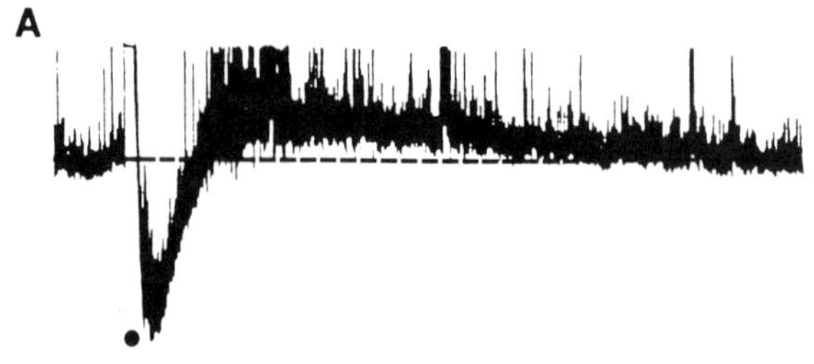

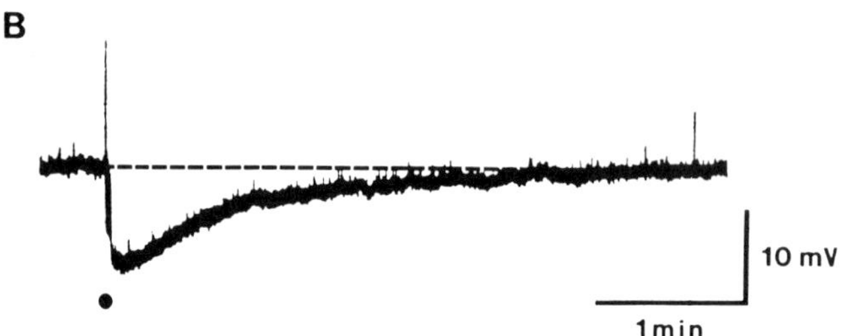

Fig. 6 A, B. High-intensity repetitive stimulation of lumbosacral dorsal roots elicited two types of potential changes in two different neurons. In **A**, the initial orthodromic burst of action potentials (vertical tracings have been truncated) was followed by a hyperpolarization which in turn was followed by a slow depolarization. In **B**, the initial burst was followed by a longer-lasting hyperpolarization. **A** 18-day-old rat, resting membrane potential (Vm) = -64 mV; **B** 23-day-old rat, Vm = -60 mV

Table 1. Effect of neonatal capsaicin treatment of rats on the slow depolarization in the spinal dorsal horn neurons

Treatment	No of cells tested	Slow EPSP present	Slow EPSP absent
Control	9	6 (66.7 %)	3 (33.3 %)
Capsaicin (50 mg/kg s.c. on day 2)	18	3 (17 %)	15 (83.0 %)

Mg^{2+} solution and tetrodotoxin, the result indicating that it is dependent on propagated action potentials and synaptic transmission. Slow hyperpolarization is usually associated with a fall in neuronal membrane resistance; its amplitude decreased with membrane hyperpolarization.

Bath application of enkephalinamides, SS, and NE reversibly hyperpolarized the same neurons having slow hyperpolarizing potentials. Naloxone and yohimbine effectively blocked the enkephalinamide-evoked and NE-evoked hyperpolarizations. However, dorsal root-elicited slow hyperpolarization was only slightly reduced by naloxone and yohimbine. Slow hyperpolarization was enhanced by bicuculline.

Discussion

Experimental evidence supports the concept that SP may function as a neurotransmitter and/or neuromodulator in synaptic transmission between primary afferent fibers and neurons within the spinal cord (Nicoll et al. 1980), although synaptic potentials mediated by the peptide have only recently been demonstrated (Urban and Randić 1983). Immunohistochemical studies have demonstrated the presence of SP within axon terminals of certain small-diameter primary afferent fibers in the superficial laminae of the dorsal horn (Hökfelt et al. 1976; Chan-Palay and Palay 1977; Barber et al. 1979). Upon electrical or chemical stimulation, Ca^{2+}-dependent release of SP from primary afferent fibers has been demonstrated (Otsuka 1978; Yaksh et al. 1980). Electrophysiological data derived largely from extracellular recordings showed that SP-induced excitation of dorsal horn neurons has a slow onset and decay (Henry et al. 1975; Randić and Miletić 1977), and intracellular recordings demonstrated that SP produces slow neuronal depolarization associated with an increase in input resistance (Krnjević 1977, Murase et al. 1982; Murase and Randić 1984) or no change (Sastry 1979; Zieglgänsberger and Tulloch 1979). In addition, by using a single-electrode voltage clamp technique we have recently shown that SP augmented a slow inward calcium-sensitive current and reduced, in a few cells, the M-like current (Murase et al. 1986).

Our findings indicate that the dorsal root-evoked slow depolarization and the SP-induced depolarization are similar in several aspects: (1) both responses cause depolarization and increase excitability of dorsal horn neurons; (2) the sizes of both responses vary in parallel when the membrane potential is shifted over a wide range; (3) both responses are markedly reduced or abolished by an analogue of SP having antagonist properties; and (4) the depression of the dorsal root-elicited slow depolarization during and after the SP-induced depolarization suggests that SP, or SP-like peptide, and the natural transmitter for the dorsal root-elicited slow depolarization bind to the same receptors. On the basis of this parallel behavior of the dorsal root-elicited response and the SP-produced depolarization, we suggested that SP, or SP-like peptide, may be an agonist that mimics in several important aspects the action of the natural transmitter for the slow depolarization potential (Urban and Randić 1984; Randić and Urban, in press).

In an attempt to investigate further the possible functional involvement of SP in a generation of the slow depolarization, both polyclonal and monoclonal antibodies to SP have been used to try to antagonize the effect of dorsal root stimulation and exogenous SP application. The present study indicated that both polyclonal and monoclonal antibodies to SP markedly suppressed the slow depolarizing response of rat dorsal horn neurons to repetitive stimulation of a dorsal root. However, the reduction of a dorsal root-induced slow depolarization observed after perfusion with SP antibodies is not fully understood. Several explanations are possible. That SP antisera acted by depressing the effect of endogenous SP released during dorsal root stimulation seems likely, since: (a) bath perfusion with a normal rabbit serum, affinity chromatography-preadsorbed SP antiserum, nonspecific mouse IgG, or nonimmune ascites fluid had no similar depressant effect; (b) fast monosynaptic and polysynaptic excitatory potentials were not affected by SP antisera; (c) the monoclonal antibody to SP had effects similar to those of the polyclonal SP antisera; and (d) the antisera were relatively specific to SP, as the depolarizing effects of CCK-8 or N-methyl-D-aspartic acid were not significantly affected.

Alternatively, SP may be only one of two or more neuromediators, structurally related or unrelated, that are released during activation of primary afferent fibers. The SP-related peptides neurokinin A and neurokinin B have recently been demonstrated in the mammalian spinal cord (Kangawa et al. 1983; Kimura et al. 1983; Maggio et al. 1983; Nawa et al. 1983). Furthermore, these peptides may be concentrated in the nerve terminals of the superficial laminae of the spinal dorsal horn (Kanazawa et al. 1984). The excitatory action of neurokinins A and B on spinal motoneurons has recently been reported (Matsuto et al. 1984). In addition, the depolarizing action of neurokinins A and B was depressed by the substance P antagonist (D-Arg^{1}, D-Pro^{2}, D-Trp^{7,9}, Leu^{11})-SP.

Much less information is available regarding possible mediators of the slow hyperpolarization. At present we can only suggest that the slow hyperpolarization appears to be a synaptic potential, that it is bicuculline-resistant, and that it is reduced only slightly by naloxone and yohimbine. The unidentified transmitter for this hyperpolarizing potential may act by increasing the potassium permeability of the membrane of dorsal horn neurons.

Acknowledgements. We would like to thank Dr. A. I. Basbaum (University of California, San Francisco) for immunohistochemistry and Dr. T. M. Jessell (Harvard Medical School) for generous donation of SP antisera. This work was supported in part by grants from the National Institute for Neurological and Communicative Disorders and Stroke (NS 17297) (DHHS/NIH No. 2 S07 RR07034-19), the National Science Foundation (BNS 8418042), and the United States Department of Agriculture.

References

Barber RP, Vaughn JE, Slemmon RJ, Salvaterra PM, Roberts E, Leeman SE (1979) The origin, distribution and synaptic relationships of substance P axons in rat spinal cord. J Comp Neurol 184 : 331–352

Chan-Palay V, Palay SL (1977) Ultrastructural identification of substance P cells and their processes in rat sensory ganglia and their terminals in the spinal cord by immunocytochemistry. Proc Natl Acad Sci USA 74 : 4050–4054

Fitzgerald M (1983) Capsaicin and sensory neurones – a review. Pain 15 : 109–130

Henry JL, Krnjević K, Morris ME (1975) Substance P and spinal neurones. Can J Physiol Pharmacol 53 : 423–432

Hökfelt T, Elde R, Johansson O, Luft R, Nilsson G, Arimura A (1976) Immunohistochemical evidence for separate populations of somatostatin-containing and substance P-containing primary afferent neurons in the rat. Neuroscience 1 : 131–136

Jancso G, Kiraly E, Jancso-Gabor A (1977) Pharmacologically induced selective degeneration of chemosensitive primary sensory neurons. Nature 270 : 741–743

JEFTINIJA S, URBAN L, RANDIĆ M (1985) Slow hyperpolarizing potentials in rat spinal dorsal horn neurons. Neurosci Abstr 11 : 1002

KANAZAWA I, OGAWA T, KIMURA S, MUNEKATA E (1984) Regional distribution of substance P, neurokinin α and neurokinin β in rat central nervous system. Neurosci Res 2 : 111–120

KANGAWA K, MINAMINO N, FUKUDA A, MATSUO H (1983) Neuromedin K and B: novel neuropeptides with smooth muscle stimulant activity identified in pig spinal cord. In: MUNEKATA E (ed) Peptide chemistry. Proceedings of the 21st Symposium on Peptide Chemistry. Protein Research Foundation, Osaka, pp 309–314

KIMURA S, OKADA M, SUGITA Y, KANAZAWA I, MUNEKATA E (1983) Novel neuropeptides, neurokinin α and β, isolated from porcine spinal cord. Proc Jpn Acad [B] 59 : 101–104

KRNJEVIĆ K (1977) Effects of substance P on central neurones in cats. In: VON EULER US, PERNOW B (eds) Substance P. Raven, New York, pp 217–230

MAGGIO JE, SANDBERG BEB, BRADLEY CV, IVERSEN LL, SANTIKARN S, WILLIAMS DH, HUNTER JC, HANLEY MR (1983) A novel tachykinin in mammalian spinal cord. Ir J Med Sci [Suppl 1] 152 : 20–21

MATSUTO T, YANAGISAWA M, OTSUKA M, KANAZAWA I, MUNEKATA E (1984) The excitatory action of the newly discovered mammalian tachykinins, neurokinin α and neurokinin β, on neurons of the isolated spinal cord of the newborn rat. Neurosci Res 2 : 105–110

MURASE K, RANDIĆ M (1983) Electrophysiological properties of rat spinal dorsal horn neurones in vitro: calcium-dependent action potentials. J Physiol (Lond) 334 : 141–153

MURASE K, RANDIĆ M (1984) Actions of substance P on rat spinal dorsal horn neurones. J Physiol (Lond) 346 : 203–218

MURASE K, NEDELJKOV V, RANDIĆ M (1982) The actions of neuropeptides on dorsal horn neurons in the rat spinal cord slice preparation: an intracellular study. Brain Res 234 : 170–176

MURASE K, RYU PD, RANDIĆ M (1986) Substance P augments a persistent slow inward calcium-sensitive current in voltage-clamped spinal dorsal horn neurons of the rat. Brain Res 365 : 369–376

NAWA H, HIROSE T, TAKASHIMA H, INAYAMA S, NAKANISHI S (1983) Nucleotide sequences of cloned cDNAs for two types of bovine brain substance P precursor. Nature 306 : 32–36

NICOLL RA, SCHENKER C, LEEMAN SE (1980) Substance P as a transmitter candidate. Annu Rev Neurosci 3 : 227–268

NORTH RA, YOSHIMURA M (1984) The actions of noradrenaline on neurones of the rat substantia gelatinosa in vitro. J Physiol (Lond) 349 : 43–55

OTSUKA M (1978) Substance P as a transmitter of primary sensory neurons. Neurosci Res Prog Bull 16 : 286–293

RANDIĆ M, MILETIĆ V (1977) Effects of substance P in cat dorsal horn neurones activated by noxious stimuli. Brain Res 128 : 164–169

RANDIĆ M, MILETIĆ V (1978) Depressant actions of methionine-enkephalin and somatostatin in cat dorsal horn neurones activated by noxious stimuli. Brain Res 152 : 196–202

RANDIĆ M, URBAN L (in press) Slow excitatory transmission in rat spinal dorsal horn and the effects of capsaicin. Acta Physiol Hung

RANDIĆ M, RYU PD, URBAN L (1986) Effects of polyclonal and monoclonal antibodies to substance P on slow excitatory transmission in rat spinal dorsal horn. Brain Res 383 : 15–27

Rosell S, Bjorkroth U, Xu J-C, Folkers K (1983) The pharmacological profile of a substance P (SP) antagonist. Evidence for the existence of subpopulations of SP receptors. Acta Physiol Scand 117 : 445–449

Sastry BR (1979) Substance P effects on spinal nociceptive neurones. Life Sci 24 : 2169–2178

Urban L, Randić M (1983) Slow excitatory transmission in rat dorsal horn: possible mediation by peptides. Neurosci Abstr 9 : 255

Urban L, Randić M (1984) Slow excitatory transmission in rat dorsal horn: possible mediation by peptides. Brain Res 290 : 336–341

Urban L, Willetts J, Randić M, Papka RE (1985) The acute and chronic effects of capsaicin on slow excitatory transmission in rat dorsal horn. Brain Res 330 : 390–396

Yaksh TL, Jessell TM, Gamse R, Mudge AW, Leeman SE (1980) Intrathecal morphine inhibits substance P release from mammalian spinal cord in vivo. Nature 286 : 155–157

Zieglgänsberger W, Tulloch IF (1979) Effects of substance P on neurones in the dorsal horn of the spinal cord of the cat. Brain Res 166 : 273–282

28 Intracellularly Recorded Responses of Neurones in Lamina II of Cat Spinal Dorsal Horn to Activation of Cutaneous Afferent Inputs

W. M. Steedman and V. Molony

Introduction

The superficial dorsal horn (Rexed's laminae I and II) is the principal area of termination of small myelinated and unmyelinated primary afferent fibres carrying information from cutaneous nociceptors (Réthelyi 1984). Horseradish peroxidase (HRP) labelling of neurones with characterized afferent inputs has demonstrated the existence of a population of cells which are excited by noxious stimulation of the skin in the outer part of lamina II and around its border with lamina I (Light et al. 1979; Bennett et al. 1980; Molony et al. 1981; Réthelyi et al. 1983; Woolf and Fitzgerald 1983). While only a small proportion appear to project to higher levels, many project to adjacent laminae from which arise long ascending tracts.

It is well established that the onward transmission of nociceptive information from the dorsal horn is subject to considerable modulation by inhibitory inputs (Wall 1980; Iggo et al. 1985). The authors' laboratory has described neurones in the outer part of lamina II which are excited by noxious and inhibited by innocuous stimulation of the skin, and has attempted to identify the mechanisms involved. This paper will focus on two particular aspects of the activity evoked by stimulation of primary afferents and recorded intracellularly from neurones in this part of the superficial dorsal horn of the cat lumbar spinal cord – firstly the inhibition evoked by activation of afferent inputs and secondly the excitatory responses to C fibre stimulation.

Inhibitory inputs from cutaneous mechanoreceptors have been reported for many different types of neurone in the dorsal horn that form part of the somatosensory system, and there is evidence for involvement of both presynaptic and postsynaptic mechanisms (Hongo et al. 1968; Calvillo 1978; Hentall and Fields 1979; Fitzgerald and Woolf 1981). Analysis of synaptic potentials has only recently become possible for the small neurones in lamina II because of the technical difficulties of making prolonged intracellular recordings, so that evidence for inhibitory mechanisms is mainly indirect. We have previously reported inhibitory hyperpolarizing potentials evoked in HRP-stained nociceptive neurones in lamina II by natural stimulation of cutaneous receptive fields and by electrical stimulation of peripheral nerves (Steedman et al. 1985). We report here further details of the mechanism of this inhibition.

Extracellular recordings from neurones located in lamina II showed regular, time-locked C-evoked discharges, whereas neurones in laminae IV and V showed irregular responses, strongly suggesting that the C input to lamina II was monosynaptic while that to laminae IV and V was polysynaptic (Fitzgerald and Wall 1980). This has been confirmed by intracellular recording, and we report here further details of the nature of the intracellularly recorded, time-locked responses of neurones in the superficial dorsal horn to C fibre stimulation.

Methods

Experiments were performed on cats anaesthetized with chloralose (60–70 mg. kg^{-1}), ventilated artificially and paralysed with gallamine triethiodide. Single-barrelled glass microelectrodes filled with 3 M KCl or with a solution of HRP were used for intracellular potential recording and for current injection. The location of the neurones within the superficial dorsal horn was determined by injection of HRP either into the neurone being recorded from or into a neurone at approximately the same depth on an adjacent track. Neurones were characterized by their responses to both innocuous and noxious stimulation of the skin. Single shock rectangular pulses were applied to the tibial and peroneal nerves at the ankle, and to the ipsilateral dorsal root from which the compound action potential could also be recorded. Membrane potential was changed by passing steady current through the microelectrode and input resistance was measured by recording the electrotonic responses to injected current pulses.

Results

All neurones included in this study were excited from the skin by noxious stimulation, generally from a small area on one or more toes. Some were nociceptive-specific, but the majority were multireceptive and excited also by innocuous mechanical stimulation. All had inhibitory cutaneous receptive fields which were more extensive and generally adjoined and often overlapped the excitatory field. As previously described (Steedman et al. 1985), excitation was associated with depolarization and firing of action potentials, each of the latter arising from an EPSP, while stimulation of the inhibitory field evoked hyperpolarization. All neurones were located in the outer part of lamina II or in the border zone with lamina I, and stained cells were characteristic of those described from several laboratories – small perikarya (maximum diameter 30 μm) and dendritic trees that arose from a small number of principal dendrites and were narrow mediolaterally but extensive rostrocaudally. Axons could not be followed for long distances but mainly terminated locally within lamina II or projected into adjacent laminae; some could be traced into Lissauer's tract.

Electrical stimulation of peripheral nerves revealed varying patterns of converging inputs carried by Aβ, Aδ and C fibres, but all had excitatory inputs carried by Aδ and /or C fibres. Excitatory responses consisted of action potentials arising singly from EPSPs. These contrasted strongly with the complex, prolonged EPSPs giving rise to multiple action potentials which were recorded from large neurones in deeper laminae.

Hyperpolarizing Responses

Hyperpolarizing responses, 8–13 mV in amplitude and 250–1500 ms in duration, were recorded in all neurones in response to stimulation of peripheral nerves. They were activated at Aβ threshold and evoked by inputs carried by fibres conducting at 45–80 m. s^{-1} along polysynaptic pathways (Steedman et al. 1985). They increased in both amplitude and duration as stimulus intensity was increased up to levels which activated Aδ and C fibres. This is illustrated in Fig. 1, where the duration of the hyperpolarization matches the period of inhibition of ongoing activity and the Aδ and C responses are seen to arise from a hyperpolarized membrane.

Figure 2 shows examples of different combinations of excitatory and inhibitory responses recorded from different neurones. The hyperpolarization was not always associated with Aβ-evoked excitation (Fig. 2A, C), and conversely Aβ-evoked excitation could be recorded in the absence of hyperpolarization (Fig. 2B). Hyperpolarizations could be evoked by stimulation of one (Fig. 2B, C) or both (Fig. 2A) of the peripheral nerves that were used.

The effect of altering the membrane potential was studied in ten neurones which had stable resting potentials of -60 to -75 mV and input resistances of 100–150 MΩ by passing current through a recording microelectrode filled with 3 M KCl. The hyperpolarizing responses to electrical stimulation of peripheral nerves were voltage-dependent, with rever-

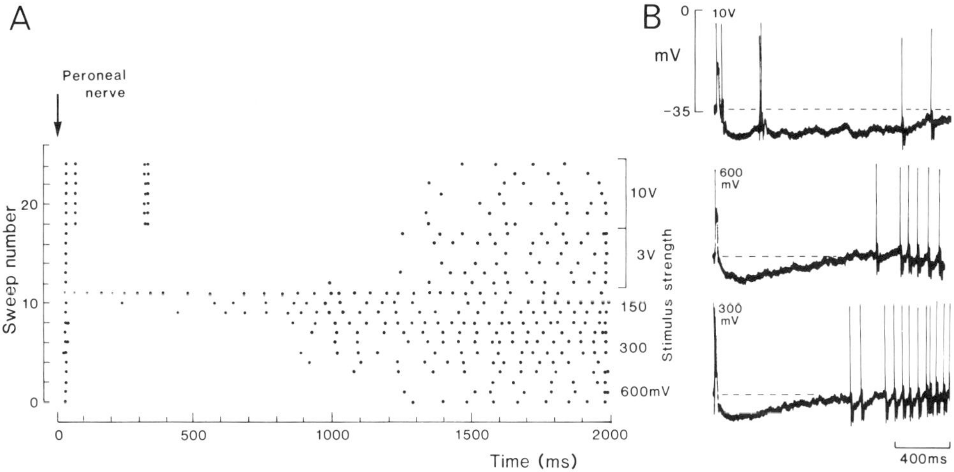

Fig. 1 A–B. The responses of a nociceptive neurone in the superficial dorsal horn to repeated single-pulse stimulation of the peroneal nerve at varying intensities. Stimulus durations were 0.2 ms up to 1V intensity and 1.2 ms at higher intensities. **A** Raster display of post-stimulus inhibition of background activity. Aβ, Aδ and C excitatory inputs could be activated. Inhibition occurred at the same threshold as Aβ excitation; its duration increased with increasing stimulus intensity, up to and above threshold for activating C fibers. **B** Intracellular recordings of responses to stimulation at the intensities indicated, showing the prolonged hyperpolarization which lasted for the same time as the inhibition of background activity. Both Aδ and C excitatory responses arose from a hyperpolarized membrane potential. (From Steedman et al. 1985)

sal potentials that ranged from -85 to -95 mV. We conclude therefore that the inhibition is postsynaptic.

Figure 3 shows the IPSP recorded from a neurone which had a small excitatory receptive field responsive to squeezing the toes in the field of distribution of the tibial nerve, and a more extensive inhibitory receptive field responsive to brushing the skin. The tibial nerve carried Aβ and C excitatory inputs and an inhibitory input activated at Aβ threshold; the peroneal nerve carried inhibitory input only.

When an Aβ excitatory response was present, the after-hyperpolarization of the action potential complicated the picture. This is illustrated in Fig. 4, where the hyperpolarizing response recorded at the resting membrane potential of -75 mV was increased in amplitude by depolarization and abolished and in part reversed by hyperpolarization. It is not known whether further hyperpolarization would have reversed the later part of the response. The

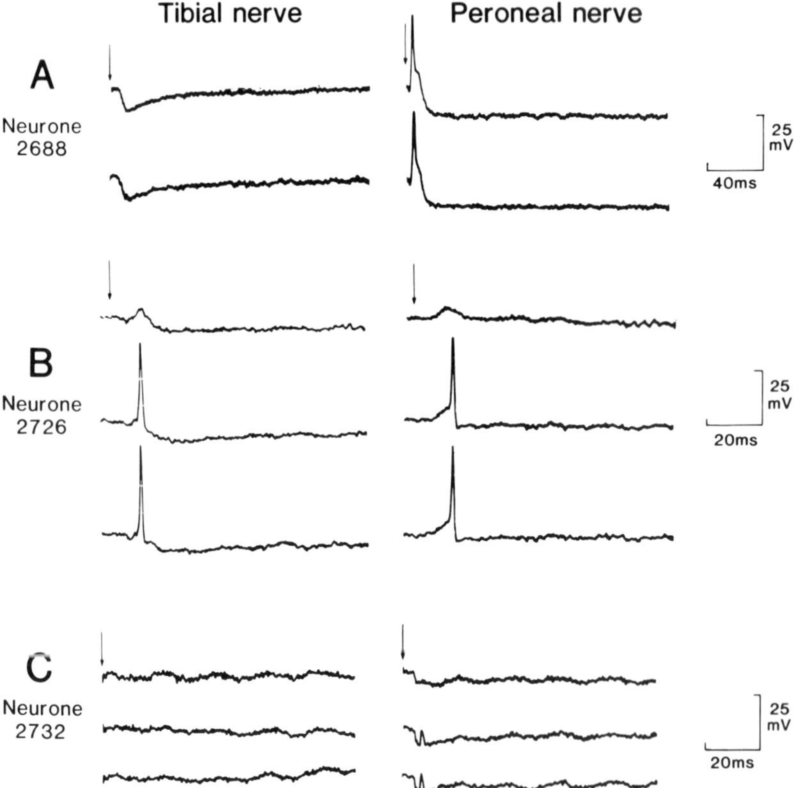

Fig. 2 A–C. Responses of three neurones in the outer part of lamina II to electrical stimulation of peroneal and tibial nerves [pulses of 200 mV (top traces, **B** and **C**) and 600 mV, 0.2 ms]. **A** Neurone 2688 was nociceptive-specific, was inhibited from both nerves and had Aβ and C excitatory inputs in the peroneal nerve. Resting potential was -40 mV. **B** Neurone 2726 was multireceptive, was inhibited from the tibial nerve only and had Aβ excitatory inputs in both nerves and a C input in the tibial nerve. Resting potential was -45 mV. **C** Neurone 2732 did not respond to stimulation of the tibial nerve and was inhibited and had Aδ and C excitatory inputs in the peroneal nerve. Resting potential was -60 mV. All three neurones had inhibitory receptive fields on the skin

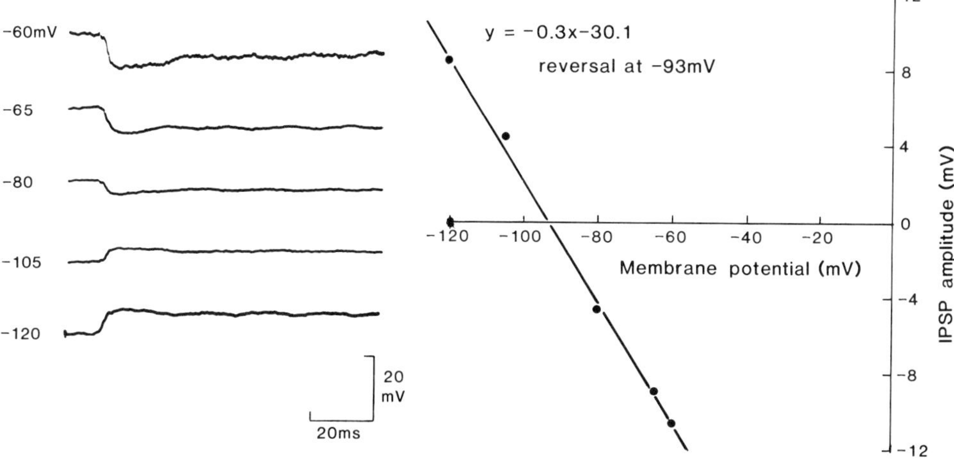

Fig. 3. Intracellular recording of the response of a nociceptive-specific neurone in the outer part of lamina II to single-shock electrical stimulation of the peroneal nerve (pulses of 150 mV, 0.2 ms) at different membrane potentials. Resting potential was -60 mV. The amplitudes of the hyperpolarizations were plotted as a function of the membrane potential

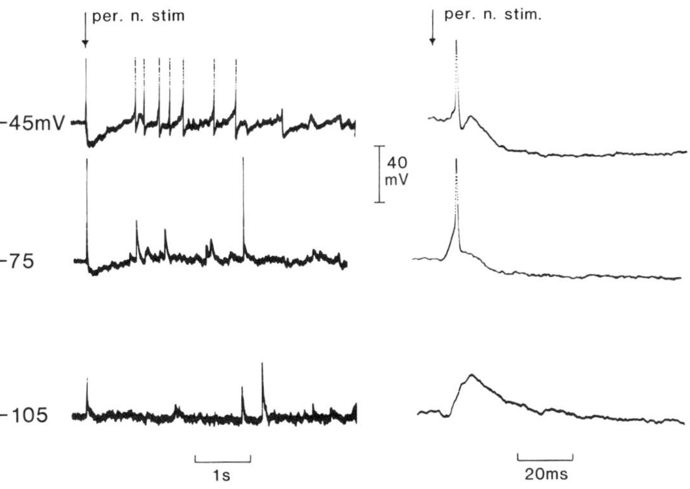

Fig. 4. Intracellular recording of the response of a multireceptive neurone in the outer part of lamina II to a single-pulse stimulation of the peroneal nerve above threshold for activation of C fibres (pulse of 8 V, 1.2 ms). Resting membrane potential was -75 mV and was changed by passage of depolarizing and hyperpolarizing current. The early part of the response is shown on an expanded time-base on the right

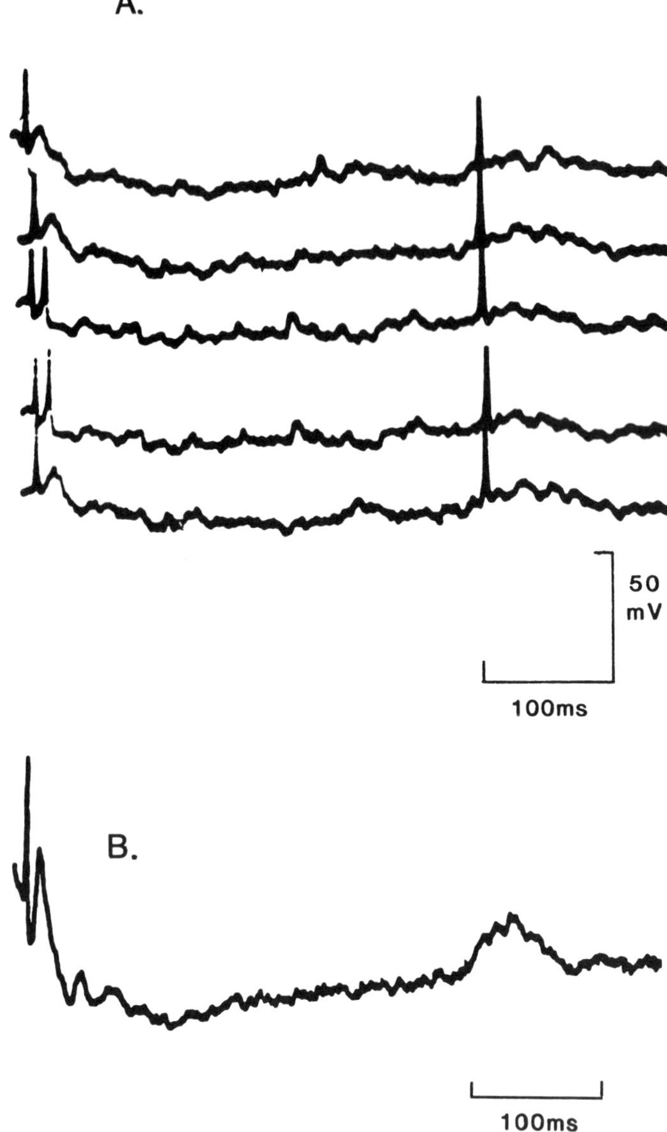

Fig. 5 A. Intracellular recording of the activity evoked in a multireceptive neurone in outer lamina II by repeated single-shock stimulation of the peroneal nerve (pulses of 3 V, 1.2 ms). This neurone could be excited only by squeezing a small receptive field on the fourth toe, but had a more extensive inhibitory field on the third and fourth toes responsive to brushing and squeezing. Resting potential was -70 mV; spikes were attenuated by the recording system. **B** Summed responses ($n = 15$; bin width = 100 μs) to stimuli subthreshold for an action potential

after-hyperpolarization of the action potential was apparently reversed at a lower potential than the IPSP. This does not preclude the possibility that both are caused by similar changes in conductance. Because current is being injected into the soma, the change in potential at the synapses mediating the inhibition, which are likely to be on the dendrites, will be lower than the recorded potential change. The ion channels responsible for the after-hyperpolarization of the action potential are probably closer to the microelectrode and therefore will be more affected by injected current.

Reversal potentials calculated for the ten neurones ranged from -85 to -95 mV. There was no evidence of chloride leakage from the high-resistance microelectrodes - the hyperpolarizing potentials were recorded throughout the entire intracellular recording period (up to 90 min). We conclude therefore that chloride and/or potassium ions are involved.

Excitatory Responses to Activation of C Fibres

In cells in which a constant-latency C fibre response was elicited by electrical stimulation of a peripheral nerve, a stimulus just below threshold for evoking an action potential evoked a compound EPSP lasting up to 100 ms with two or more superimposed short-lived EPSPs each lasting 10–15 ms. As the stimulus strength was raised the amplitude and duration of the compound EPSP increased, and a single, regularly occurring, time-locked action potential arose from one of the short-lasting EPSPs (Fig. 5). The intracellular recordings show a single, time-locked action potential arising regularly in response to each stimulus (Fig. 5A). Figure 5B shows the summed EPSP collected for 15 responses to stimuli subthreshold for an action potential. Further increase in stimulus strength evoked more action potentials, each arising from a single distinct wave in the EPSP. These short-lived and regular responses contrasted sharply with the prolonged series of EPSPs on which were superimposed multiple action potentials that were recorded from a multireceptive neurone in lamina IV (Fig. 6).

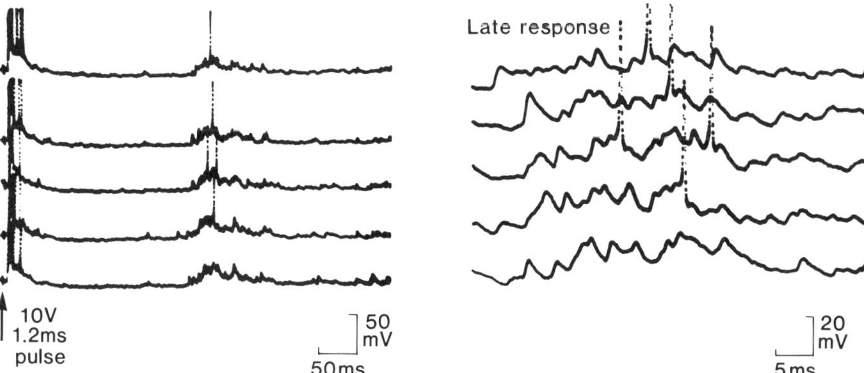

Fig. 6. Intracellular recording of the activity evoked in a multireceptive neurone in lamina IV by repeated single-shock electrical stimulation of the peroneal nerve. The late C fibre response is shown on an expanded time-base on the right. Resting potential was -70 mV. (From Steedman et al. 1985)

Conclusions

To summarize, hyperpolarizing responses were: (1) Recorded from both multireceptive and nociceptive-specific neurones and also from neurones with converging inputs carried by different fibre groups. (2) Distinct from the after-hyperpolarization of the action potential. (3) Evoked at Aβ threshold but increased in amplitude and duration with increasing stimulus intensity up to C levels. (4) Voltage-dependent, reversing (at least in part) at −85 to −95 mV.

We conclude that there is a pathway by which afferent input from the skin can inhibit postsynaptically nocireceptive neurones in the superficial dorsal horn, probably by increasing the conductance to potassium and/or chloride ions. This would reduce the effectiveness of the excitatory input by moving the membrane away from firing threshold and by lowering the membrane resistance. There is evidence that hyperpolarizations induced in neurones in lamina II in spinal cord slices result from increased potassium conductance (North and Yoshimura 1984).

Similar hyperpolarizations have been recorded from neurones in lamina II in response to stimulation of various areas of the brain stem (Light et al. 1986; Mokha, personal communication). Light et al. (1986) showed that these were voltage-dependent, associated with a small conductance increase, and reversed with a moderate amount of hyperpolarizing current. It is perhaps reasonable to suggest that these descending pathways and the pathways from cutaneous afferents involve a common interneurone or transmitter.

Réthelyi (1984) has described elaborate patterns of arborization of C fibres in the outer part of lamina II, each in an area narrow mediolaterally and extensive rostrocaudally with clusters of terminals in a position to provide multiple inputs to one neurone. Neurones stained in the outer part of lamina II have similar dendritic tree orientations. We would therefore suggest, on the basis of the ultrastructural evidence together with the physiological evidence we have presented, that the C fibre input to these cells has two components: 1. Weak inputs from a number of C fibres. These result in a compound EPSP which increases in amplitude and duration as more fibres with different conduction velocities are activated and therefore depolarizes the neurone closer to firing threshold. 2. Strong inputs from a small number of C fibres each with multiple endings on the neurone. Spatial summation results in the discrete EPSPs from which the action potentials arise, these being superimposed on the compound EPSP described above.

The effectiveness of these noxious excitatory inputs is dependent on the level of membrane potential of the neurone and therefore on the extent of concurrent activation of a cutaneous inhibitory receptive field which hyperpolarizes the membrane away from its firing threshold. Peripheral afferents thus interact within the superficial dorsal horn and modulate transmission of nociceptive information to other parts of the nervous system.

Acknowledgements. This work was supported by a Wellcome Trust grant to A. Iggo and W. M. Steedman. Thanks are due to Heather Hunter, Aileen Leask, John Greenhorn, Colin Warwick and Anne Stirling-Whyte for assistance. Animals were held in the Wellcome Animal Research Unit of the Faculty of Veterinary Medicine.

References

Bennett GJ, Abdelmoumene M, Hayashi H, Dubner R (1980) Physiology and morphology of substantia gelatinosa neurons intracellularly stained with horseradish peroxidase. J Comp Neurol 194 : 809–827

Calvillo O (1978) Primary afferent depolarization of C fibers in the spinal cord of the cat. Can J Physiol Pharmacol 56 : 154–157

Fitzgerald M, Wall PD (1980) The laminar organization of dorsal horn cells responding to peripheral C fiber stimulation. Exp Brain Res 41 : 36–44

Fitzgerald M, Woolf CJ (1981) Effects of cutaneous nerve and intraspinal conditioning on C fiber afferent terminal excitability in decerebrate spinal rats. J Physiol (Lond) 318 : 25–39

Hentall ID, Fields HL (1979) Segmental and descending influences on intraspinal thresholds of single C fibers. J Neurophysiol 42 : 1527–1537

Hongo T, Jankowska E, Lundberg A (1968) Post-synaptic excitation and inhibition from primary afferents in neurones of the spinocervical tract. J Physiol (Lond) 199 : 569–592

Iggo A, Steedman WM, Fleetwood-Walker S (1985) Spinal processing: anatomy and physiology of spinal nociceptive mechanisms. Philos Trans R Soc Lond [Biol] 308 : 235–252

Light AR, Casale EJ, Menétrey DM (1986) The effects of focal stimulation in nucleus raphe magnus and periaqueductal gray on intracellularly recorded neurons in spinal laminae I and II. J Neurophysiol, 56 : 555–571

Light AR, Trevino DL, Perl ER (1979) Morphological features of functionally defined neurons in the marginal zone and substantia gelatinosa of the spinal dorsal horn. J Comp Neurol 186 : 151–172

Molony V, Steedman WM, Cervero F, Iggo A (1981) Intracellular marking of identified neurones in the superficial dorsal horn of the cat spinal cord. QJ Exp Physiol 66 : 211–223

North RA, Yoshimura M (1984) The actions of noradrenaline on neurones of the rat substantia gelatinosa in vitro. J Physiol (Lond) 349 : 43–55

Réthelyi M (1984) Synaptic connectivity in the spinal dorsal horn. In: Davidoff RA (ed) Handbook of the spinal cord, vols 2 and 3. Dekker, New York, pp 137–177

Réthelyi M, Light AR, Perl ER (1983) Synapses made by nociceptive laminae I and II neurons. In: Bonica JJ, et al. (eds) Advances in pain research and therapy. Raven, New York, pp 111–118

Steedman WM, Molony V, Iggo A (1985) Nociceptive neurones in the superficial dorsal horn of cat lumbar spinal cord and their primary afferent inputs. Exp Brain Res 58 : 171–182

Wall PD (1980) The role of substantia gelatinosa as a gate control. In: Bonica JJ (ed) Pain. Raven, New York, pp 205–231

Woolf CJ, Fitzgerald M (1983) The properties of neurones recorded in the superficial dorsal horn of the rat spinal cord. J Comp Neurol 221 : 313–328

29 Afferent C Fibre Function in the Dorsal Horn: Brief and Prolonged Excitation

C. J. Woolf

Unmyelinated primary afferent C fibres resemble myelinated sensory afferent A fibres in possessing peripheral receptive fields within which an adequate stimulus produces a graded depolarization of the peripheral afferent terminal. The depolarization in both types of afferent is transformed into action potentials such that the interspike interval encodes the amplitude of the stimulus. The major physiological features which differentiate C fibres from A fibres are that (1) their conduction velocity is lower, (2) the majority of C fibres require intense peripheral stimuli to be activated and (3) they can be activated by mechanical, chemical and thermal stimuli either uni- or polymodally. A consequence of the properties of their peripheral terminals is that afferent C fibres register the onset, location and duration of potentially damaging stimuli to superficial and deep tissue (Lynn and Carpenter 1982; Mense and Meyer 1985).

C fibres terminate in the superficial laminae of the dorsal horn of the spinal cord in a highly somatotopically ordered way. The C fibre terminals from an area of skin innervated by a cutaneous nerve lie contiguous to the C fibre terminals innervating the adjacent skin (Swett and Woolf 1985) and in this way the high-threshold body surface is represented two-dimensionally in the horizontal plane of lamina II. The spatial architecture of the central terminals of primary afferents provides a framework for the generation of the somatotopically organized receptive fields of second-order dorsal horn neurones whose dendrites make synaptic contacts with the afferent terminals (Woolf and Fitzgerald 1986). It is rare, however, for neurones to be mono- or polysynaptically activated exclusively by afferent C fibres (Light et al. 1979; Bennett et al. 1980; Woolf and Fitzgerald 1983), the commonest pattern is a convergence of A and C fibre input. There are two ways of unravelling which component of a peripheral-stimulus-evoked discharge in a dorsal horn neurone is due to C fibre input and which to A fibres. The first is to use natural stimuli that predominantly or exclusively activate only one type of afferent, and the second is to use electrical stimuli that successively activate Aβ, Aδ and C afferents in a peripheral nerve.

As a result of studies from a large number of laboratories using extra- and intracellular recordings in rats, cats and primates, it is clear that both A and C primary afferent fibres evoke fast (10–20 ms duration) depolarizations in dorsal horn neurones. Figure 1 illustrates examples of the activity evoked in a dorsal horn neurone in the rat lumbar spinal cord by brushing the skin (which activates myelinated hair follicle afferent fibres), by pinching the skin (which stimulates low- and high-threshold myelinated afferents and high-mechano-threshold C afferents) and by heating the skin (which almost exclusively activates C fibres). Short-duration ($<$ 20 ms) excitatory post-synaptic potentials reflect, with a temporal spread for A and C fibres, the peripheral activation of primary afferents and in this way provide the central nervous system with a "picture" of the inputs currently impinging upon the periphery. The purpose of this paper is to present evidence that C fibres, in addition to this classical role, have at least one other major function whereby they modulate, over periods of seconds and minutes, the excitability of dorsal horn neurones. The importance of this second function of C fibres is that it may be responsible for some of the major sensory disorders that follow peripheral tissue injury.

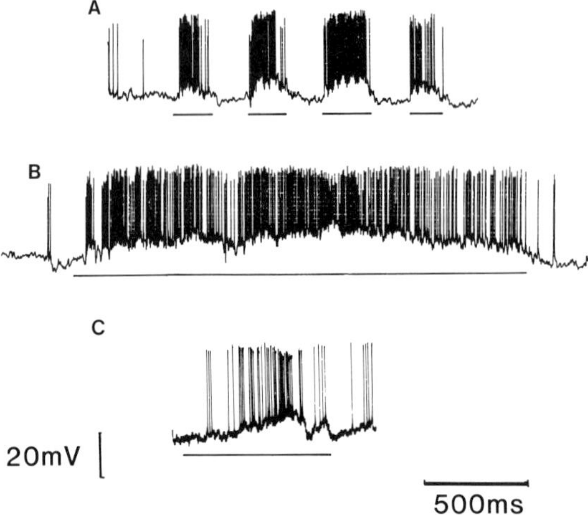

Fig. 1 A–C. Intracellular recordings from a dorsal horn neurone in lamina V of the rat lumbar spinal cord. **A** The response to repeated brushing of the cells cutaneous receptive field. **B** The effect of a sustained pinch to the receptive field. **C** The effect of briefly heating the skin to 50 °C. The solid lines indicate the duration of the cutaneous stimuli

Alterations in the Function of the Spinal Cord Evoked by Peripheral Injury

Acute or chronic peripheral inflammatory lesions produce marked alterations in the flexion reflex in decerebrate rats. The threshold for initiating this withdrawal reflex by stimulating the skin falls and its responsiveness increases. Essentially, the peripheral injury transforms the high-threshold phasic flexion reflex into a low-threshold tonic reflex (Woolf, 1983b, 1984; Woolf and McMahon 1985). An electrophysiological study of the cutaneous receptive fields of flexor alpha-motoneurones in decerebrate-spinal rats has shown that the injury-induced expansion of their receptive fields is not immediately reversed by a sensory block at the site of the injury with local anaesthesia (Woolf 1983b). Somehow the afferent barrage generated by the tissue-damaging stimulus has triggered a change within the spinal cord that is not dependent upon an ongoing afferent input. A major point of this finding is that in addition to the sensitization of high-threshold receptors that peripheral injury may produce (Meyer et al. 1985), the injury also produces a change centrally, within the spinal cord.

C-Fibre-Induced Excitability Changes in the Spinal Cord

We have shown in decerebrate-spinal rats that it is possible to mimic the effects of peripheral injury by a brief (20 s) conditioning stimulus to peripheral nerves, but only provided the strength of the stimulus is sufficient to activate C fibres (Wall and Woolf 1984). Stimulation of the sural nerve (a cutaneous nerve) for 20 s at 1 Hz produces up to a 10-min increase in the excitability of the flexion reflex elicited by a standard pinch to the toes, while stimulation of the gastrocnemius-soleus nerve produces a facilitation of the reflex that persists for up to 90 min (Fig. 2A). Pretreating the conditioning nerves proximal to the site of stimulation with the C fibre neurotoxin capsaicin completely blocks the excitability increase (Woolf and Wall 1986a) and uncovers an A fibre afferent-mediated inhibition (Fig. 2B).

Mustard oil, a chemical irritant that produces an intense burning sensation when applied to the skin in man, has been found by a single unit analysis of cutaneous afferent fibres to excite only the slowly conducting C fibres (Woolf and Wall 1986a). The application of mustard oil to a small patch of skin on the rat hindlimb produces a very marked and prolonged increase in the excitability of the flexion reflex (Fig. 2C). The duration of this facilitation outlasts the firing in the chemosensitive afferents by a factor of at least 10.

The intra-articular injection of a small volume of mustard oil also produces a very prolonged facilitation of the flexion reflex (Fig. 3A) (Woolf and Wall 1986a). When this injection is followed by an intra articular injection of lignocaine it fails to suppress the facilitation (Fig. 3B), even though this injection of the local anaesthetic is sufficient to prevent the facilitation if it precedes the injection of the mustard oil (Fig. 3C). These findings reinforce the idea that the activation of afferent C fibres produces a marked alteration in the excitability of the spinal cord and that once the process has been initiated it does not require a continuing afferent input. One implication of this is that any peripheral stimulus of sufficient strength to activate afferent C fibres will produce a change in the way the spinal cord responds to subsequent inputs for long periods after cessation of the original stimulus. The duration of such changes appears, moreover, to depend upon the tissue innervated by the C fibres, since the unmyelinated afferents in muscle or joint nerves produce more prolonged facilitations than cutaneous C fibres (Woolf and Wall 1986a). These differences may reflect the different chemical constituents present within the primary afferents (McMahon et al. 1984).

The Location of C-Fibre-Induced Prolonged Excitations

Conditioning stimuli to the sural and to the gastrocnemius-soleus nerve identical to those that produce prolonged facilitations of the flexion reflex do not alter the amplitude of the Ia monosynaptic reflex in the flexor alpha-motoneurones, nor do they alter the central terminal excitability of the cutaneous afferent fibres that initiate the reflex (Cook et al.

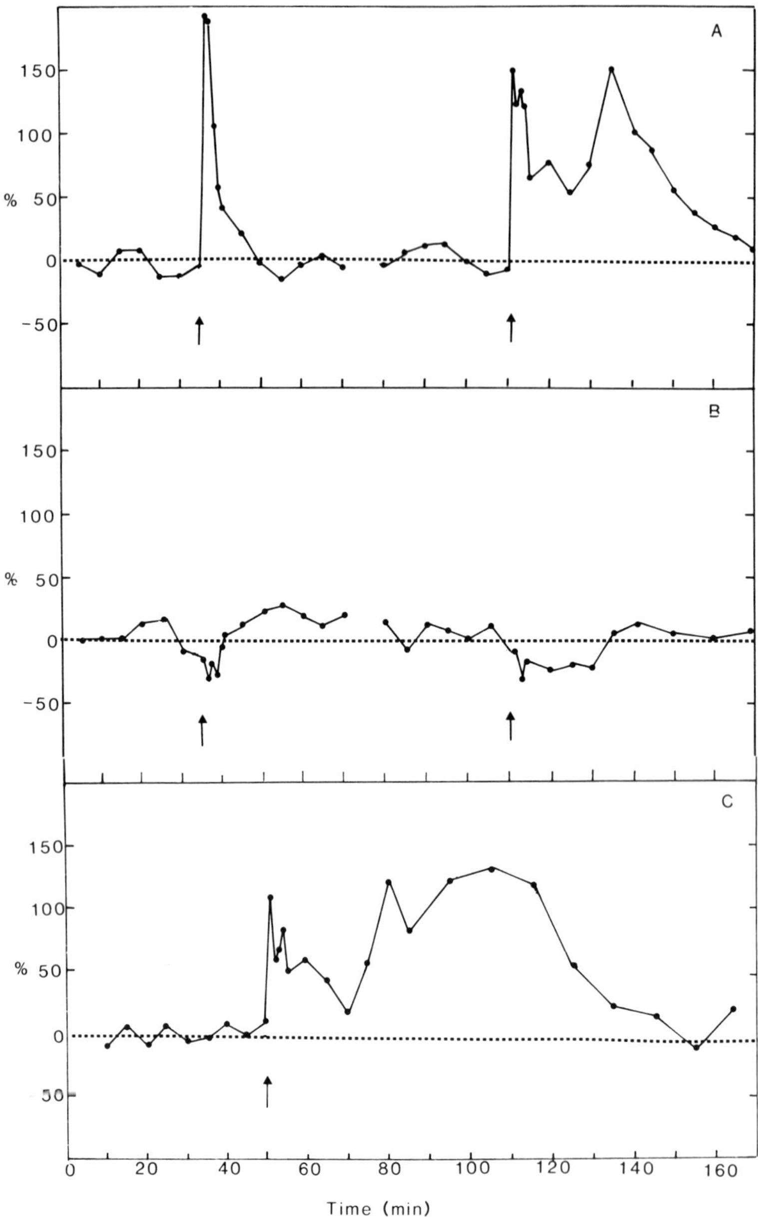

Fig. 2 A–C. Changes in the excitability of the flexion reflex provoked by peripheral conditioning stimuli in the decerebrate-spinal rat. The excitability of the reflex is expressed as the percentage deviation from the preconditioning baseline. At each point a standard mechanical stimulus (150 g) was applied to the middle three toes for 3 s and the total number of spikes evoked in a flexor alpha-motoneurone counted. **A** C-fibre-strength conditioning stimuli (1 Hz, 20 s) were applied to the sural nerve (left trace) and to the gastrocnemius-soleus nerve (right trace) at the times indicated by the arrows. **B** The effect of pretreating the nerve 14 days earlier with capsaicin. **C** The increased excitability of the flexion reflex resulting from the application of 100 μl mustard oil to the skin on the dorsal surface of the hindpaw. (Adapted with permission from Woolf and Wall 1986a)

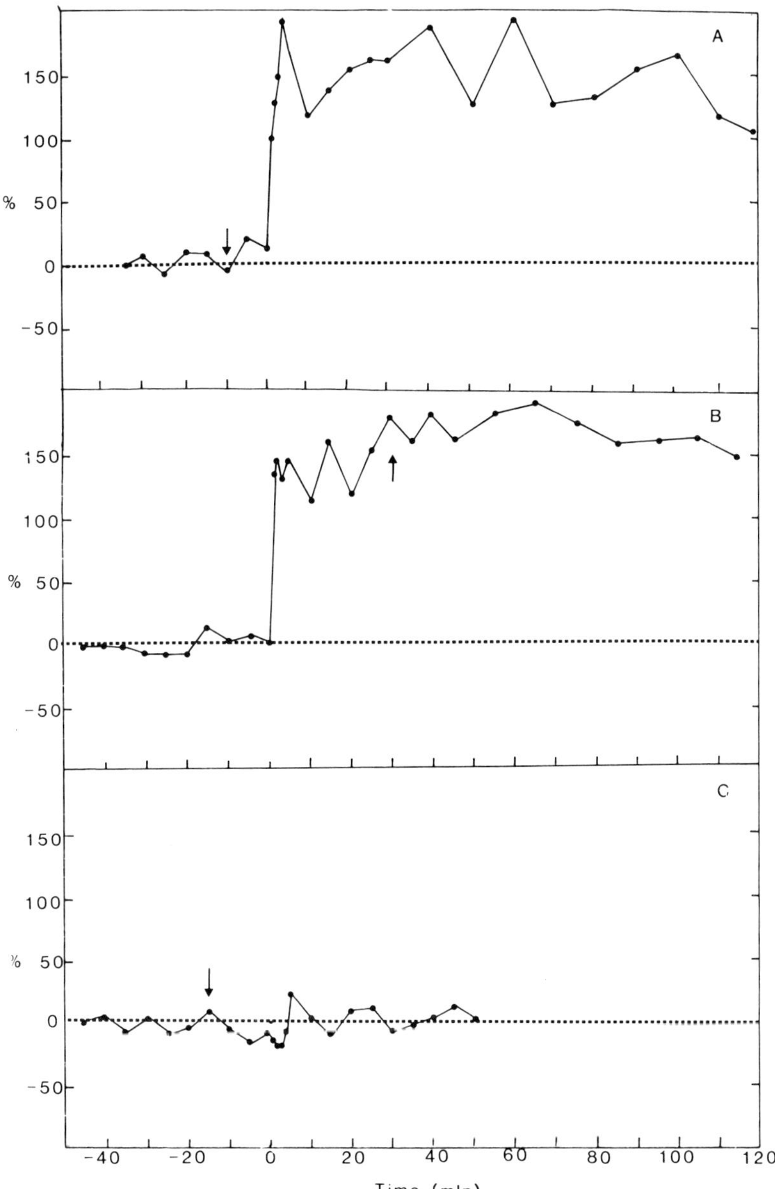

Fig. 3 A–C. The effect of intra articular (knee joint) injections of mustard oil on the excitability of the flexion reflex. **A** At the time indicated by the arrow 1 μl saline was injected which had no effect; at time 0 10 minutes after the saline injection a similar volume of mustard oil was injected, producing a marked and sustained increase in the reflex. **B** Following the injection of mustard oil at time 0, 1 μl 5% lignocaine was injected (arrow) but failed to alter the reflex facilitation. If the injection of the local anaesthetic preceded the mustard oil injection, (as in **C**), the facilitation did not occur. (Reproduced with permission from Woolf and Wall 1986a)

1986). It is therefore unlikely that the modifiability of the flexion reflex is the consequence of a change either in the amount of transmitter released by the test afferent input or in the excitability of the motoneuronal membrane. The change must be occurring somewhere in the chain of interneurones that transfer high-threshold cutaneous inputs to the flexor motoneurones (Cook and Woolf 1985).

To examine this we have looked at the effect of a standard C-fibre-strength conditioning stimulus (1 Hz for 20 s) to the gastrocnemius-soleus nerve on the receptive field properties of dorsal horn neurones (Cook et al. 1987). Three categories of neurones were examined: those cells with somata in lamina I that could be antidromically activated by stimulating the contralateral dorsolateral funiculus (McMahon and Wall 1983), those with axons lying in the contralateral ventrolateral quadrant (which are likely to be spinothalamic and spinoreticular cells) and those that could not be antidromically activated. Stimulation of the gastrocnemius-soleus nerve at C but not A fibre strength produced an expansion in the receptive fields in 85 % of the cells tested (Fig. 4). The peak of the expansion occurred at 17 min after the conditioning volley with a return to baseline at 49 min.

In addition to an alteration in the size of the receptive fields, the responsiveness of the receptive field was also altered in 35 % of the neurones. This included the appearance of low threshold inputs in three of ten cells that formerly only responded to intense peripheral stimuli (i.e. nociceptive specific cells can become wide dynamic range cells). These results show that some C fibre inputs can induce a modification of the cutaneous receptive fields of

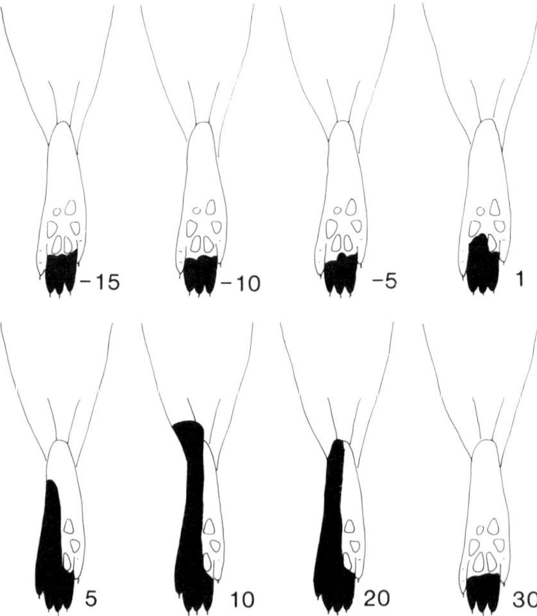

Fig. 4. Changes in the cutaneous receptive field of a lamina I neurone with an axon in the contralateral dorsolateral funiculus produced by a C-fibre-strength conditioning stimulus to the gastrocnemius-soleus nerve (1 Hz, 20 s). The numbers refer to the time in minutes relative to the conditioning stimulus. The size of the receptive field was stable prior to the conditioning stimulus, but increased substantially in size for 20 min following the C fibre input

dorsal horn neurones that outlasts the conditioning input for tens of minutes. Some of these changes may underly the alterations observed in the flexion reflex, but the fact that the C fibre conditioning stimuli also altered dorsal horn neurones with axons projecting to the brain indicates that these C-fibre-induced changes may also modify sensation.

Fast and Slow C-Fibre-Evoked Excitations

The fast monosynaptic excitatory post-synaptic potentials (EPSPs) produced by C fibres in dorsal horn neurones must be the result of the release of a fast transmitter from the C fibre terminals. The best-studied prototypes of fast transmitters within the central nervous system are the excitatory amino acids. There is a growing body of evidence pointing to a role for these putative transmitters in small-diameter afferents. For example, glutamate-binding sites are concentrated in lamina II (Monaghan and Cotman 1985) and kynurenic acid, an amino acid antagonist, blocks C-fibre-evoked activity in dorsal horn neurones in vitro (Schneider and Perl 1985).

If the excitatory amino acids glutamate and aspartate, or similar compounds, mediate fast C-fibre-evoked EPSPs, what may be responsible for the long-lasting C-fibre-mediated facilitations? Good candidates for such a role are the neuropeptides contained within C afferents, which characteristically have a slow onset and prolonged action (Urban and Randić 1984). When the neuropeptides in the central terminals of C fibres are depleted by peripheral nerve section, the afferents maintain their ability to activate spinal cord neurones directly but lose the capacity to produce prolonged facilitations (Wall and Woolf 1986). Intrathecal injections of substance P and calcitonin-gene-related peptide produce a prolonged synergistic increase in the excitability of the flexion reflex similar to that produced by C fibre conditioning stimuli (Woolf and Wiesenfeld-Hallin 1986). A particularly interesting finding is that low doses of systemic morphine that do not modify C-fibre-evoked discharges in flexor motoneurones can prevent the prolonged C-fibre-induced facilitations of the flexion reflex (Woolf and Wall 1986b). Morphine may therefore have two actions. At low doses it may block the prolonged C-fibre-induced facilitations, possibly by preventing the release of neuropeptides while at high doses it may block, presumably postsynaptically, the fast C-fibre-evoked EPSPs. The former action could then be responsible for the analgesic effects of morphine, while the latter could be an example of its antinociceptive effect.

Intracellular Recordings of C-Fibre-Evoked Activity in the Rat Dorsal Horn

In order to examine the cellular mechanisms of C-fibre-evoked changes on dorsal horn neurones we have begun an analysis of C-fibre-induced fast depolarizations (10–20 ms) and of slower changes (1 s to several minutes) using intracellular recordings from deep dorsal horn neurones in vivo (King et al. 1986). In the decerebrate-spinal rat preparation, we studied ten wide-dynamic-range neurones (e.g. Fig. 1) with a long-latency depolarization only evoked when the sciatic nerve was stimulated at a strength sufficient to activate unmyelinated afferents (>2 mA at 500 μs) (Fig. 5). After completion of the electrophysiological analysis the neurones were ionophorised with horseradish peroxidase and their location and morphology established (Fig. 5).

Single electrical stimuli to the sciatic nerve at C fibre strength characteristically produced in these neurones a short-latency depolarization, due to A fibre input, followed by a second delayed depolarization representing the summed effects of many C fibre inputs. Repeated stimulation of the sciatic nerve at 1 Hz resulted in substantial changes in the responses of eight of the ten neurones. With each successive stimulus, the late depolarization evoked by

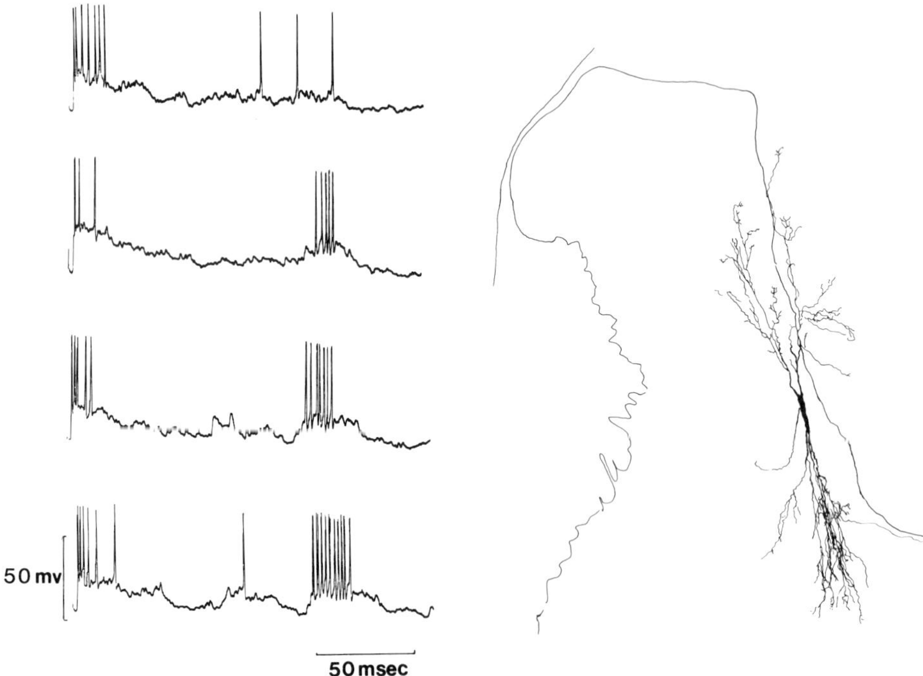

Fig. 5. Intracellular recordings from a neurone in the deep dorsal horn illustrating from top to bottom the effect of four repetitive stimuli to the sciatic nerve at C fibre strength at 1 Hz. Note the "wind up" of the late evoked response and the associated prolonged depolarization. The camera lucida reconstruction illustrates the location and appearance of the neurone

the C fibre input increased substantially in amplitude and duration. In some neurones this resulted in a progressive increment in the number of action potentials evoked by the standard stimulus (Fig. 5), a phenomenon first observed with extracellular studies in the cat by Mendell in 1966 and termed by him "wind up". In other neurones the depolarization produced by the repeated C fibre strength was sufficiently great (>20 mV) to produce attenuation or complete block of the action potentials. This may explain the progressive response decrement seen in some neurones using extracellular recordings (Woolf 1983a). These results show that when C fibres are repeatedly stimulated, the relationship between stimulus and response is not fixed because of the long-lasting effects (of at least 1 s) produced by each stimulus. After a brief (10-s) train of C-fibre-strength stimuli the membrane potential in several neurones remained depolarized for tens of seconds in a manner similar to the depolarization observed by stimulation of the dorsal root in the in vitro rat spinal cord slice preparations (Urban and Randić 1984). Such long-lasting (several minutes) postsynaptic depolarizations produced by C fibre inputs could produce an expansion and alteration in the receptive fields of dorsal horn neurones by recruiting subthreshold inputs from the subliminal fringe of the neurones to a level where they begin to evoke action potentials. The actual mechanisms responsible for the very prolonged (several hours) changes we have observed are currently being investigated.

Conclusions

C fibres may be considered, therefore, to have at least two central functions. Firstly, they have the capacity to deliver to the central nervous system an accurate representation of the location, the temporal properties and the intensity of peripheral noxious stimuli. Secondly, some C fibres have the capacity to "sensitize" the central nervous system to noxious and innocuous inputs in a less tightly spatially and temporally ordered way by producing prolonged increases in the excitability of second-order neurones. The sensitization of dorsal horn neurones following peripheral noxious stimuli that activate C fibres could act to increase the avoidance of further peripheral injury by increasing the gain and sensitivity of the flexion withdrawal reflex, so that even low intensity stimuli evoke the withdrawal response. The sensory accompaniment in man of a C-fibre-induced central sensitization could be increased pain following mild noxious stimuli (hyperalgesia) and pain produced by formerly non-painful stimuli (allodynia).

Many studies have shown that peripheral injury results in a sensitization of peripheral nociceptors in the immediate vicinity of the injury (see Lynn 1977). However, peripheral sensitization is unable to explain all the sensory and behavioural changes that result from peripheral injury (e.g. Meyer et al. 1985) and studies on ventrobasal thalamic neurones following carrageenin inflammation in the rat have revealed changes in the properties of the neurones that cannot be accounted for simply by the changes that the inflammation produces in primary afferents (Benoist et al. 1985). A central mechanism has to be invoked. Our data point to involvement of afferent C fibres in the generation of central sensitization.

References

BENNETT GJ, ABDELMOUMENE MA, HAYASHI H, DUBNER R (1980) Physiology and morphology of substantia gelatinosa neurons intracellularly stained with horseradish peroxidase. J Comp Neurol 194 : 809–827

BENOIST JM, KAYSER V, GAUTRON M, GUILBAUD G (1985) Changes in responses of ventrobasal thalamic neurones during carrageenin induced inflammation in the rat. In: FIELDS HL, DUBNER R, CERVERO F (eds) Advances in pain research and therapy, vol 9. Raven, New York, pp 295–303

COOK AJ, WOOLF CJ (1985) Cutaneous receptive field and morphological properties of hamstring flexor alpha-motoneurones in the rat. J Physiol (Lond) 364 : 249–263

COOK AJ, WOOLF CJ, WALL PD (1986) Prolonged C-fibre mediated facilitation of the flexion reflex is not due to changes in afferent terminal or motorneurone excitability. Neurosci Lett 70 : 91–96

COOK AJ, WOOLF CJ, WALL PD, MCMAHON SB (1987) Dynamic receptive field plasticity in the dorsal horn of the rat spinal cord following C-primary afferent input. Nature (in press)

KING A, THOMSON SWN, WOOLF CJ (1986) Intracellular recordings from wide dynamic range neurones in the deep dorsal horn of the rat spinal cord. J Physiol (Lond) (in press)

LIGHT AR, TREVINO DL, PERL ER (1979) Morphological features of functionally defined neurons in the marginal zone and substantia gelatinosa of the spinal dorsal horn. J Comp Neurol 186 : 151–172

LYNN B (1977) Cutaneous hyperalgesia. Br Med Bull 33 : 103–107

LYNN B, CARPENTER SE (1982) Primary afferent units from hairy skin of the rat hindlimb. Brain Res 238 : 29–43

MCMAHON SB, WALL PD (1983) A system of rat spinal cord lamina I cells projecting through the contralateral dorsolateral funiculus. J Comp Neurol 214 : 217–223

MCMAHON SB, SYKOVA E, WALL PD, WOOLF CJ, GIBSON SJ (1984) Neurogenic extravasation and substance P levels are low in muscle compared to skin in the rat hindlimb. Neurosci Lett 52 : 235–240

MENDELL LM (1966) Physiological properties of unmyelinated fibre projections to the spinal cord. Exp Neurol 16 : 316–332

MENSE S, MEYER H (1985) Different types of slowly conducting afferent units in cat skeletal muscle and tendon. J Physiol (Lond) 363 : 403–417

MEYER RA, CAMPBELL JN, RAJA SN (1985) Peripheral neural mechanisms of cutaneous hyperalgesia. In: FIELDS HL, DUBNER R, CERVERO F (eds) Advances in pain research and therapy, vol 9. Raven, New York, pp 53–71

MONAGHAN DT, COTMAN CW (1985) Distribution of N-methyl-D-aspartate sensitive L-[^{3}H]-glutamate-binding sites in rat brain. J Neurosci 5 : 2909–2919

SCHNEIDER SP, PERL ER (1985) Kynurenic acid antagonises synaptic and aminoacid excitation of hamster spinal dorsal horn neurons in vitro. Soc Neurosci Abstr 11 : 217

SWETT J, WOOLF CJ (1985) The somatotopic organization of primary afferent terminals in the superficial laminae of the dorsal horn of the rat spinal cord. J Comp Neurol 231 : 66–77

URBAN L, RANDIĆ M (1984) Slow excitatory transmission in rat dorsal horn. Possible mediation by peptides. Brain Res 290 : 336–342

WALL PD, WOOLF CJ (1984) Muscle but not cutaneous C-afferent input produces prolonged increases in the excitability of the flexion reflex in the rat. J Physiol (Lond) 356 : 443–458

WALL PD, WOOLF CJ (1986) The brief and the prolonged facilitatory effects of unmyelinated afferent input on the rat spinal cord are independently influenced by peripheral nerve section. Neuroscience 17 : 1199–1205

WOOLF CJ (1983a) C-primary afferent fibre mediated inhibitions in the dorsal horn of the decerebrate-spinal rat. Exp Brain Res 51 : 283–290

WOOLF CJ (1983b) Evidence for a central component of post-injury pain hypersensitivity. Nature 306 : 686–688

WOOLF CJ (1984) Long-term alterations in the excitability of the flexion reflex produced by peripheral tissue injury in the chronic decerebrate rat. Pain 18 : 325–343

WOOLF CJ, FITZGERALD M (1983) The properties of neurones recorded in the superficial dorsal horn of the rat spinal cord. J Comp Neurol 221 : 313–328

WOOLF CJ, FITZGERALD M (1986) The somatotopic organization of cutaneous afferent terminals and dorsal horn neuronal receptive fields in the superficial and deep laminae of the rat lumbar spinal cord. J Comp Neurol 251 : 517–532

WOOLF CJ, MCMAHON SB (1985) Injury-induced plasticity of the flexor reflex in chronic decerebrate rats. Neuroscience 16 : 395–404

WOOLF CJ, WALL PD (1986a) The relative effectiveness of C-primary afferent fibres of different origins in evoking a prolonged facilitation of the flexor reflex in the rat. J Neurosci 6 : 221–232

WOOLF CJ, WALL PD (1986b) Morphine-sensitive and morphine-insensitive actions of C-fibre input on the rat spinal cord. Neurosci Lett 64 : 221–225

WOOLF CJ, WIESENFELD-HALLIN Z (1986) Substance P and calcitonin gene-related peptide synergistically modulate the gain of the nociceptive flexor withdrawal reflex in the rat. Neurosci Lett 66 : 226–230

30 Somatic and Visceral Inputs to the Superficial Dorsal Horn (Laminae I–III) of the Lower Thoracic Spinal Cord of the Cat

J. E. H. Tattersall and F. Cervero

Introduction

Previous studies have shown that primary afferent fibres innervating viscera terminate in laminae I and V of the thoracic spinal cord (Cervero and Connell 1984; De Groat 1986). It has also been reported that neurones which receive convergent somatic and visceral inputs ("viscerosomatic neurones") are found in laminae I and V of the dorsal horn and also in the ventral horn, but are almost completely absent from laminae II, III and IV (see Cervero and Tattersall 1986). The existence of a distinct group of neurones in lamina I which relay their specific nociceptive drives to supraspinal regions (Cervero et al. 1976, 1979b; Willis 1985) suggests that this area of the spinal cord could play an important role in the processing of somatic and visceral nociceptive information.

In the present study, we have examined in some detail the extent of viscerosomatic convergence onto neurones in laminae I, II and III of the thoracic cord. We have also studied the cutaneous receptive field properties of neurones in these laminae, with particular emphasis on the comparison of receptive field properties between somatic and viscerosomatic neurones in lamina I.

Methods

Experiments were performed on 14 cats which were anaesthetised with chloralose (60 mg/kg I.V.) and paralysed with gallamine. Extracellular single-unit recordings were made from a total of 85 neurones in the right side of the grey matter of the 11th thoracic segment of the spinal cord. An ipsilateral dorsal rootlet was stimulated electrically while searching for neurones. All of the recorded neurones had cutaneous receptive fields.

Somatic afferent fibres were activated by natural stimulation of their receptive fields or by electrical stimulation through intradermal electrodes. Visceral afferent fibres were activated by electrical stimulation of the ipsilateral greater splanchnic nerve, as described previously (Cervero 1983a,b).

The locations of the recording sites of neurones were determined from iontophoretically deposited spots of pontamine sky blue, as described previously (Molony 1978; Cervero et al. 1979a).

Results

Recordings were made from 85 neurones in laminae I–III of the thoracic spinal cord. These were classified into two types according to their responses to somatic and visceral stimulation: (i) somatic neurones, driven only by somatic inputs, and (ii) viscerosomatic neurones, driven by both somatic and visceral inputs.

Locations of Recording Sites

Figure 1 shows the locations of the recording sites of 60 somatic and 25 viscerosomatic neurones. The somatic neurones were distributed throughout the three laminae studied, in contrast to the viscerosomatic cells, all of which were recorded in lamina I or in the immediately adjacent white matter.

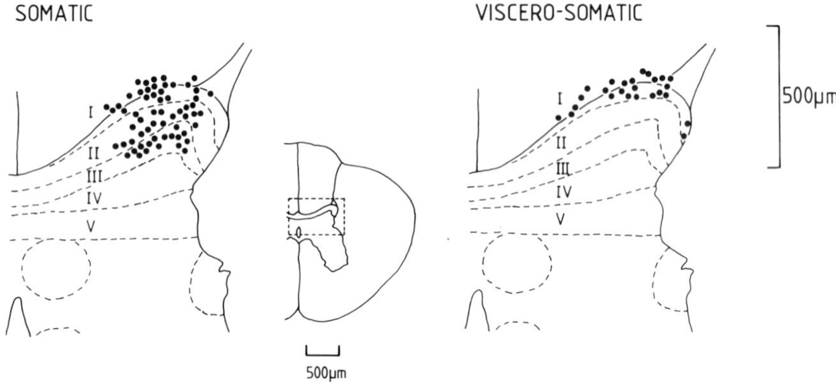

Fig. 1. Locations of the recording sites of 60 somatic neurones (left) and 25 viscerosomatic cells (right). The locations have been pooled on standard transverse sections of the lower thoracic spinal cord. The inset shows a transverse section of the entire grey matter

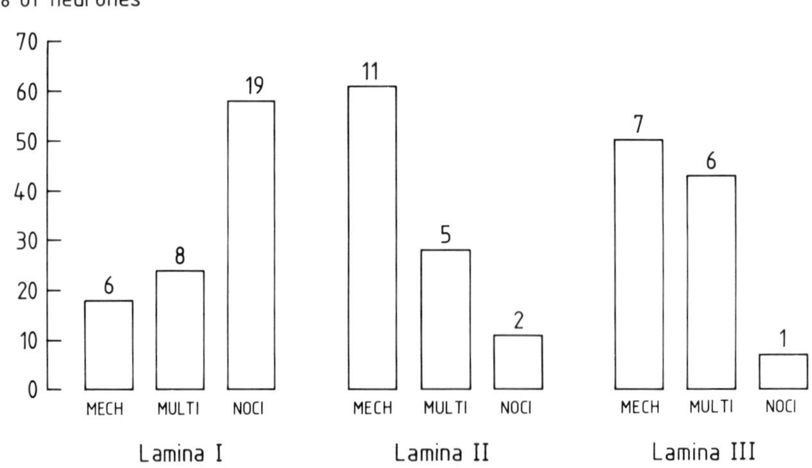

Fig. 2. Cutaneous receptive field properties of neurones in laminae I, II and III. Neurones were classified as mechanoreceptive (MECH), multireceptive (MULTI) or nociceptive (NOCI). The figures above the bars indicate numbers of neurones in each sample

Cutaneous Receptive Field Properties

The cutaneous receptive fields were fully characterised for 65 of the neurones in our sample, and these were classified according to the types of natural stimuli (hair movement, touch or pinch) which were effective in exciting the neurones. All receptive fields were ipsilateral to the recording site. The results are shown in Fig. 2.

The majority (58 %) of neurones in lamina I were nocireceptive. In contrast, only 11 % of cells were nocireceptive in lamina II and only 7 % in lamina III. Most lamina II neurones (61 %) were mechanoreceptive, while in lamina III there were approximately equal proportions of mechanoreceptive (50 %) and multireceptive (43 %) neurones.

Cutaneous Receptive Field Sizes

The areas of the cutaneous receptive fields of 65 neurones were measured. These were arbitrarily divided into small (< 4 cm^2), medium (4–10 cm^2) or large (> 10 cm^2). The results are shown in Fig. 3.

The distribution of receptive field sizes was similar in all three laminae. The majority of neurones had small receptive fields, a smaller number had medium-sized fields, and very few had large receptive fields.

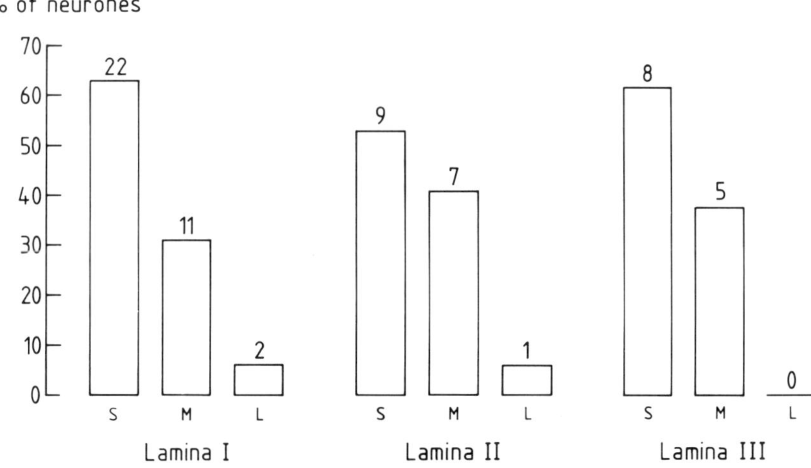

Fig. 3. Cutaneous receptive field sizes of neurones in laminae I, II and III. Receptive fields were classified as small (S), medium (M) or large (L). The figures above the bars indicate numbers of neurones in each sample

Cutaneous Receptive Fields of Lamina I Neurones

The cutaneous receptive fields of somatic and viscerosomatic neurones in lamina I are compared in Fig. 4. All somatic lamina I neurones in our sample received specific cutaneous inputs: the majority (76 %) were nocireceptive and the remainder were mechanoreceptive. In contrast, half of the viscerosomatic neurones were multireceptive, 37 % were nocireceptive and 13 % were mechanoreceptive.

The sizes of the cutaneous receptive fields also differed between the two groups of neurones. Nearly all (88 %) of the lamina I somatic cells had small receptive fields, whereas a large proportion of viscerosomatic neurones had medium (50 %) or large (11 %) receptive fields.

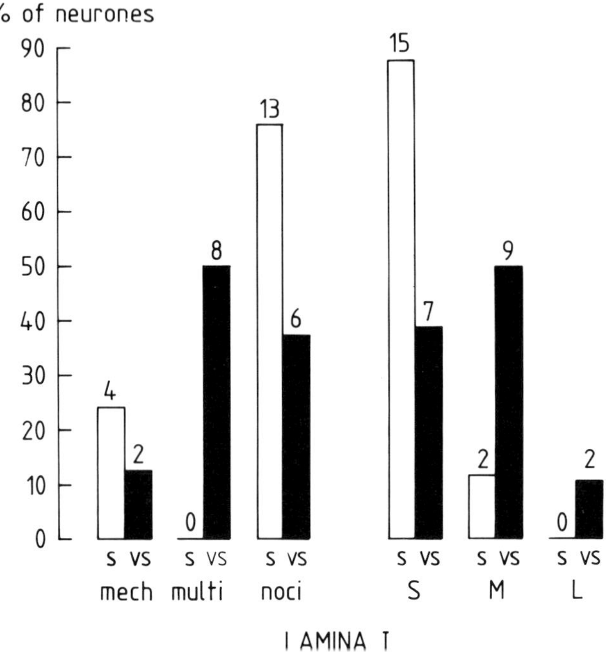

Fig. 4. Cutaneous receptive field properties (left) and sizes (right) of neurones in lamina I. Open bars represent somatic neurones, filled bars show viscerosomatic cells. The figures above the bars indicate numbers of neurones in each sample

Discussion

Studies using transganglionic transport of horseradish peroxidase (HRP) through visceral nerves have demonstrated a consistent pattern of termination of visceral afferent fibres in the spinal cord (Cervero and Connell 1984; De Groat 1986). The only dorsal horn areas which receive visceral afferent projections are lamina I and lamina V (see Cervero and Tattersall 1986).

Previous studies have already demonstrated convergence of cutaneous, muscle and visceral afferent inputs onto lamina I neurones, including those which project in the spinothalamic tract (Cervero 1983a,b; Craig and Kniffki 1985; Willis 1985). In the present study, we have confirmed the existence of extensive viscerosomatic convergence onto neurones in lamina I. Our results also confirm previous reports that laminae II and III receive little or no visceral input. The presence of substantial numbers of viscerosomatic neurones in lamina I, together with our finding that most of these neurones receive somatic nociceptive inputs – either exclusively or in combination with low-threshold mechanoreceptive inputs – provides support for the "convergence-projection theory" of referred visceral pain (Ruch 1946). The cutaneous receptive field properties of viscerosomatic neurones in lamina I were similar to those of viscerosomatic neurones in the rest of the spinal cord (Cervero and Tattersall 1985).

A further finding in our study was that viscerosomatic neurones in lamina I tended to have larger cutaneous receptive fields than did somatic cells in this lamina. This difference between somatic and viscerosomatic neurones has been found previously in other laminae (Cervero and Tattersall 1985), and presumably means that the somatic representation of the viscerosomatic neurones is less precise than that of somatic neurones, a feature which may help to explain the relatively diffuse nature of visceral pain.

All of the somatic lamina I neurones in our sample, which comprised about half of the total number of cells recorded in this lamina, received specific cutaneous inputs, and the vast majority of these were nocireceptive. It would appear, therefore, that lamina I in the thoracic cord contains a significant population of neurones which relay purely somatic nociceptive information.

We conclude from this study that lamina I is an important area for the processing and relaying of convergent inputs from somatic and visceral afferent fibres, and that it nevertheless preserves a specific nociceptive somatic relay.

Acknowledgements. We would like to thank Mr. Steven Allen for technical assistance. This work was supported by the Medical Research Council.

References

CERVERO F (1983a) Somatic and visceral inputs to the thoracic spinal cord of the cat: effects of noxious stimulation of the biliary system. J Physiol (Lond) 337 : 51–67

CERVERO F (1983b) Supraspinal connections of neurones in the thoracic spinal cord of the cat: ascending projections and effects of descending impulses. Brain Res 275 : 251–261

CERVERO F, CONNELL LA (1984) Distribution of somatic and visceral primary afferent fibres within the thoracic spinal cord of the cat. J Comp Neurol 230 : 88–98

CERVERO F, IGGO A, OGAWA H (1976) Nociceptor driven dorsal horn neurones in the lumbar spinal cord of the cat. Pain 2 : 5–24

CERVERO F, IGGO A, MOLONY V (1979a) An electrophysiological study of neurones in the substantia gelatinosa Rolandi of the cat's spinal cord. J Exp Physiol 64 : 297–314

CERVERO F, IGGO A, MOLONY V (1979b) Ascending projections of nociceptor-driven Lamina I neurones in the cat. Exp Brain Res 35 : 135–149

CERVERO F, TATTERSALL JEH (1985) Cutaneous receptive fields of somatic and viscerosomatic neurones in the thoracic spinal cord of the cat. J Comp Neurol 237 : 325–332

CERVERO F, TATTERSALL JEH (1986) Somatic and visceral sensory integration in the thoracic spinal cord. Prog Brain Res 67 : 189–205

CRAIG AD, KNIFFKI KD (1985) Spinothalamic lumbosacral Lamina I cells responsive to skin and muscle stimulation in the cat. J Physiol (Lond) 365 : 197–221

DE GROAT WC (1986) Spinal cord projections and neuropeptides in visceral afferent neurones. Prog Brain Res 67 : 165–187

MOLONY V (1978) Fine glass microelectrodes for recording from small neurones in the spinal cord of the cat. J Physiol (Lond) 284 : 27–28P

RUCH TC (1946) Visceral sensation and referred pain. In: FULTON JF (ed) Howell's textbook of physiology, 15th edn. Saunders, Philadelphia pp 385–401

WILLIS WD (1985) The pain system. Karger, Basel

31 Fine Afferent Fibres from Viscera and Visceral Pain: Anatomy and Physiology of Viscero-Somatic Convergence

F. Cervero

Introduction

The innervation of internal organs is mediated almost entirely by fine nerve fibres. The efferent component of this innervation is made up of axons of pre- and postganglionic neurones of the sympathetic and parasympathetic systems. All of these axons are either thin myelinated (B) or unmyelinated (C) fibres. The afferent side of visceral innervation is also mediated by small myelinated (Aδ) and unmyelinated (C) fibres. Only a small number of thick myelinated afferent fibres (Aβ) are present in visceral nerves and are believed to be connected with mesenteric pacinian corpuscles. The analysis of visceral sensory systems can therefore be regarded as a convenient way of studying the role of fine afferent fibres in the processing of sensory information.

In this article the functions of fine afferent fibres from viscera will be reviewed in the context of their contribution to visceral sensation and visceral pain. Further information on some of the points discussed in this paper can be obtained from other recent reviews of the neurophysiological mechanisms of visceral pain (Cervero 1983, 1985; Cervero and Tattersall 1986; Foreman 1986).

Fine Afferent Fibres and Visceral Sensation

It has long been known that most afferents in visceral nerves are either unmyelinated or small myelinated fibres. Earlier estimates of 80% or more of all visceral afferent fibres being unmyelinated have been confirmed by modern electron-microscopic studies of visceral nerves which show ratios of 10 : 1 in favour of unmyelinated fibres (Kuo et al. 1982). It is also well known that most of the myelinated afferent fibres in visceral nerves are of fine diameter and that many of them become unmyelinated as they approach their peripheral target organs (Iggo 1958). Similarly, the efferent innervation of viscera is also mediated, to a large extent, by unmyelinated efferent fibres of the autonomic nervous system.

Large numbers of unmyelinated afferent fibres are also present in somatic nerves, but in most of these nerve trunks they are accompanied by many thick myelinated afferent fibres connected to a variety of cutaneous sensory receptors, the vast majority of which are sensitive mechanoreceptors. Therefore, the very large preponderance of afferent C fibres in visceral nerves and the almost complete absence of large myelinated afferents in these nerves are the most distinctive features of the peripheral organization of visceral sensory systems. Correlations between the kind and range of sensory experiences evoked from viscera and the CNS mechanisms involved in the processing of visceral afferent signals can provide valuable insights into the sensory role of fine afferent fibres.

Visceral Sensation and Visceral Pain

Most internal organs have a dual afferent innervation. Some visceral afferent fibres join sympathetic nerves, such as the splanchnic nerves, whereas other afferent fibres from the same viscera course in parasympathetic nerves, such as the vagus and pelvic nerves. Clinical, behavioural and neurophysiological studies have demonstrated that most forms of visceral sensation (and especially visceral pain) are mediated by visceral afferent fibres running in sympathetic nerves. Afferent fibres in parasympathetic nerves do not seem to be concerned, in most cases, with visceral sensations but rather with the reflex regulation of visceral function [see Cervero and Tattersall (1986) for a full discussion]. This generalization applies, with few exceptions, to pain from upper abdominal viscera, but it is important to point out that non-painful visceral sensations or visceral pain from thoracic or pelvic organs may be elicited by the stimulation of afferent fibres in somatic or parasympathetic nerves.

Although visceral sensation is commonly equated with visceral pain, there are some distinct sensory experiences from internal organs that are clearly non-painful. In some cases, non-painful visceral sensations are expressed as sensory awareness of internal organs, most commonly in the form of feelings of distension (e.g. gastric distension after a heavy meal, bladder distension prior to micturition or rectal distension prior to defecation). It is interesting to note that these sensory experiences are usually the lower end of a graded sensation leading to pain. Thus, the pain of, for example, gastric, urinary or rectal distension is only quantitatively different from the non-painful sensations evoked by mild distension of these viscera [see for instance the report by Nathan (1981)]. From a neurophysiological point of view, it is tempting to establish a parallel between these graded sensory experiences and the behaviour of mechanosensitive afferent fibres from the same viscera (Jänig and Morrison 1986) which are believed to react to innocuous and noxious levels of distension by progressive increases in the frequency of their responses (i.e. an "intensity-encoding" mechanism). In contrast, viscera from which pain is the only sensory experience that can be evoked, such as the heart or the biliary system, appear to be innervated by specific nociceptors similar to those found in somatic tissues (Cervero 1985; but see Malliani 1982).

Visceral Afferent Projection to the Spinal Cord

Visceral pain from upper abdominal viscera is mediated almost exclusively by afferent fibres in sympathetic nerves that reach the lower thoracic spinal cord via the sympathetic chain and the "rami communicantes". All visceral afferent fibres that enter the lower thoracic spinal cord join the sympathetic chain by way of the splanchnic nerves. These visceral afferent fibres have their cell bodies in the thoracic spinal ganglia and their central branches enter the spinal cord through the dorsal roots. According to Kuo et al. (1982), the greater splanchnic nerve of the cat contains no more than 3000–3500 afferent fibres, less than 20 %

of the total number of fibres in this nerve. The vast majority of these afferents (2000–3000) are unmyelinated; 250–400 are Aδ fibres and 120–350 are Aβ fibres. Thus, the visceral afferent input to the spinal cord, including all afferent fibres that signal pain from upper abdominal viscera, is entirely mediated by a small number of afferents, 90 % of which are unmyelinated.

Using transganglionic transport of horseradish peroxidase (HRP) through the splanchnic nerves, it has been possible to estimate the proportions of visceral primary afferent fibres in the lower thoracic spinal ganglia (Cervero et al. 1984). Fewer than 7 % of all dorsal root ganglion cells in the T8 and T9 ganglia were found labelled with HRP via the ipsilateral splanchnic nerves. Thus, even in the main area of projection of the splanchnic nerve, the actual number of afferent fibres that reach the spinal cord is very small. It therefore follows that visceral pain is mediated by the activation of very few visceral afferent fibres. This leaves little scope for fine discrimination and offers a possible explanation for the diffuse nature of visceral pain.

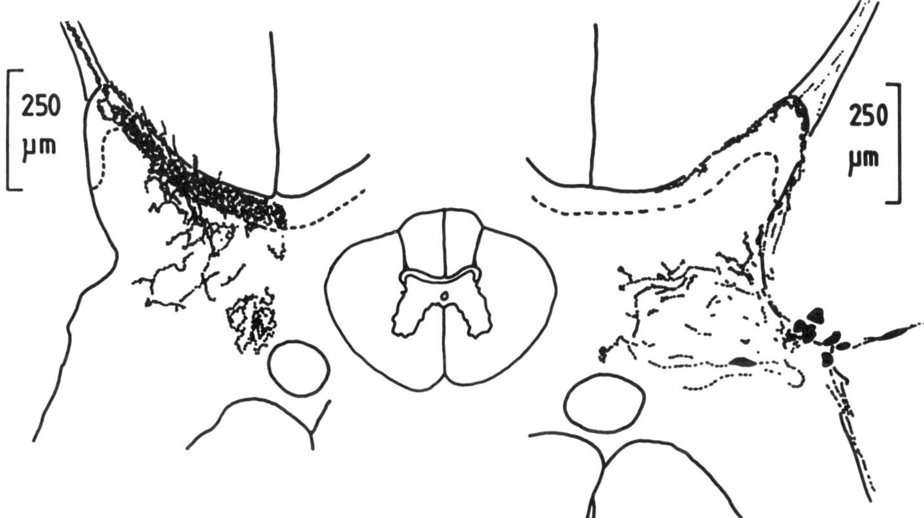

Fig. 1. Reconstruction from three (left) and from seven (right) 80µm transverse serial sections of the projections of somatic (left) and visceral (right) afferent fibres to the T9 segment of the spinal cord. HRP was applied to the intercostal nerve of the T9 segment (left) and to the splanchnic nerve (right). Note the absence of a visceral afferent projection to the substantia gelatinosa, whose ventral border is indicated by the dotted line. (Modified from Cervero and Connell 1984)

The pattern of termination of visceral afferent fibres within the spinal cord has been examined in a variety of animal species (cats, monkeys and rats) and in sacral, lumbar and thoracic regions of the cord (for references see de Groat 1986). It is clear from all these HRP studies that visceral afferent fibres display a consistent pattern of termination throughout the spinal cord, with areas of projection in laminae I and V but sparing the intermediate dorsal horn (Fig. 1). The density of the visceral projection to the dorsal horn is substantially lower than that of the somatic projection (Cervero and Connell 1984), showing that the few visceral afferents which reach the spinal cord do not branch extensively within the cord. The substantia gelatinosa (lamina II) does not receive a direct visceral projection, which calls into question the generally accepted belief that most afferent C fibres terminate in the substantia gelatinosa of the dorsal horn and suggests that this region of the cord deals only with the processing of cutaneous sensory information.

Viscero-Somatic Convergence in the Spinal Cord

Visceral pain is often dull, aching and ill-localized. A characteristic feature of most forms of visceral pain is the referral of the sensation to the skin and other superficial structures innervated by the same spinal cord segments that receive the input from the originating viscus. Therefore, neurophysiological interpretations of visceral pain are based on the convergence of inputs from somatic and visceral structures onto sensory neurones whose activation leads to the experience of somatic pain (Ruch 1946).

There is considerable experimental support for the occurrence of viscero-somatic convergence onto spinal cord neurones (Cervero and Tattersall 1986). Two types of spinal cord neurone can be distinguished according to the presence or absence of an excitatory visceral input. Some neurones can be excited by stimulation of cutaneous and subcutaneous afferent fibres but do not receive excitatory inputs from visceral afferent fibres (somatic neurones). Other cells respond to visceral as well as to somatic stimulation (viscero-somatic neurones). Figure 2 shows representative examples of both types of neurone.

Somatic neurones are mainly located in laminae II, III and IV of the dorsal horn whereas viscero-somatic neurones are located in laminae I and V of the dorsal horn and in the ventral horn. This agrees with the anatomical data on the mode of termination of somatic and visceral fibres in the spinal cord and provides further evidence for a lack of involvement of the substantia gelatinosa (lamina II) in the processing of visceral sensory information.

The majority of somatic neurones are mechanoreceptive, i.e. activated only by low-threshold mechanoreceptors, whereas most viscero-somatic cells are driven by nociceptors either specifically (nocireceptive) or in addition to their low threshold inputs (multireceptive). Many of the viscero-somatic neurones in laminae V, VII and VIII are strongly excited by stimulation of subcutaneous tissues, particularly muscle. This offers an explanation for the clinically relevant observation that visceral pain, when referred to a somatic location, more often takes the form of muscle cramp than of cutaneous pain. As for the nature of the visceral input to viscero-somatic neurones, it has been reported that noxious intensities of visceral stimulation are required in order to activate these neurones.

Visceral sensory information reaches supraspinal structures via the projections of some viscero-somatic neurones whose axons join the spino-thalamic and spino-reticular tracts (Foreman 1986). In spite of the low numbers of visceral afferents entering the thoracic spinal cord, a large proportion of thoracic neurones are viscero-somatic, which indicates extensive divergence of the visceral input to the CNS. Also, 80% of viscero-somatic neurones have medium-sized or large receptive fields, suggesting that the spatial discrimination of referred visceral sensations is poorer than that of somatic sensations from the same area of skin.

All these functional properties of viscero-somatic neurones support the main postulates of the "convergence-projection" theory of referred visceral pain (Ruch 1946) and strongly indicate a divergent and diffuse central organization of the visceral input to the spinal cord involving viscero-somatic convergence onto neurones with somatic nociceptive drives from large receptive fields.

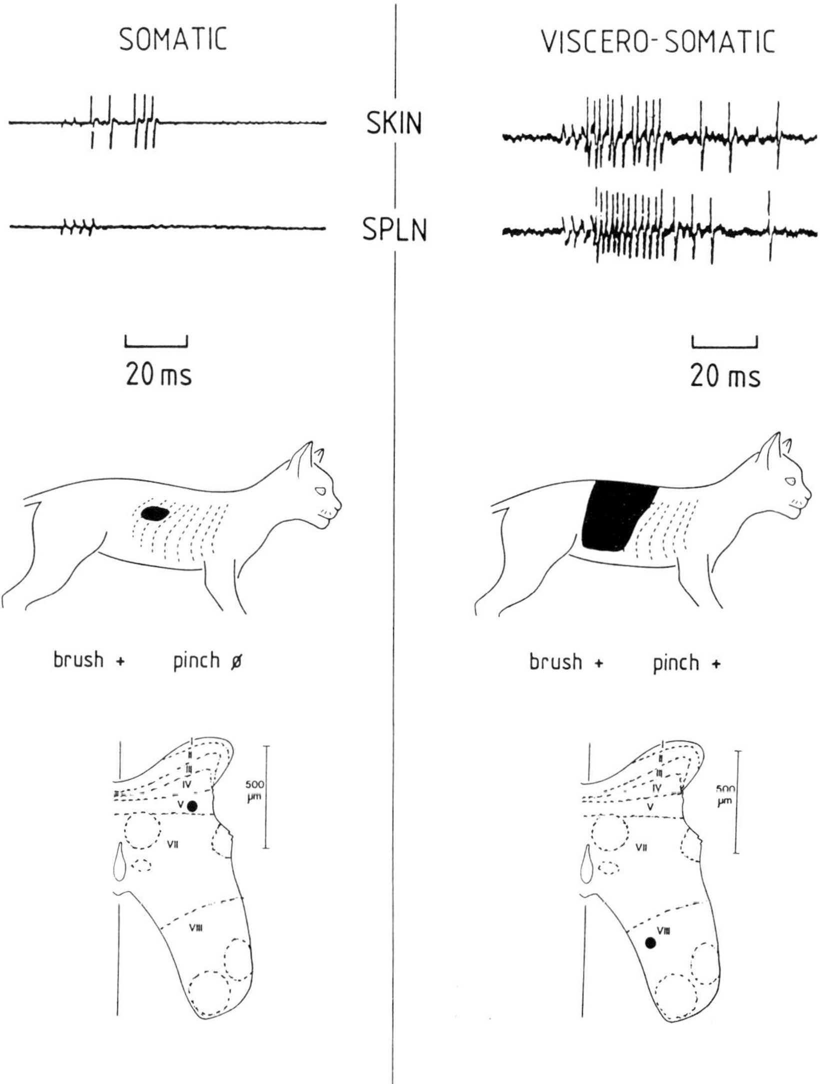

Fig. 2. Responses of a somatic neurone (left) and a viscero-somatic neurone (right) to electrical stimulation of their cutaneous receptive fields (top traces) and of the splanchnic nerve (SPLN; lower traces). The cutaneous receptive fields of both neurones and the locations of the recording sites are also shown. (From Cervero and Tattersall 1986)

Spinal and Supraspinal Integration of Visceral Sensory Information

Facilitatory and inhibitory interactions have been demonstrated between somatic and visceral inputs onto viscero-somatic neurones (Tattersall et al. 1986b). The response of these neurones to somatic and visceral volleys can be powerfully inhibited by a preceding visceral or somatic stimulus. This inhibition can last up to 1 s and is not affected by spinalization, indicating a spinal organization of the network responsible for the inhibition. It is conceivable that such segmental inhibition could play a role in the enhancement of contrast between the different inputs to viscero-somatic neurones and in the detection of sudden changes in activity through any of their peripheral drives.

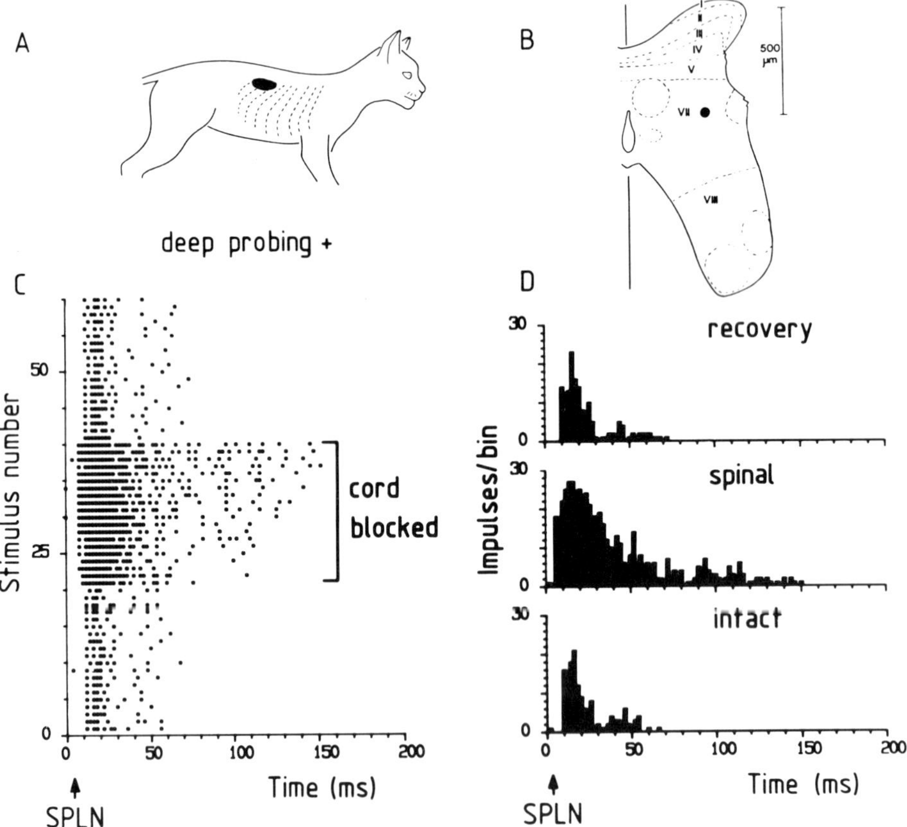

Fig. 3 A-D. Viscero-somatic neurone in the thoracic spinal cord showing tonic descending inhibition. The cell was excited by probing of deep, subcutaneous tissues **(A)** and was located in lamina VII **(B)**. **C** A dot-raster display of the responses of the neurone to electrical stimulation of the ipsilateral splanchnic nerve (SPLN) before, during and after reversible spinalization. **D** The same data presented in histogram form, bin width 2 ms. (From Tattersall et al. 1986a)

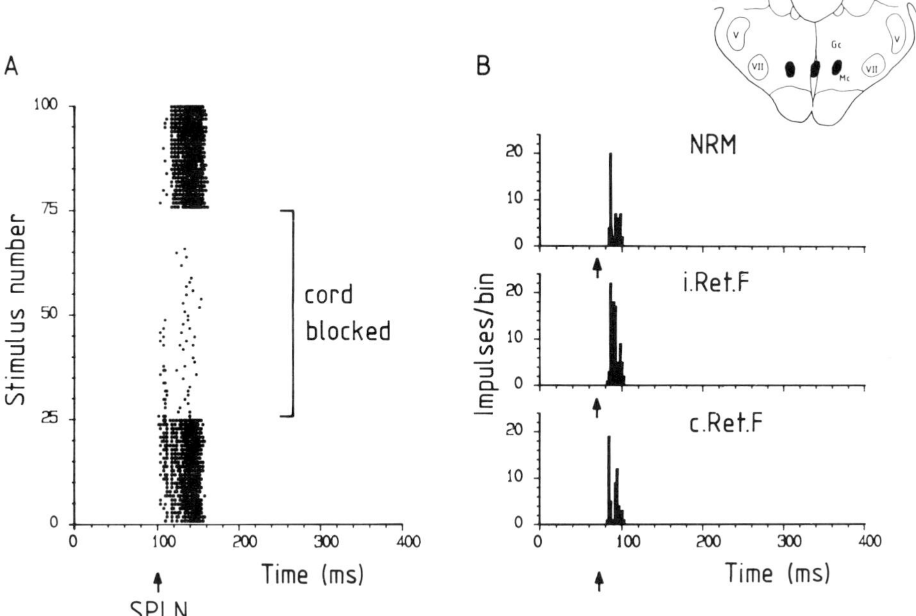

Fig. 4 A, B. Viscero-somatic neurone of the thoracic spinal cord with a supraspinal excitatory input and phasic excitation from the brain stem. **A** A dot-raster display of the responses of the neurone to electrical stimulation of the splanchnic nerve (SPLN) before, during and after reversible spinalization. **B** Peristimulus time histograms (25 sweeps, bin width 2 ms) of the responses of the neurone to electrical stimulation of the nucleus raphe magnus (NRM) and the ipsilateral and contralateral reticular formation (Ret.F.). The inset shows the locations of the stimulating electrodes. (From Tattersall et al. 1986b)

Viscero-somatic neurones in the spinal cord are also subjected to substantial descending control from supraspinal areas. This involves descending inhibition of peripheral inputs as well as descending excitation of some of the neurones. The latter phenomenon is probably responsible for the considerable divergence of the visceral input, which results in many spinal cord cells being able to respond to the activation of the few visceral afferents that reach the thoracic spinal cord.

Using the technique of reversible spinalization with a cold block, it has been possible to distinguish two kinds of tonic descending effects on viscero-somatic neurones (Tattersall et al. 1986a). About half of the neurones increased the intensity of their responses to visceral and to somatic stimulation in the spinal state and developed or increased their background activity (Fig. 3). This indicates that these cells were under tonic descending inhibition of both somatic and visceral afferent inputs. Many of these neurones were located in or close to lamina V of the dorsal horn.

The other half of the viscero-somatic neurones studied showed reduced or abolished visceral responses in the spinal state (Fig. 4). Therefore, the visceral input to these neurones seems to be mediated or reinforced by a neuronal link that involves supraspinal regions. Many neurones in this group were located in the ventral horn.

Neurones under tonic descending inhibition can also be inhibited by phasic stimulation of brain stem locations such as the nucleus raphe magnus (NRM) and adjacent areas of the reticular formation (Ret.F.). This inhibition can also be evoked by selective chemical stimulation with DL-homocysteic acid of cell bodies located in these brain stem areas. In contrast, viscero-somatic neurones under descending excitation respond with an excitation followed by a period of inhibition to electrical stimulation of the NRM and Ret.F. (Fig. 4), but can only be inhibited by selective chemical stimulation of cell bodies in these regions. Therefore, these cells are under descending inhibition mediated by axons with cell bodies in the NRM and Ret.F. and under descending excitation mediated by axons which pass through these locations but whose cell bodies are located elsewhere, probably in more rostral areas of the brain stem (Tattersall et al. 1986b).

Summary and Conclusions

Visceral pain from upper abdominal viscera is mediated by the activation of a few visceral afferent fibres, the vast majority of which are unmyelinated. The spinal cord projections of these visceral afferent fibres converge onto neurones driven by inputs from the skin and from deep somatic structures such as muscle, tendons and ligaments. These neurones can only be excited by noxious levels of visceral stimulation and some of them have axons that project to supraspinal levels via spino-reticular and spino-thalamic pathways. All these observations may offer a neurophysiological explanation for the referral of visceral pain to somatic structures.

In addition, the visceral input to the spinal cord generates extensive divergence within the CNS, sometimes involving long supraspinal loops. This divergent input can activate many different systems which will trigger the general reactions characteristic of visceral pain: a diffuse and ill-localized pain referred to somatic regions, visceral reflexes and altered autonomic control of viscera and an increase in somatic reflexes resulting in prolonged muscle spasms.

The organization of visceral sensory systems can be compared to that of a trip-wire alarm mechanism, i.e. a few peripheral sensors whose activation results in generalized responses. Therefore, the sensory functions of fine afferent fibres seem to be closely linked to the mechanisms of arousal and alertness in which the experience of an aversive sensation is only a component of the total response of the system to its peripheral activation.

References

Cervero F (1983) Mechanisms of visceral pain. In: Lipton S, Miles J (eds) Persistent pain, vol 4. Grune & Stratton, London, pp 1-19

Cervero F (1985) Visceral nociception: peripheral and central aspects of visceral nociceptive systems. Philos Trans R Soc Lond [Biol] 308 : 325-337

Cervero F, Connell LA (1984) Distribution of somatic and visceral primary afferent fibres within the thoracic spinal cord of the cat. J Comp Neurol 230 : 88-98

Cervero F, Tattersall JEH (1986) Somatic and visceral sensory integration in the thoracic spinal cord. Prog Brain Res 67 : 189-205

Cervero F, Connell LA, Lawson SN (1984) Somatic and visceral primary afferents in the lower thoracic dorsal root ganglia of the cat. J Comp Neurol 228 : 422-431

De Groat WC (1986) Spinal cord projections and neuropeptides in visceral afferent neurones. Prog Brain Res 67 : 165-187

Foreman RD (1986) Spinal substrates of visceral pain. In: Yaksh TL (ed) Spinal afferent processing. Plenum, New York, pp 217-242

Iggo A (1958) The electrophysiological identification of single nerve fibres with particular reference to the slowest conducting vagal afferent fibres in the cat. J Physiol (Lond) 142 : 110-126

Jänig W, Morrison JFB (1986) Functional properties of spinal visceral afferents supplying abdominal and pelvic organs with special emphasis on visceral nociception. Prog Brain Res 67 : 87-114

Kuo DC, Yang GCH, Yamasaki DS, Krauthamer GH (1982) A wide field electron microscopic analysis of the fiber constituents of the major splanchnic nerve in cat. J Comp Neurol 210 : 49-58

Malliani A (1982) Cardiovascular sympathetic afferent fibres. Rev Physiol Biochem Pharmacol 94 : 11-74

Nathan PW (1981) Gastric sensations: report of a case. Pain 10 : 259-262

Ruch TC (1946) Visceral sensation and referred pain. In: Fulton JF (ed) Howell's textbook of physiology, 15th edn. Saunders, Philadelphia

Tattersall JEH, Cervero F, Lumb BM (1986a) Effects of reversible spinalization on the visceral input to viscero-somatic neurones in the lower thoracic spinal cord of the cat. J Neurophysiol 56 : 785-796

Tattersall JEH, Cervero F, Lumb BM (1986b) Viscero-somatic neurones in the lower thoracic spinal cord of the cat: excitations and inhibitions evoked by splanchnic and somatic nerve volleys and by stimulation of brain stem nuclei. J Neurophysiol 56 : 1411-1423

32 Stimulus-Response Properties of Lumbosacral Spinal Neurons to Graded Colorectal Distension in the Rat

T.J. Ness and G.F. Gebhart

Introduction

Spinal neurons important to the transmission of nociceptive information arising from somatocutaneous structures have been well characterized (e.g., Willis and Coggeshall 1978). Comparatively little is known, however, about the response characteristics of spinal neurons involved in the transmission of deep pain of visceral origin. Indeed, the neurophysiologic bases of visceral sensation in general, and visceral nociception in particular, are poorly understood (see Cervero 1983 for review). Afferent fibers which encode visceral nociceptive information have been generally considered to travel exclusively in conjunction with motor fibers of the sympathetic nervous system (e.g., splanchnic nerves). Visceral afferent fibers traveling in association with motor fibers of the parasympathetic nervous system, in contrast, have not been considered to play a role in visceral nociception. These concepts are increasingly being questioned (e.g., Mei 1983), and accumulating evidence suggests that pelvic visceral sensations, including nociception, are conveyed by pelvic sacral parasympathetic nerves to the lumbosacral spinal cord.

Visceral pain has not been as extensively investigated as somatocutaneous pain, in part because of the incompletely understood and more complex (and controversial) nature of the relevant neuroanatomy, but also because of the greater difficulty in developing quantifiable, reproducible methods for producing visceral pain. Simply defining a noxious visceral stimulus has been a continuing problem. For example, many organs can be cut or crushed without evoking pain. However, distension of hollow visceral organs is known to be painful to humans and constitutes an experimentally satisfactory noxious visceral stimulus (e.g., Cervero 1982).

In animals, pain can only be inferred from the reflex reactions that accompany nociception – changes in heart rate, blood pressure, respiration, etc. – and such pseudaffective reflexes have been well documented in man and animals alike. Although pain may not be both the necessary and sufficient condition which evokes these reflexes, studies complementary to the present investigation have established that colorectal distension in the awake rat evokes pseudaffective pressor and visceromotor reflexes and rapidly leads to learned avoidance behavior (Ness and Gebhart 1986). These observations are consistent with interpretation of the distending stimulus as nociceptive. The objective of the electrophysiologic studies reported here was to characterize spinal neuronal responses to graded colorectal distension in the rat. The rat was chosen for study because it is widely employed in complementary neurochemical, pharmacologic, and behavioral investigations of nociception.

Methods

Rats were initially anesthetized with sodium pentobarbital (45–50 mg/kg ip) and venous (femoral), arterial (femoral), and tracheal cannulae were inserted. Before starting the vertebral laminectomy, rats were paralyzed with pancuronium bromide (0.4 mg/kg iv and 0.2 mg/kg/h thereafter) and mechanically ventilated for the remainder of the experiment. Blood pressure and rectal core temperature were continuously monitored. Anesthesia during the course of the experiment was maintained with halothane (0.5%) and 67% N_2O:33% O_2. The vertebral column was firmly clamped rostral and the ischia caudal to a laminectomy exposing the lumbosacral spinal cord. A second, smaller laminectomy was made over the cervical spinal cord for insertion of stimulating electrodes into the ventral ipsilateral and contralateral spinal cord for antidromic invasion of neurons in lumbosacral segments. The dura was opened, and the spinal cord covered with warmed mineral oil and agar for stabilization of the spinal cord during recording.

Tungsten microelectrodes (0.5–1.2 MΩ) were used for single-unit recording in the L6-S1 spinal segments, midline to 0.5 mm lateral, and 0.2–1.4 mm from the cord dorsum. Areas lateral in the L6–S1 spinal cord (e.g., parasympathetic nucleus) were not examined. Antidromic stimulation in the contralateral cervical spinal cord and colorectal distension (75–85 mmHg pressure) were used as search stimuli. Colorectal distension was produced by inflation with air of a 7-to 8-cm-long flexible latex balloon inserted via the anus into the rectum and distal colon. Intracolonic distending pressures were monitored continuously with a Century Technology low-volume pressure transducer. Stimulus-response functions to graded colorectal distension (typically 20–100 mmHg) were generated and least squares linear regressions determined for each neuron, allowing estimation of threshold distending pressures to neuronal response. Neurons were also characterized with respect to convergent somatocutaneous receptive fields, antidromic invasion from the cervical spinal cord, and response to the intra-arterial administration of bradykinin (1 μg in 50 μl normal saline). Neuronal responses to colorectal distension were carefully differentiated from distension-associated responses due to mechanical stimulation of cutaneous perianal receptive fields or proprioceptors in muscles/tendons related to tail movement. All colorectal distensions were 20 s in duration and were given at 4-min intervals. To quantify spinal neuronal responses to colorectal distension and bradykinin, the total number of unit discharges were counted during a preselected interval, starting with the onset of the distending stimulus or bradykinin injections. All data are reported as the mean ± standard error of the mean.

At the end of an experiment, electrolytic lesions to mark spinal recording and antidromic stimulation sites were made. Animals were killed with an overdose of pentobarbital iv or inhaled halothane (>5% concentration). Spinal cord tissue was fixed in formalin and recording and stimulation sites reconstructed histologically from 40-μm sections stained with cresyl violet or hematoxylin-eosin.

Results

Neurons in the medial L6-S1 spinal segments responsive to colorectal distension were the focus of the present study. Many of the spinal neurons were established by antidromic invasion from the contralatral cervical spinal cord (C1) to project rostrally and also to have convergent perianal/scrotal cutaneous receptive fields. Neuronal responses were categorized based upon their initial response to a 20-s, 75-to 85-mmHg colorectal distension. Most

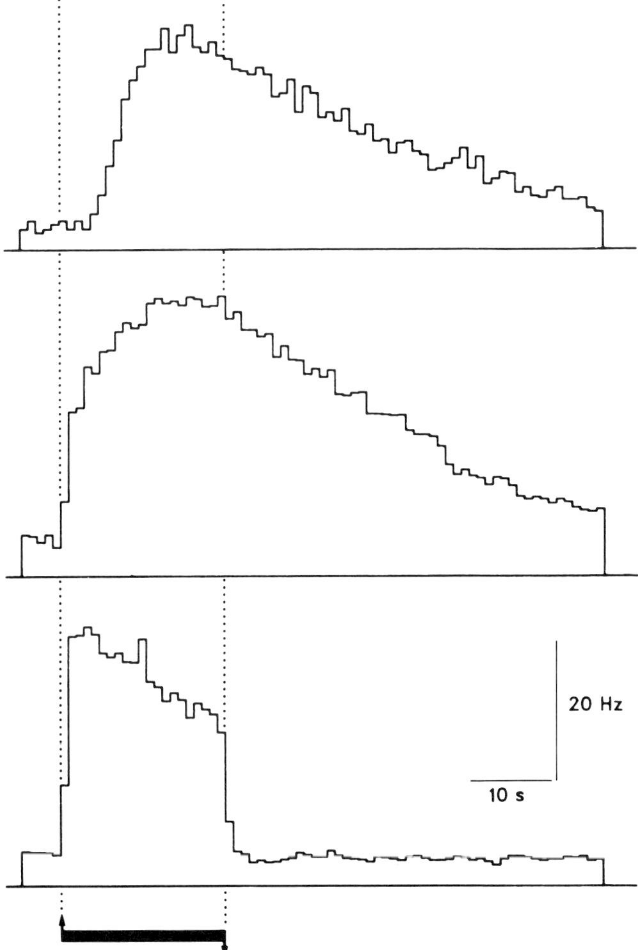

Fig. 1. Mean responses of neurons excited by colorectal distension. Neurons were classified based upon their initial response to a 20-s, 75- to 85-mmHg distending stimulus (filled horizontal bar). Peristimulus time histograms (1 s bin width) represent three types of neurons excited by colorectal distension: neurons having short latencies to response onset and termination temporally related to stimulus onset and termination; neurons having a short latency to response onset and a sustained response to the distending stimulus; and neurons having a long latency to response onset and a sustained response to the distending stimulus (bottom to top). Recording loci for neurons represented here are given in Fig. 2 - 4

neurons excited by colorectal distension responded at short latency (1 s) to the onset of the distending stimulus. One subgroup of these neurons exhibited an abrupt return to baseline upon stimulus termination; the other subgroup exhibited a sustained response which continued for 4–120 s following stimulus termination. A smaller, third subgroup of neurons excited by colorectal distension also exhibited a sustained response following stimulus termination, but were characterized by a long latency to response following stimulus onset. The mean responses of neurons in these three subgroups are portrayed in Fig. 1. A final group of neurons were inhibited by colorectal distension.

Neurons Excited by Colorectal Distension at Short Latency

The two subgroups of neurons excited by colorectal distension at short latency were more commonly encountered than other categories of neurons responsive to colorectal distension. An example of a neuron responding at short latency with an abrupt termination of the response coincident with stimulus termination is shown in Fig. 2. Neurons in this first subgroup (n = 10) responded within 1 s of stimulus onset and abruptly returned to baseline

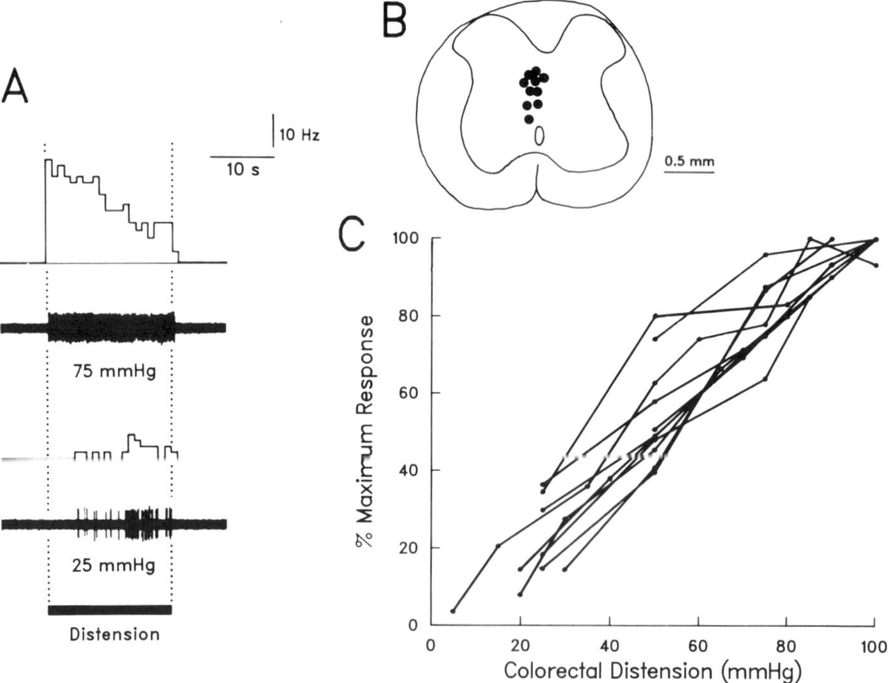

Fig. 2 A–C. Stimulus-response characteristics of neurons having short latencies to response onset and termination temporally related to the onset and termination of colorectal distension. **A** Peristimulus time histograms (1 s bin width) and oscillographic tracings illustrating the response of a neuron to two intensities of 20-s colorectal distension. **C** Stimulus-response functions of neurons (n = 10) whose recording sites are shown in **B**

within 1–2 s upon stimulus termination. Responses were either maintained at a steady rate during colorectal distension or exhibited a slow adaptation during the 20 s period of distension. The mean maximum response to 75–85 mmHg colorectal distension was 42.2 ± 7.4 imp/s; six of these 10 neurons were spontaneously active (10.3 imp/s). Eight of eight neurons tested were antidromically invaded from the contralateral cervical spinal cord and thus presumably convey information rostrally. Nine neurons had convergent scrotal/perianal cutaneous receptive fields which were generally small in size (~ 1 cm^2) and restricted to the ipsilateral anus/scrotum. Five of these nine neurons responded to cutaneous stimuli in a manner consistent with their classification on that basis as class 3 spinal neurons (i.e., responsive only to noxious stimuli); two were class 2 neurons. Stimulus-response functions for these neurons are shown in Fig. 2, as are the recording loci in the medial lumbosacral spinal cord. Neuronal thresholds for response to colorectal distension were estimated by extrapolation of the linear portion of the stimulus-response function to the abcissa. Least squares analysis of these stimulus-response functions yielded extrapolated thresholds for neuronal response near 0 mmHg.

The second subgroup of neurons (n = 12) excited by colorectal distension at short latency (1 s) exhibited a sustained response which outlasted the period of colorectal distension. An example of a neuron typical of this subgroup is illustrated in Fig. 3. Neuronal activity typically accelerated during colorectal distension, reaching a mean maximum of 49.6 ± 9.2 imp/s immediately before termination of 20 s distension. Excitation produced by distension in this subgroup of neurons continued for an additional 41.6 ± 10.4 s (range 4–120 s) after stimulus termination. Eight of these 12 neurons were spontaneously active (4.6 imp/s). Five of nine neurons tested had long ascending projections as demonstrated by antidromic

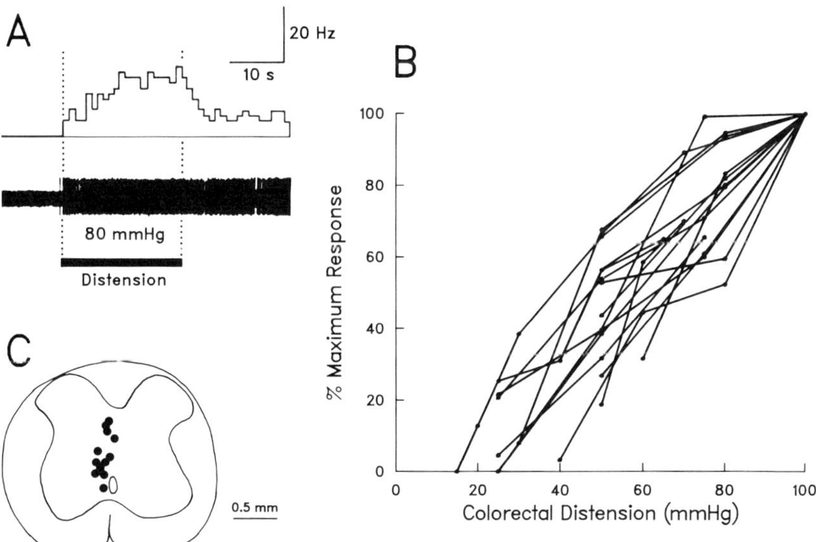

Fig. 3 A–C. Stimulus-response characteristics of neurons having a short latency to response onset and a sustained response to colorectal distension. **A** Peristimulus time histogram (1 s bin width) and oscillographic tracing illustrating the response of a neuron to 20-s, 80-mmHg colorectal distension. **B** Stimulus-response functions of neurons (n = 12) whose recording sites are shown in **C**

invasion from the cervical spinal cord; four of the total 12 neurons had convergent scrotal/perianal cutaneous receptive fields and were excited only by noxious pinch in the cutaneous receptive field (i.e., class 3). Neuronal thresholds for response of this subgroup of neurons to colorectal distension were estimated from least squares line analyses of their stimulus-response functions (Fig. 3B), yielding an extrapolated threshold for neuronal response of 14.7 ± 5.2 mmHg.

Thus, most neurons examined responded at short latency to colorectal distension. This group was divisible into two distinctly different subgroups. One subgroup ceased responding coincident with stimulus termination and have apparent thresholds of response to colorectal distension near 0 mmHg. The second subgroup exhibited an accelerating response during the period of colorectal distension which was sustained following termination of the distending stimulus. This subgroup have apparent thresholds of response to distension near 15 mmHg.

Neurons Excited by Colorectal Distension at Long Latency

A third group of neurons (n = 4) excited by colorectal distension exhibited relatively long latencies to respond to the distending stimulus (mean 7.5 s, range 6–12 s). An example of such a neuron is portrayed in Fig. 4. The neurons comprising this group exhibited accelerating responses during colorectal distension, attaining maximum responses (38 ± 6.5 imp/s) near or after termination of 20 s distension. Responses of these neurons were sustained for an additional mean 83.8 s (range 20–240 s) following stimulus termination. The latency to respond to colorectal distension appeared to be related to the intensity of the distending stimulus; the latency to respond was longer at lesser intensities of colorectal distension. None of the neurons examined exhibited rostral projections or convergent cutaneous receptive fields. Stimulus-response functions to graded colorectal distension in this small subgroup of neurons yielded an extrapolated response threshold of near 7 mmHg.

Neurons Inhibited by Colorectal Distension

A small sample of neurons (n = 4) were also encountered which were inhibited by colorectal distension. Examples are given in Fig. 5. Obviously, it was possible to study inhibition of neuronal activity by colorectal distension only in spontaneously active neurons. Since the rates of spontaneous activity were variable and different between neurons, it was difficult to establish latencies to inhibition reliably. It is apparent from examination of Fig. 5, however, that a relation exists between the distending pressure, the latency to onset of inhibition, and the duration of inhibition of neuronal activity.

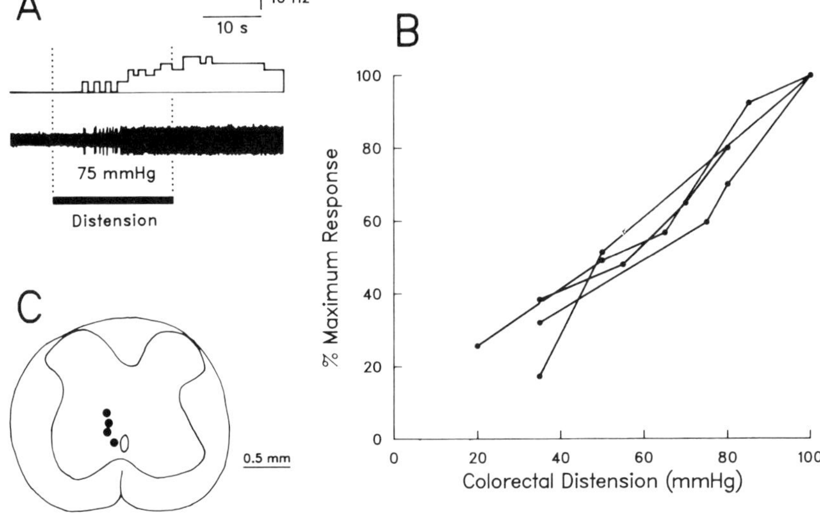

Fig. 4 A–C. Stimulus-response characteristics of neurons having a long latency to response onset and a sustained response to colorectal distension. **A** Peristimulus time histogram (1 s bin width) and oscillographic tracing illustrating the response of a neuron to 20-s, 75-mmHg colorectal distension. **B** Stimulus-response functions of neurons whose recording sites are shown in **C**

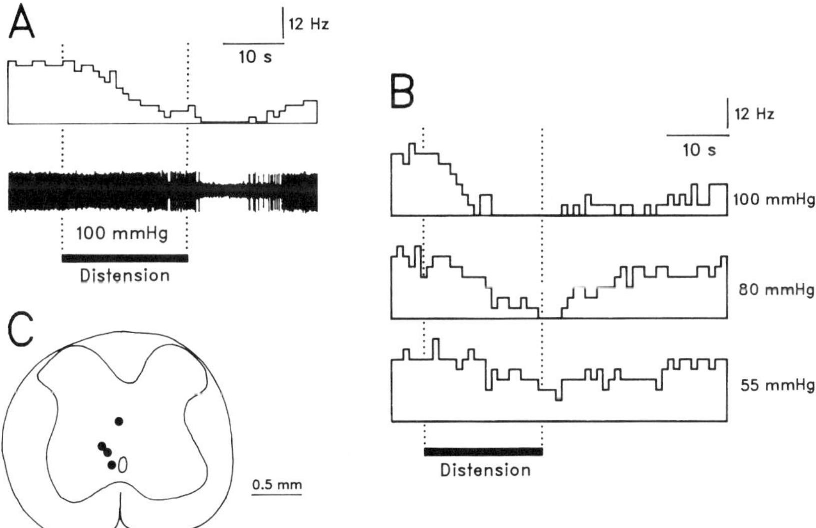

Fig. 5 A–C. Examples of neurons inhibited by colorectal distension. **A** Peristimulus time histogram (1 s bin width) and oscillographic tracing illustrating inhibition of spontaneous activity by 20-s, 100-mmHg colorectal distension. **B** Peristimulus time histograms (1 s bin width) of a neuron inhibited by different intensities of colorectal distension, suggesting a relation between the distending pressure, the latency to onset of inhibition, and the duration of inhibition of neuronal activity. **C** Recording sites of neurons inhibited by colorectal distension

Bradykinin Sensitivity

Additional support for the contention that neurons responsive to colorectal distension are involved in nociceptive processing is provided by chemosensitivity to the algesic peptide bradykinin. Intra-arterial injections were made into the abdominal aorta near its bifurcation. In the examples shown in Fig. 6, it can be seen that the latency to onset of bradykinin-induced excitation was short. Of the 26 neurons excited by colorectal distension reported here, 14 were tested and 11 were excited by bradykinin. Neurons inhibited by colorectal distension could also be inhibited by bradykinin administration. As shown in Fig. 6, responses to bradykinin were typically greater than produced by presumptive noxious colorectal distension. Intraarterial dye injections at the end of several experiments confirmed that bradykinin had been administered into the primary blood supply of the descending colon and rectum.

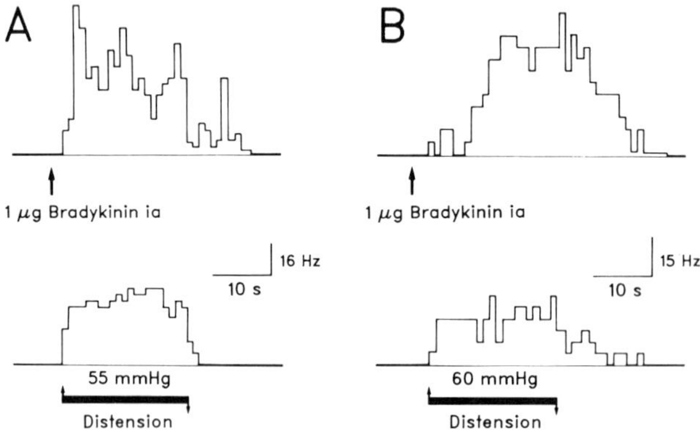

Fig. 6 A, B. Examples of neuronal responses to the intra-arterial (ia) injection of bradykinin. Neurons in **A** and **B** both responded to colorectal distension at short latencies; the neuron in **B** exhibited a sustained response. In both **A** and **B**, responses to bradykinin are shown to occur within seconds following its intra-arterial administration and to be greater than produced by presumptive noxious colorectal distension (55–60 mmHg)

Discussion

The present study describes three different subgroups of neurons in the medial lumbosacral spinal cord of the rat excited by colorectal distension. A fourth group of neurons was inhibited by colorectal distension. Many of the neurons excited at short latency by the distending stimulus were demonstrated to have long ascending projections as determined by antidromic activation in the ventrolateral cervical spinal cord and thus may be important to the rostrad transmission of visceral sensation. A role for these neurons in spinal nociceptive transmission is suggested by their relatively high thresholds of response to colorectal distension, responses to bradykinin, and convergence of nociceptive input from cutaneous receptive fields. Somatovisceral convergence onto rostrally projecting neurons, interpreted in the context of the convergence-projection theory of Ruch (see Cervero 1983), gives an explanation for reports of referred pain experienced in the perineum and other sacral dermatomes (Ritchie 1973; Swarbrick et al. 1980). The responses of many of these neurons are qualitatively similar to spinal dorsal horn neurons mediating nociceptive transmission from somatocutaneous structures. These findings suggest that a group of neurons in the medial lumbosacral spinal cord, including the area defined as lamina X, encode for visceral nociception and demonstrate, further, that information about distension of the gut transmitted to the medial lumbosacral spinal cord is involved not only in local short-loop reflexes, but also in long-loop reflexes and/or higher level processing of visceral sensations.

There is clinical and experimental evidence that distension of the colon and rectum, either due to pathological conditions or effected by a distending balloon, is extremely painful in humans. Pain has been reported when the volume/pressure inside the gut exceeds normal levels (e.g., at distending pressures of roughly 25 mmHg; see Blumberg et al. 1983). Investigations in animals have also utilized distension of hollow viscera (e.g., gall bladder and urinary bladder), the reported thresholds for activation of pseudaffective cardiovascular reflexes ranging between 20 and 50 mmHg (Cervero 1982; Schondorf et al. 1983). Similarly, colorectal distension evokes pseudaffective cardiovascular and visceromotor responses in rats at intracolonic pressures ≥20 mmHg (Ness and Gebhart 1986). This same stimulus has been demonstrated to increase significantly the latency of rats to "step down" in a passive avoidance paradigm and, further, not to be abolished by section of thoracolumbar visceral afferents ("sympathetic afferents") (Ness and Gebhart 1986). Taken together, these results provide support for the use of controlled colorectal distension as a noxious visceral stimulus in the rat. Typically, visceral chemical pain induced by the intraperitoneal administration of phenylquinone, acetic acid, hypertonic saline, etc. has been used in writhing models in the rat. As a model, writhing is somewhat less than satisfactory since (1) it is attenuated not only by analgetic but also by nonanalgetic drugs, and (2) rats cannot escape the stimulus, thus raising ethical concerns. Moreover, there is no physiologic/anatomic analysis of the writhing response to chemical stimulation of the peritoneal cavity. The development of a reliable, humane model of visceral pain which could be performed in either an anesthetized or waking, unrestrained animal would represent an improvement over presently employed models.

The electrophysiologic results reported here implicate neurons in the medial lumbosacral spinal cord in visceral nociceptive transmission. Two subgroups of neurons excited by colorectal distension had apparent mean thresholds of response between 7 and 15 mmHg colorectal distension, distending pressures near those reported as painful in humans and which also produce pseudaffective reflexes and avoidance behavior in rats. The short-latency, sustained-response subgroup of neurons is similar in many ways to spinal nociceptive neurons excited by cutaneous nociceptive stimuli (e.g., radiant heat). The apparent thresholds of response are at intensities believed noxious. Neuronal responses accelerate during the application of a controlled noxious stimulus and outlast the period of stimulation. It is well known that many spinal nociceptive neurons exhibit "wind-up" upon repeated stimulation. Although not quantitatively evaluated in the present study, the 4-min interval between repeated colorectal distension was selected on the basis of preliminary studies suggesting that too frequent colorectal distension can lead to unstable, enhanced neuronal responses to the distension. Thus, in many ways these neurons are similar to class 2 and/or class 3 spinal nociceptive neurons characterized in somatocutaneous systems.

Neurons which were excited by colorectal distension but quickly returned to baseline coincident with stimulus offset were commonly encountered. These neurons appear most similar to mechanoreceptors described for somatocutaneous structures, referred to as "tension receptors" in the walls of hollow organs (see Mei 1983) and also shown to exist in lumbosacral visceral afferents (Clifton et al. 1976). It should be noted, however, that these neurons appear to encode both non-noxious and noxious intensities of distension. It would appear, based upon the demonstration of long ascending projections, that neurons responding to colorectal distension at short latency, including those exhibiting sustained responses, subserve multiple functions. These neurons are likely components of cardiovascular and visceromotor reflexes as well as important second-order neurons leading to conscious sensation of colonic and rectal events. Because of their sustained and relatively high threshold for response to distension, the short-latency, sustained-response neurons are the most likely candidates for involvement in visceral nociceptive transmission. Neurons responding to colorectal distension at long latency, but having sustained responses, are probably not involved in the rostrad transmission of nociceptive information. Since none of these neurons were found to project as far as the cervical spinal cord, they are probably involved in local processing of colorectal information and/or short-loop reflexes. Neurons inhibited by colorectal distension may similarly be involved in reflex responses to colorectal distension (sphincter control, etc.).

In summary, the functional categorization of neurons in the medial lumbosacral spinal cord responsive to colorectal distension suggest that these neurons have probable roles in sensory transmission, including nociception, as well as involvement in vegetative aspects of visceral function. These results are, to the best of our knowledge, the first such reported for the rat and support the contention that visceral nociceptive processing occurs in the lower lumbar and sacral spinal cord.

Acknowledgements. The technical assistance of M. Burcham and A. Giner, and the secretarial assistance of T. Fuhrmeister are gratefully acknowledged. This work was supported by USPHS awards NS 19912, DA 02879, and T32 AMO1295.

References

Blumberg H, Haupt P, Jänig W, Kohler W (1983) Encoding of visceral noxious stimuli in the discharge patterns of visceral afferent fibers from the colon. Pflügers Arch 198 : 33–40

Cervero F (1982) Afferent activity evoked by natural stimulation of the biliary system in the ferret. Pain 13 : 137–151

Cervero F (1983) Mechanism of visceral pain. In: Lipton S, Miles J (eds) Persistent pain: modern methods of treatment, vol 4. Grune & Stratton, London, pp 1–19

Clifton GL, Coggeshall RE, Vance WH, Willis WD (1976) Receptive fields of unmyelinated ventral root afferent fibers in the cat. J Physiol (Lond) 256 : 573–600

Mei N (1983) Sensory structures in the viscera. In: Ottoson D (ed) Progress in sensory physiology, vol 4. Springer Berlin Heidelberg, New York, pp 1–42

Ness TJ, Gebhart GF (1986) Behavioral, cardiovascular, electrophysiologic and viseromotor responses to noxious colorectal distension in the rat. Neurosci Abstr 12 : 223

Ritchie J (1973) Pain from distension of the pelvic colon by inflating a balloon in the irritable colon syndrome. Gut 14 : 125–132

Schondorf R, Laskey W, Polosa C (1983) Upper thoracic sympathetic neuron response to input from urinary bladder afferents. Am J Physiol 245 : R311–R320

Swarbrick ET, Bat L, Hegarty JE, Williams CB, Dawson AM (1980) Site of pain from the irritable bowel. Lancet 2 : 443–446

Willis WD, Coggeshall RE (1978) Sensory mechanisms of the spinal cord. Plenum, New York, pp 129–160

33 The Physiology and Anatomy of Spinal Laminae I and II Neurons Antidromically Activated by Stimulation in the Parabrachial Region of the Midbrain and Pons

A. R. Light, E. Casale, and M. Sedivec

Three years ago Daniel Menétrey, Eugene Casale, and I were looking at the descending effects of stimulating in the parabrachial region on neurons in laminae I and II of the lumbar spinal cord. The parabrachial region is located at the junction between the midbrain and pons and surrounds the axons which become the superior cerebellar peduncle (the brachium conjunctivum). This region is extremely complex and has been implicated in a variety of functions, including autonomic reflexes such as cardiovascular control and respiration, and sensory functions such as taste and temperature (see for example, Fulwiler and Saper 1984).

During the course of our experiments we were surprised to find that quite a few lamina I neurons were antidromically activated by our electrodes in the parabrachial region, rather than inhibited as we had expected. We then initiated a series of studies to examine this phenomenon more closely.

Methods

Cats were anesthetized with sodium pentobarbital (i.p., 35 mg/kg) and maintained with this drug (i.v., 5–15 mg for each supplemental dose) for the duration of the experiment. For neurophysiologic recording from the lumbosacral region, cats were placed in a stereotaxic head holder and spinal frame, a laminectomy performed, a cannula inserted into the trachea for artificial respiration, and a bilateral pneumothorax made. The dorsal roots to L6–S1 were separated and placed on bipolar stimulating electrodes. Monopolar microelectrodes (10 megohm at 1000Hz) were inserted into the brain stem and thalamus and used to test for antidromic activation of spinal cord neurons. These electrodes were placed under stereotaxic control into the parabrachial region just dorsal to the brachium conjunctivum at the level of the pontomedullary junction and 3.75 mm lateral to midline. In all experiments one electrode was placed contralateral to the spinal cord recording site, and in many experiments another electrode was placed ipsilaterally. Stimulation intensity was 80 V at 0.1 ms during search procedures. In a few experiments, the stimulating electrode was moved in order to determine the lowest threshold stimulating site. These studies established that current spread to the spinothalamic tract was unlikely to occur. Some of the most effective antidromic activation sites in the contralateral brain stem are demonstrated in Fig. 1. In most experiments an electrode was placed in the contralateral medial or lateral thalamus.

Spinal cord neurons were recorded with glass micropipettes filled with 0.1 M Tris (pH 7.6), 0.5 M KCL, and 4 % horseradish peroxidase (HRP). The S1, L7, and L6 segments were searched for dorsal horn neurons. The search stimulus was stimulation once per second of the dorsal roots at an intensity sufficient to activate all classes of primary afferents. When a neuron was isolated extracellularly it was tested to determine the type of natural stimulation which excited it when applied to the receptive field, which was on the leg or foot. Once a neuron was classified, it was tested to determine whether it could be antidromically activated from the brain stem or thalamic regions. Criteria for antidromic activation included invariant latency, collision within a critical period, and ability to follow trains of 300-Hz sti-

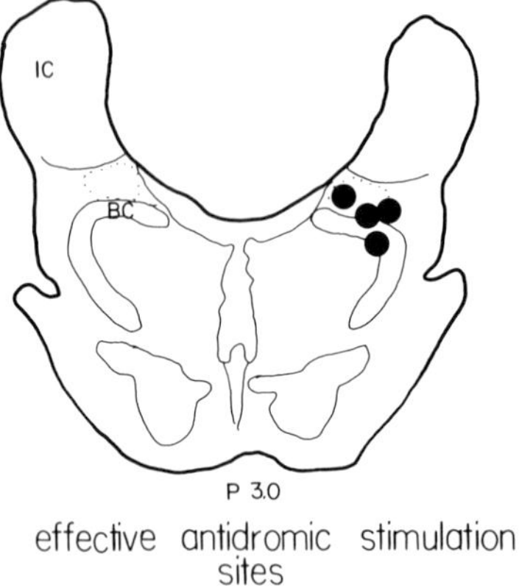

Fig. 1. Locations from which four lumbar spinal lamina I neurons were antidromically activated with the lowest thresholds. Filled circles indicate the locations of lesions made with the stimulating electrodes placed at the site of lowest threshold. The section is from the pontomedullary junction, at posterior 3.0 according to the Berman atlas. IC, inferior colliculus; BC, brachium conjunctivum

mulation with invariant latency. This last criterion often proved too stringent for extracellularly recorded neurons, as was verified by intracellular recordings in several neurons. This will be discussed later (see Fig. 3). Following extracellular characterization, the neurons were impaled for intracellular recording. Following these recordings, HRP was iontophoresed from the electrode. Recorded neurons were separated by at least 2 mm. After the recording session, the cats were perfused with paraformaldehyde/glutaraldehyde and the brain and spinal cord were removed and fixed overnight. The spinal cord was sectioned sagittally on a Vibratome at 50μm and the sections were reacted with 3.3'-diaminobenzidine + H_2O_2 and scanned with a microscope. Selected sections were reacted with osmium and embedded in plastics between teflon-coated coverslips. Neurons were reconstructed using a Nikon microscope and drawing tube.

Results

A total of 58 neurons were recorded which were antidromically activated from the parabrachial region. All but three of these were activated from the contralateral brain stem. In a sample of 26 tested neurons, 13 were activated only from the contralateral brain stem, three only from the ipsilateral brain stem, and 10 from both. The latencies from the two sides were often very different, with the contralateral one being shorter in most cases. Seven of the 58 neurons were also activated from the contralateral medial or lateral thalamus. The latency difference between activation from the thalamus and the brain stem suggested that the conduction velocity slowed down considerably between the brain stem and thalamus. Most of the antidromically activated neurons were nociceptive-specific (39 responded only to noxious pinch, 10 to both noxious pinch and noxious heat), with only five being multireceptive (responding to innocuous stimuli and higher frequency response to noxious stimuli). All of these neurons had discrete receptive fields, usually on the foot or leg confined to one hindlimb. None responded exclusively to innocuous mechanical stimulation. In addition, three neurons which were antidromically activated from the contralateral parabrachial region responded only to innocuous cooling of discrete receptive fields on the hindlimb. One antidromically activated neuron could not be activated by stimulation of the skin. (All 58 units were tested with all stimuli.) Electrical dorsal root stimulation activated 35 units with components associated only with A fibers, while 20 units exhibited components associated with both A and C fiber stimulation. Three units were activated only by stimulation at C fiber intensity, with two of these responding only to innocuous cooling and one responding only to noxious pinch. Most of the units responding to noxious stimulation demonstrated no or little ongoing discharge in the absence of stimulation, although a few demonstrated 1–10/s ongoing discharge. These units were difficult to antidromically activate due to collision of antidromic action potentials with ongoing discharges. All of the units responding to innocuous cooling demonstrated 1–10/s ongoing discharge.

The most impressive finding in these studies was the sheer number of superficial dorsal horn neurons which could be antidromically activated by stimulation in the parabrachial region. In 11 experiments in which more than one antidromically activated neuron was isolated, 89 nociceptive specific neurons were isolated, and of these 49 were antidromically

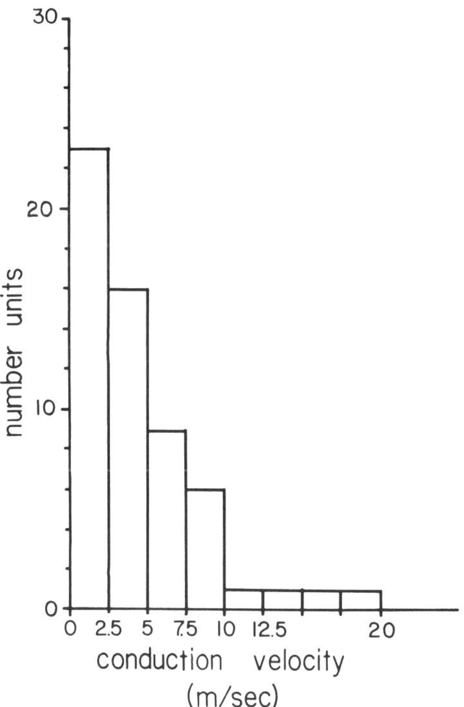

Fig. 2. Histogram of conduction velocities of the 58 neurons reported. Conduction velocity was calculated by dividing the conduction distance by the latency of the antidromic action potential evoked by stimulation in the parabrachial region

activated from the parabrachial region. Thus, 55% of the nociceptive-specific neurons recorded in the superficial dorsal horn were antidromically activated from this region of the brain stem.

The calculated conduction velocities of the ascending axons of the antidromically activated neurons were quite low. The overall average was 4.3 m/s; the range was 0.7 to 23.2 m/s. The average was 3.8 m/s for the nociceptive-specific neurons; 10.9 m/s for the multireceptive neurons; and 3.9 m/s for the innocuous cooling cells. Figure 2 indicates the distribu-

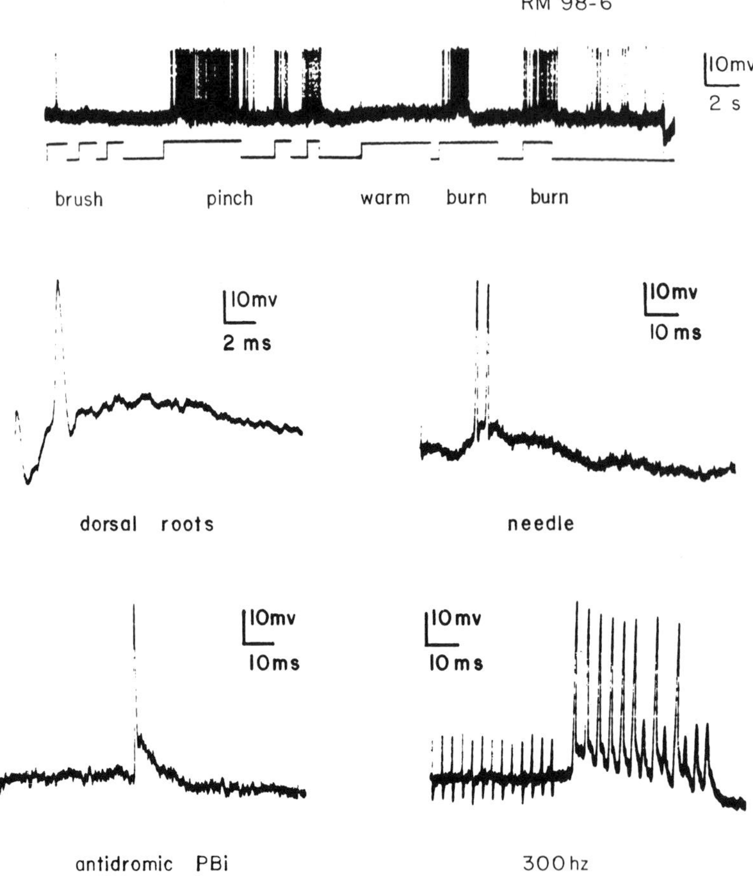

Fig. 3. Intracellular recording of a lamina I neuron which was antidromically activated by stimulation in the ipsilateral parabrachial region. The conduction velocity from this site was 7.4 m/s. The top trace shows the response to natural stimulation of the receptive field which was on the ventral-lateral part of the foot. The middle trace shows the response of this neuron to electrical stimulation of the dorsal roots (left) and electrical stimulation through needle electrodes placed in the receptive field in the foot (right). The bottom trace demonstrates the antidromic action potentials elicited by stimulation in the ipsilateral parabrachial region. The left-hand trace illustrates the results of a single stimulation, and the right-hand trace indicates the results of a train of stimuli delivered at 300 Hz. The spikes at the beginning of the trace are the shock artifacts. Note that action potentials 7,9,11–13 are much reduced in amplitude but are still all-or-none in character and, thus, may represent the initial segment (IS) action potentials

tion of conduction velocities with a histogram. As this figure indicates, many of the neurons had conduction velocities which would be consistent with that of unmyelinated axons.

Many neurons were also recorded intracellularly. Figure 3 illustrates data from one such neuron. The top trace indicates the neuron's response to natural stimulation of its receptive field, which was a 1.5-cm ovoid on the lateral side of the foot. As this figure indicates, the neuron did not respond to brushing with a soft camel-hair brush, but responded vigorously to pinch with flat forceps. It also did not respond to warming (holding a hot glass probe 5 mm from the skin), but did respond to noxious heat (touching the hot glass probe to the skin). As was the case in nearly all neurons, the somadendritic action potential failed when 300 Hz stimulation was delivered to the parabrachial region. However, the initial segment (IS) action potential faithfully followed all delivered stimuli. Neurons with slower conduction velocities tended to show more somadendritic failures than those with faster conduc-

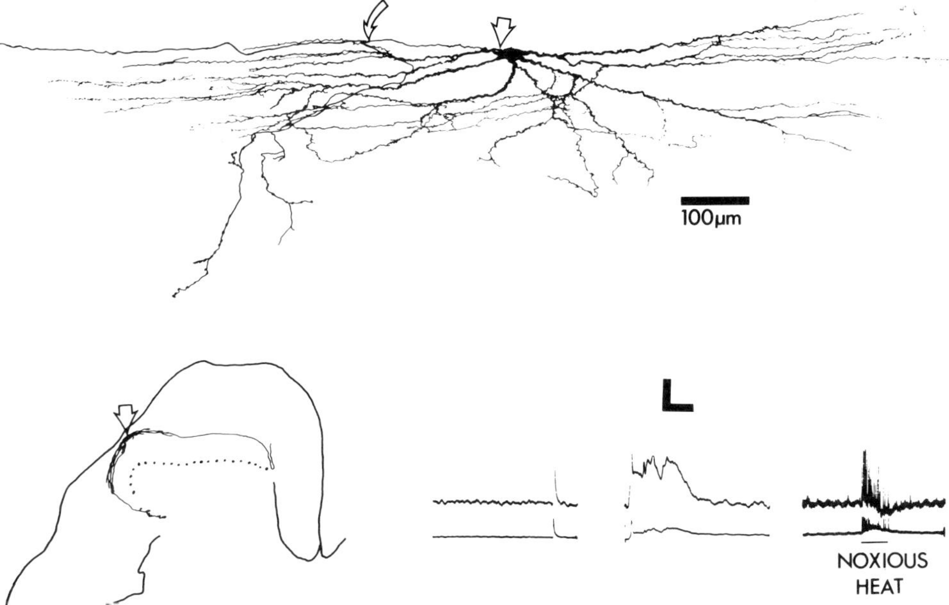

Fig. 4. Reconstruction (from 30 sagittal sections, 50 μm thick) of a lamina I neuron which was antidromically activated by stimulation of the contralateral parabrachial region. Note extensive dendritic spread and distribution of terminal axon collaterals to laminae I and V. The latency for the antidromic action potential was 410 ms. Given the conduction distance of 300 mm, the conduction velocity was 0.7m/s. The receptive field was on the foot and toes. Insert at left indicates the orientation of this neuron in the transverse plane. Note that the dendrites follow the outline of lamina I and the main axon also follows the outline of lamina I medially. The axon collaterals follow lamina I laterally and eventually reach lamina V. Inserts at bottom indicate the antidromic action potential, and intracellular recordings during electrical stimulation of the dorsal roots at Aα, Aδ, and C intensity, and during noxious heating of the receptive field. The arrow in the middle panel indicates the component of the EPSP which was evoked only by recruitment of C dorsal root fibers. The top and bottom traces in each panel are high-gain, AC-coupled and low-gain, DC-coupled traces respectively. The horizontal calibration bar in the left panel indicates 50 ms; in the middle panel, 20 ms; and in the right panel 0.5 s. The vertical calibration bars indicate 10 mV for each of the top traces and 50 mV for each of the bottom traces

tion velocities. Intracellular recordings like these verified that many neurons which would not follow 300 Hz stimulation when recorded extracellularly, had IS action potentials which followed 500 Hz stimulation faithfully.

Eleven cells were labeled by intracellular injection of HRP. Eight of these were in lamina I and three were in the outer part of lamina II (IIo). All of the labeled neurons were nociceptive-specific. Figure 4 illustrates a lamina I neuron which was intracellularly labeled. This neuron was a large Waldeyer cell with dendrites which ran rostral and caudal for several millimeters and transverse dendrites which wrapped around the dorsal horn. The conduction velocity for this neuron was surprisingly low, particularly in light of the relatively large diameter axon which was found to stem from this neuron. The initial portion of the axon was probably myelinated, as was indicated by the presence of darker staining at thinner areas which have been shown in the past to be nodes of Ranvier. The axon initially

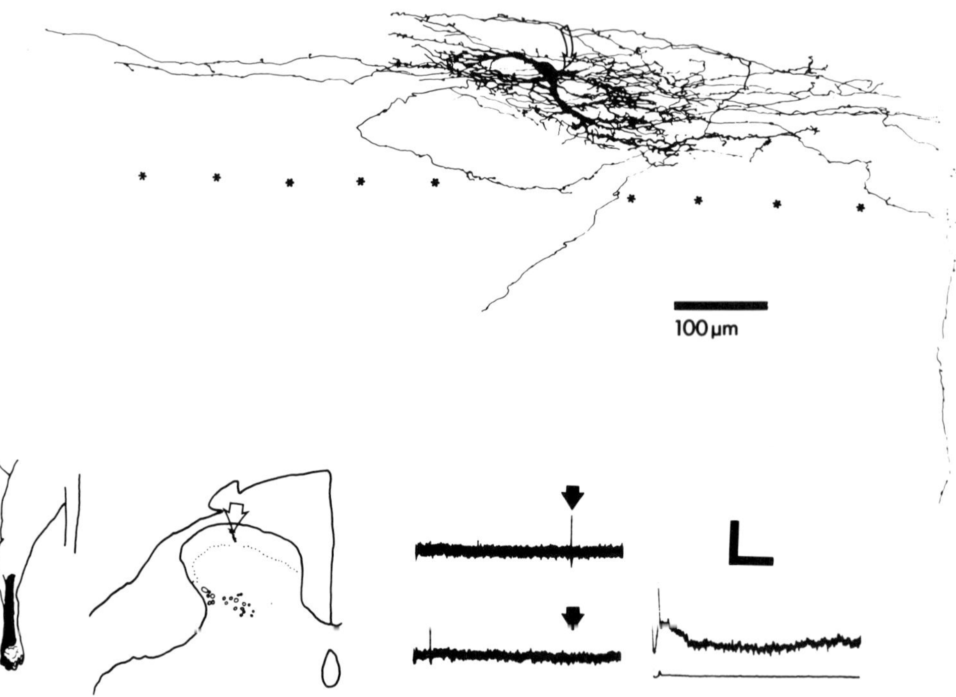

Fig. 5. Reconstruction (from seven sagittal sections, 50 μm thick) of a lamina II neuron which was antidromically activated from the contralateral parabrachial region with a latency of 375 ms. The conduction velocity of this neuron was 0.7 ms. Note the relatively restricted spread of dendrites and the extensive local collateralization of the axon, as well as axon projections to deeper laminae. The receptive field was on the heel and lower leg. Insert at left indicates the orientation of this neuron in the transverse plane. Inserts at right and far right indicate the extracellularly recorded antidromic action potential (arrow, top trace) and the lack of the antidromic action potential following collision (arrow, bottom trace), and the response to electrical stimulation of the dorsal roots during intracellular recording. The calibration for the right panel is 4 mV, 50 ms, while the calibration for the far right panel is 4 mV, 20 ms for the top trace and 50 mV for the bottom trace

coursed caudally and laterally before turning rostrally and medially and was followed to the midline where the reaction product faded. This neuron issued an axon collateral which terminated in laminae I and V. Axon collaterals were seen on most of the intracellularly labeled neurons which had been identified by antidromic activation from the parabrachial region.

Figure 5 illustrates a lamina II neuron which had been identified as projecting to the parabrachial region and which was labeled by intracellular injection of HRP. This neuron was a small neuron and is typical of many substantia gelatinosa neurons. Its axon branched many times and issued terminal collaterals within the vicinity of the cell body. In addition, some axon collaterals penetrated into deeper laminae of the dorsal horn where en passant and terminal enlargements were identified.

Discussion

The present study indicates that a large proportion of the recordable neurons in lamina I project at least as far rostrally as the parabrachial region in the rostral pons. The physiological properties of projecting neurons were similar to those reported previously for lamina I cells in general (Light et al. 1979). The precise termination of these projecting neurons cannot be determined with the present techniques. The axons of most presumably terminate somewhere below the thalamus, since only seven of the 58 recorded neurons could be additionally activated by stimulation in the thalamus. In addition, current spread to the spinothalamic tract can be ruled out because of empirical observations that moving the stimulating electrode 2 mm from the optimal stimulation region resulted in inability to activate the unit even at the highest stimulation strengths available. The probability that at least some of the recorded neurons terminated near the vicinity of the antidromic stimulating electrode is enhanced by the anatomical observation that many lamina I neurons terminate in the parabrachial region.

During the last 3 years, several anatomical papers have been published on the topic of the projection of lamina I neurons to the parabrachial region of the midbrain. These include retrograde and anterograde tracing studies by Wiberg and Blomqvist (1984) and similar studies by Panneton and Burton (1985) and Cechetto et al. (1985). These studies in cat and rat indicate that many lamina I neurons project to a small region that lies just dorsal to the brachium conjunctivum (superior cerebellar peduncle) at the junction of the pons and midbrain both ipsilaterally and contralaterally. The study by Panneton and Burton (1985) also indicates that few of the lamina I neurons which project to the parabrachial region also project to the thalamus. The results of the present study support these findings and demonstrate that most of the neurons projecting to the parabrachial region are nociceptive-specific.

This latter finding also agrees with a recent report by Hylden et al. (1986) in which lamina I, nociceptive-specific neurons were antidromically activated from a region of the mesencephalon which is quite close to the parabrachial region stimulated in the present study. The

Hylden et al. (1986) report is also similar to the present report in that the axons were slowly conducting and that few neurons could be additionally antidromically activated from the thalamus. One difference is that in the present study neurons were found projecting to the parabrachial region which responded only to innocuous cooling.

Conclusion

The present report suggests the following:

1. A large proportion of nociceptive lamina I neurons have long axons which project at least as far rostral as the parabrachial region of the pons and midbrain.
2. The parabrachial region may contain a region which receives and relays predominantly nociceptive-specific information and innocuous cooling information.
3. Lamina I and II neurons which project at least as far rostral as the midbrain have local axon collaterals in the spinal cord which may participate in the local integration of nociceptive information.

Acknowledgement. This research was supported by PHS, NINCDS grant NS16433

References

Cechetto DF, Standaert DG, Saper CB (1985) Spinal and trigeminal dorsal horn projections to the parabrachial nucleus in the rat. J Comp Neurol 240 : 153–160

Fulwiler CE, Saper CB (1984) Subnuclear organization of the efferent connections of the parabrachial nucleus in the rat. Brain Res Rev 7 : 229–259

Hylden JLK, Hayashi H, Dubner R, Bennett GJ (1986) Physiology and morphology of the lamina I spinomesencephalic projection. J Comp Neurol 247 : 505–515

Light AR, Trevino DL, Perl ER (1979) Morphological features of functionally defined neurons in the marginal zone and substantia gelatinosa of the spinal dorsal horn. J Comp Neurol 186 : 151–171

Panneton WM, Burton H (1985) Projections from the paratrigeminal nucleus and the medullary and spinal dorsal horns to the peribrachial area in the cat. Neuroscience 15 : 779–797

Wiberg M, Blomqvist A (1984) The spinomesencephalic tract in the cat: its cells of origin and termination pattern as demonstrated by the intraaxonal transport method. Brain Res 291 : 1–18

34 Functional Properties of Subnucleus Caudalis Lamina I Neurons Projecting to Nucleus Submedius

J. O. Dostrovsky, J. G. Broton, and N. K. Warma

Introduction

The spinothalamic tract and the portion of the trigeminothalamic tract which originates in the trigeminal subnucleus caudalis (SNC) are believed to be the primary pathways involved in conveying pain- and temperature-related information to thalamus (Dubner et al. 1978; Willis 1985). The cells of origin of these pathways are located primarily in laminae I, V, VII and VIII of the spinal cord (Willis 1985) and laminae I, V–VIII of SNC (Shigenaga et al. 1983). The main sites of termination of these tracts are the ventrobasal complex (VB), nucleus centralis lateralis (CL) and posterior nucleus (Burton and Craig 1983; Ralston 1984).

Recently Craig and Burton (1981) described an additional thalamic termination site for spinothalamic and trigeminothalamic tract neurons: nucleus submedius (Sm). Nucleus submedius is a small region immediately ventrolateral to the central medial nucleus and on the dorsal border of the ventromedial nucleus. This projection has been demonstrated in cat, rat, raccoon and monkey (Mantyh 1983; Burton and Craig 1983; Ralston 1984). The cells of origin are located exclusively in lamina I of the spinal cord dorsal horn and of SNC. In addition, neurons in Sm project quite specifically to a small region of the ventrolateral aspect of the orbital cortex in the cat (Craig et al. 1982). This region of cortex has a direct projection to the periaqueductal gray, a reciprocal projection to Sm and cortical projections to regions associated with the somatosensory system (Craig et al. 1982). Craig and Burton (1981) also mention having found neurons in Sm which respond to a noxious stimulus. On the basis of these findings, the fact that lamina I contains almost exclusively nociceptive-specific neurons and thermal neurons, and circumstantial evidence from various clinical reports, they suggested that Sm may be specifically involved in nociception.

The major aim of the present study was to characterize the response properties of SNC neurons that project to Sm. A brief report of this study has been published (Dostrovsky and Broton 1985).

Methods

Experiments were performed on 36 cats anesthetized with either chloralose or sodium pentobarbital. Details of animal preparation and maintenance have been described previously (Dostrovsky et al. 1983). A craniotomy was performed to expose the cortex overlying the thalamus. A fine-tipped glass-coated tungsten microelectrode was inserted vertically through thalamus so that its tip was in Sm. In order to determine the location of Sm, the same electrode was first stereotaxically introduced at A9.0, L5.0 and subsequently moved in a series of 0.5- or 1 mm steps in the mediolateral and rostrocaudal directions in order to determine, by single- and multiunit recordings, the location of the rostral, dorsal and ventral borders of the ventroposteromedial nucleus (VPM). Use was made of the somatotopy of VPM (Vahle-Hinz and Gottschaldt 1983) to estimate the position of a given track within VPM. The same electrode was then inserted 1 mm lateral to the midline at the rostrocaudal level of the rostral border of VPM and at a depth approximately midway between the dorsal and ventral borders of VPM. Although recordings were obtained from this medial track they were of no help in placing the electrode because the neurons in and around Sm did not appear to respond consistently to peripheral stimulation.

Recordings of neurons in SNC were obtained with glass-coated tungsten microelectrodes of the same type used for thalamic (Sm) stimulation. The electrode was inserted slowly into SNC while Sm was stimulated (usually at about 30 μA; 130 μA max, 0.1–0.2 ms, 10 Hz). When a unit was found which responded to thalamic stimulation, specific criteria were used to determine whether it was antidromically propagated: constant latency even with increased intensity, ability to follow two pulses at short intervals (<3 ms) and, when technically possible, collision of antidromic and orthodromic spikes at intervals shorter than the predicted collision interval (Lipski 1981). In addition, in later experiments the Sm electrode was moved up or down by up to 1 mm while the recording electrode was in lamina I to search for antidromic responses and to determine the depth corresponding to lowest stimulation threshold. The cell was then further studied to determine its responses to a variety of mechanical and thermal stimuli (application of a brush, wooden probe, flat forceps, serrated forceps, innocuous warming and cooling, and noxious warming and sometimes cooling) delivered to the orofacial region.

At the end of the experiment the stimulation site in thalamus was marked by passing a current of 10 μA for 10 s. An additional lesion was usually made 2 mm above the first lesion. In many experiments a recording site in the SNC was marked. The cat was then perfused with saline followed by 10 % buffered formalin and finally by 10 % formalin in 10 % sucrose. The head was removed and immersed in the latter solution and subsequently the brain was blocked in the stereotaxic coronal plane and placed in 30 % sucrose. The brain was then sectioned, mounted on chrome alum-coated slides and stained with cresyl violet.

Results

Characteristics of Antidromically Activated Neurons

A total of 79 SNC neurons were activated by stimulation within the contralateral Sm or on its borders. Each was activated at a constant latency and had a clear threshold for activation. This latency remained constant as the intensity of stimulation was increased. In addition, collision of the antidromic and orthodromic spikes at the appropriate collision interval was confirmed for all 35 neurons tested. For 26 cells the minimum interval between two stimuli at which the antidromic unit could still follow was determined and ranged from 0.8 to 2.2 ms. Figure 1A shows the location of an electrode track through Sm and the locations within Sm from where five SNC neurons could be antidromically evoked. Figure 1 also gives examples of the data collected from one of these neurons (N2) which was antidromically activated at a latency of 6.8 ms and followed two pulses at 1.8 ms (Fig. 1D). Figure 1E shows

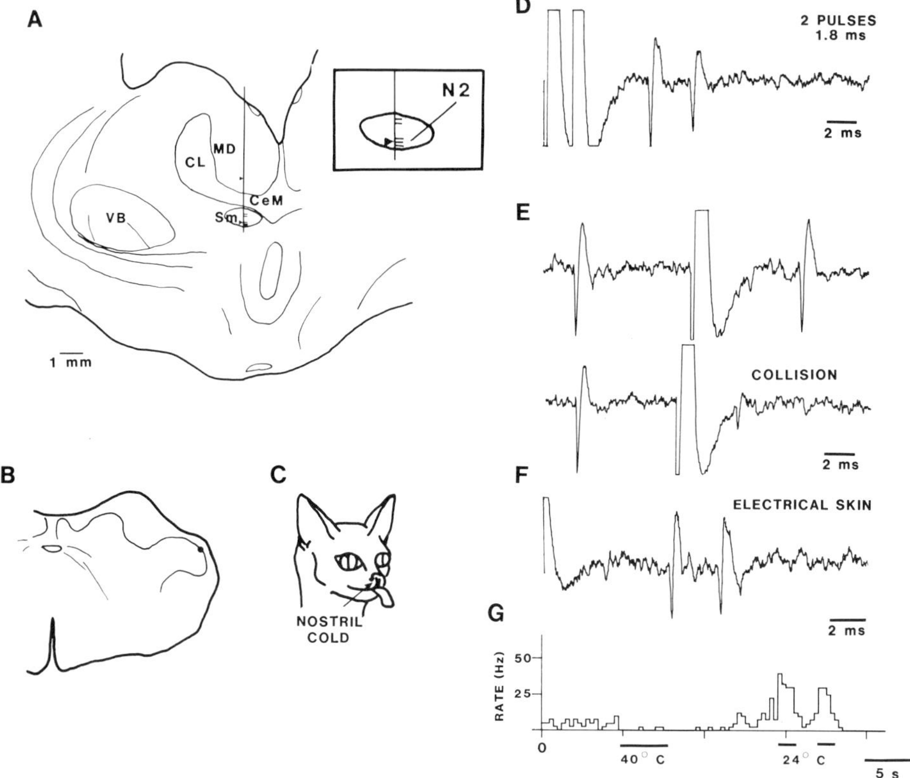

Fig. 1 A–G. This composite figure illustrates the type of data collected in these experiments. **A** The location in Sm (see inset) from where five SNC neurons could be antidromically activated (lowest threshold sites). **B** The recording site of unit N2 in lamina I of subnucleus caudalis. **C** The receptive field of this unit (in the nostril). **C** Digitized oscilloscope trace illustrating the ability of this neuron to follow two stimuli at an interval of 1.8 ms (note that the interval between the action potentials is significantly longer than 1.8 ms due to the decrease in the conduction velocity of the second spike which follows within the relative refractory period of the first). **E** Collision at intervals less than 7.2 ms. **F** Response of this neuron to electrical stimulation within its receptive field. **G** An event histogram showing the decrease in spontaneous rate by injection of warm water (40 °C) into the nostril and excitation by insertion of a cool metal probe at 24 °C into the nostril during the times indicated

an example of collision of the antidromic spike with an orthodromically occurring action potential when the interval between the occurrence of the orthodromically evoked spike and stimulation in Sm was less than 7.2 ms. Figure 2 is a histogram of the distribution of antidromic latencies. The mean latency of activation was 5.2 ms, which roughly corresponds to a conduction velocity of 4.8 m/s.

The mean threshold for antidromic activation was 35 ± 26 μA (0.1 ms pulse width) and ranged from a minimum of 2.5 μA to a maximum of 130 μA. In many cases the stimulating electrode was moved up and down in order to determine the depth where the minimum threshold occurred and how quickly the current threshold changed with distance from optimal site. Figure 3 shows the relationship of current threshold to depth for three neurons.

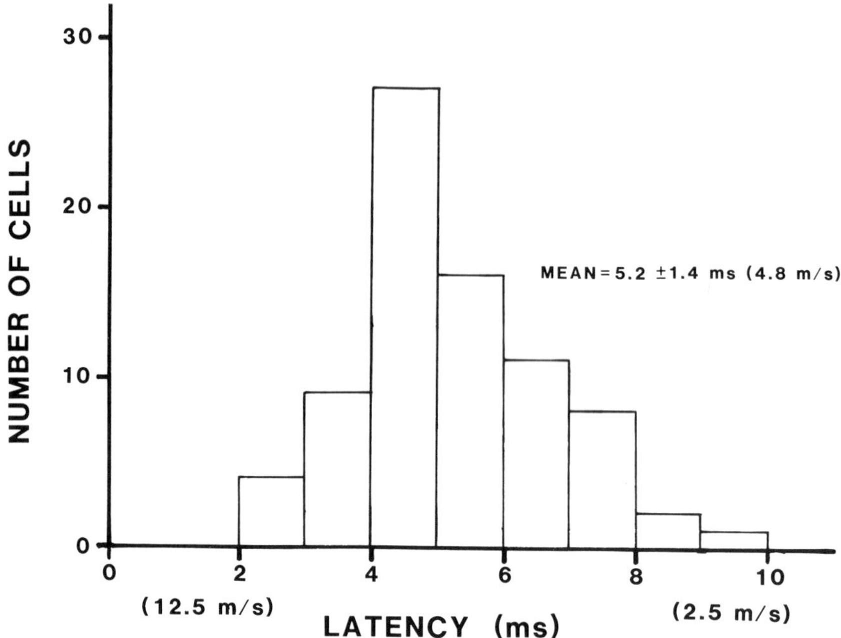

Fig. 2. Latency distributions of neurons in SNC antidromically activated by stimulation in or at the lateral edge of Sm (n = 79). The approximate mean, minimum and maximum conduction velocities are provided for reference

Location of Antidromically Activated Neurons

On the basis of location of lesions, micromanipulator readings and the presence at the recording site of neurons activated by cooling the skin (see Dostrovsky and Hellon 1978), all of the neurons reported here were located in or very close to lamina I. In many experiments we did not continue the electrode penetration once we reached the magnocellular layer (lamina III–IV) as evidenced by large-amplitude multiunit responses to low-threshold mechanical stimulation. However, in those experiments where we continued down to lamina V–VI, no antidromically activated neurons could be found even though we had successfully found such neurons above in lamina I. An example of the recording site of an antidromically activated neuron is shown in Fig. 1B.

Response Characteristics

Of the 79 neurons identified as antidromically activated from Sm, 43 could be classified according to their cutaneous inputs. No differences were noted in the characteristics of

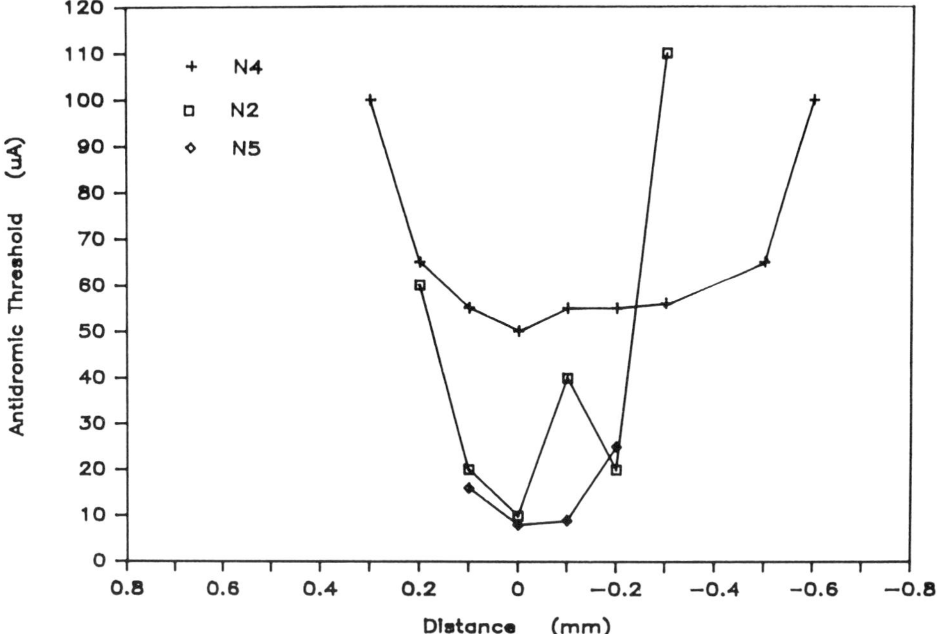

Fig. 3. Plots of antidromic threshold vs depth of the Sm electrode for the three antidromically activated cells, including the one illustrated in Fig. 1 (N2)

neurons recorded in chloralose- and pentobarbital-anesthetized cats. Most (81%) of the neurons were found to be cold neurons. These had properties as described previously by Dostrovsky and Hellon (1978). All displayed spontaneous activity which could be inhibited by slightly warming the receptive field with a radiant heat lamp. Some cold neurons could also be weakly activated by strong mechanical stimuli, but such responses may have been due to thermal changes induced by the mechanical stimulus. An example of the responses of a cold cell to warming and cooling the receptive field is given in Fig. 1G. The distribution of the antidromic latencies of cold cells was very similar to that of the whole population (Fig. 2) and had a mean of 5.1 ms.

Six (14%) of the neurons were classified as nociceptive-specific. All were activated by nociceptive mechanical stimulation of the tip of the nose. Most were spontaneously active, and only one was activated also by noxious skin heating. These neurons were antidromically activated by stimulation at the caudal (four cases), lateral (one case) or dorsal (one case) border of Sm and had a mean antidromic latency of 4.9 ms. It is possible that some of these may have been cold or warm neurons (Dostrovsky and Hellon 1978) with slight mechanical sensitivity but whose receptive field was within the nasal cavity and thus not readily accessible to application of thermal stimuli.

Two cells were encountered which had large well-isolated action potentials but for which no receptive field could be found.

Discussion

The findings of this study confirm in the cat the anatomical studies indicating the existence of a pathway from the superficial SNC to Sm (Craig and Burton 1981). The latencies of activation from Sm were on the average slightly longer than those found for the majority of SNC neurons activated from VPM in the study of Hu et al. (1981), but almost identical with the values reported by Dostrovsky and Hellon (1978) for SNC cold neurons antidromically activated from thalamus. The estimated mean conduction velocity of approximately 5 m/s is slightly higher than the mean value of 3.7 m/s that Craig and Kniffki (1985) reported for cat lamina I spinothalamic neurons. All of the neurons were in or close to lamina I, in agreement with the anatomical findings (Craig and Burton 1981), and in all those instances where we searched for neurons at greater depths none were found.

It is unlikely that the antidromic responses we observed resulted from activation of axons terminating in VPM or CL because the current thresholds were low and the increase in threshold as the Sm electrode was moved up or down was substantial (see Fig. 3). On the basis of these observations and results from other studies (Ranck 1975), current spread was probably less than 200 μm in most cases. This does not rule out activation of fibers of passage. However it is unlikely that ascending axons destined for structures other than Sm pass through this region (Burton and Craig 1983; Craig, personal communication).

The existence of many cold neurons with projections to Sm suggests that Sm may be involved in the processing of innocuous thermal information. Little is known about the thalamic representation of temperature. Poulos and colleagues (Auen et al. 1980; Poulos and Benjamin 1968) and Landgren (1960) have reported the existence of some neurons that respond to innocuous cooling of the tongue and which are located medial to VB but did not provide details of the exact recording sites. Dostrovsky and Hellon (1978) were able to antidromically activate some temperature-sensitive neurons (cold cells) in the SNC by stimulation in the region of VPM. In a few experiments they were also able to trace axons (using microstimulation mapping) of individual cold cells medially into the region of Sm but were unable to determine anatomically the exact termination sites (unpublished observations).

Only a small number of antidromically activated nociceptive neurons were found. These were activated at Sm sites near the caudal end of the nucleus or on its dorsal or lateral edge, but in view of the small sample size it is not clear whether this is a significant observation. These results raise the possibility that the nucleus receives both temperature and nociceptive information and that these sensibilities may be segregated in different parts of Sm. Craig et al. (1982) have reported that Sm can be subdivided into three regions, of which Sm_d and Sm_v are present at the levels stimulated in this study. It is tempting to speculate that Sm_d may be involved in nociception, as suggested by Craig and Burton (1981), and Sm_v in temperature sensation, although the resolution of the present study is not fine enough to provide definitive evidence for this.

In summary, these results have confirmed the existence of a projection from the superficial layers of the SNC to Sm. Furthermore, they indicate that innocuous thermal information is relayed to this region. The results also suggest that some nociceptive information reaches Sm, but unequivocal nociceptive inputs to this region remain to be demonstrated in further studies.

Acknowledgements. We wish to thank Mary Teofilo for excellent technical assistance. This study was supported by a grant from USNIDR DEO5404. JGB is an NIH postdoctoral fellow.

References

AUEN EL, POULOS DA, HIRATA H, MOLT JT (1980) Location and organization of thalamic thermosensitive neurons responding to cooling the cat oral-facial regions. Brain Res 191 : 260–264

BURTON H, CRAIG AD, JR (1983) Spinothalamic projections in cat, raccoon and monkey: a study based on anterograde transport of horseradish peroxidase. In: MACCHI G, RUSTIONI A, SPREAFICO R (eds) Somatosensory integration in the thalamus. Elsevier, New York, pp 17–41

BURTON H, CRAIG AD, Jr, POULOS DA, MOLT J (1979) Efferent projections from temperature sensitive recording loci within the marginal zone of the nucleus caudalis of the spinal trigeminal complex in the cat. J Comp Neurol 183 : 753–778

CRAIG AD, JR, BURTON H (1981) Spinal and medullary lamina I projection to nucleus submedius in medial thalamus: a possible pain center. J Neurophysiol 45 : 443–466

CRAIG AD, JR, KNIFFKI K-D (1985) Spinothalamic lumbosacral lamina I cells responsive to skin and muscle stimulation in the cat. J Physiol (Lond) 365 : 197–221

CRAIG AD, JR, WIEGAND SJ, PRICE JL (1982) The thalamocortical projection of the nucleus submedius in the cat. J Comp Neurol 206 : 28–48

DOSTROVSKY JO, BROTON JG (1985) Antidromic activation of neurons in the medullary dorsal horn from stimulation in nucleus submedius. Soc Neurosci Abstr 11 (1) : 217

DOSTROVSKY JO, HELLON RF (1978) The representation of facial temperature in the caudal trigeminal nucleus of the cat. J Physiol (Lond) 277 : 29–47

DOSTROVSKY JO, SHAH Y, GRAY BG (1983) Descending inhibitory influences from periaqueductal gray, nucleus raphe magnus and adjacent reticular formation. II. Effects on medullary dorsal horn nociceptive and nonnociceptive neurons. J Neurophysiol 49 : 948–960

DUBNER R, SESSLE BJ, STOREY AT (1978) The neural basis of oral and facial function. Plenum, New York

HU JW, DOSTROVSKY JO, SESSLE BJ (1981) Functional properties of neurons in cat trigeminal subnucleus caudalis (medullary dorsal horn). I. Responses to oral-facial noxious and nonnoxious stimuli and projections to thalamus and subnucleus oralis. J Neurophysiol 45 : 173–192

LANDGREN S (1960) Thalamic neurones responding to cooling of the cat's tongue. Acta Physiol Scand 48 : 255–267

LIPSKI J (1981) Antidromic activation of neurones as an analytical tool in the study of the central nervous system. J Neurosci Methods 4 : 1–32

MANTYH PW (1983) The spinothalamic tract in the primate: a re-examination using wheat-germ agglutinin conjugated to horseradish peroxidase. Neuroscience 9:847–862

POULOS DA, BENJAMIN RM (1968) Response of thalamic neurons to thermal stimulation of the tongue. J Neurophysiol 31:28–43

POULOS DA, BURTON H, MOLT JT, BARRON KD (1979) Localization of specific thermoreceptors in spinal trigeminal nucleus of the cat. Brain Res 165:144–148

RALSTON HJ III (1984) Synaptic organization of spinothalamic tract projections to the thalamus, with special reference to pain. In: KRUGER L, LIEBESKIND JC (eds) Advances in pain research and therapy, vol 6. Raven, New York, pp 183–195

RANCK JB Jr (1975) Which elements are excited in electrical stimulation of mammalian central nervous system: a review. Brain Res 98:417–440

SHIGENAGA Y, NAKATANI Z, NISHIMORI T, SUEMUNE S, KURODA R, MATANO S (1983) The cells of origin of cat trigeminothalamic projections especially in the caudal medulla. Brain Res 277:201–222

VAHLE-HINZ C, GOTTSCHALDT KM (1983) Principal differences in the organization of the thalamic face representation in rodents and felids. In: MACCHI G, RUSTIONI A, SPREAFICO R (eds) Somatosensory integration in the thalamus. Elsevier, New York, pp 125–145

WILLIS WD (1985) The pain system. Karger, Basel (Pain and headache, vol 8)

35 Neurons in the Rostral Spinal Trigeminal Nucleus Excited by Stimulation of the Middle Meningeal Artery and Superior Sagittal Sinus

K. D. Davis and J. O. Dostrovsky

Introduction

Vascular headaches are thought to develop following a disturbance in cranial vascular tone (Wolff 1972). Both the middle meningeal artery (MMA) and the superior sagittal sinus (SS) are pain-sensitive structures (Northfield 1938; Penfield and McNaughton 1940; Ray and Wolff 1940; Feindel et al. 1960) which may be involved in mediating vascular head pain. It is well established that the trigeminal (V) nerve innervates both the MMA and the SS (McNaughton 1938; Penfield and McNaughton 1940; Feindel 1954; Feindel et al. 1960; Kimmel 1961), and recent anatomical studies (Mayberg et al. 1984; Steiger and Meakin 1984; O'Connor and van der Kooy 1986) indicate that the cell bodies of these sensory primary afferents are located in the ophthalmic division of the V ganglion. Unfortunately, the central terminals of the MMA and SS primary afferents were not located in these studies. However, using electrophysiological techniques we have recently located a population of V subnucleus caudalis (SNC) neurons which were excited by stimulation of the MMA and also by cutaneous nociceptors in the periorbital skin (Davis and Dostrovsky 1986 a). These data provide support for the hypothesis that the referral of vascular headaches to the ophthalmic region of the face is due to the convergence of cutaneous and vascular afferents onto central neurons in the spinal nucleus of V. An alternative hypothesis to explain referred vascular head pain requires individual axons which dichotomize to innervate cutaneous and vascular structures. This is an unlikely explanation, since anatomical studies have revealed that the primary afferents which innervate dural (Borges and Moskowitz 1983) or cerebral (McMahon et al. 1985; O' Connor and van der Kooy 1986) arteries are not axon collaterals of V ophthalmic cutaneous afferents.

In the present study we provide further support for the convergence theory of referred pain by reporting the existence of cells at more rostral regions of the nucleus of spinal V which are excited by MMA and /or SS stimulation and which also have periorbital receptive fields (RFs).

Methods

Experiments were performed on 21 adult cats weighing 2.5 - 3.5 kg and anesthetized with either intravenous alpha-chloralose (60 mg/kg) or sodium pentobarbital (35 mg/kg). Mean arterial pressure, expired CO_2 and rectal temperature were monitored and maintained within their physiological range (see Davis and Dostrovsky 1986 b). The animal's head was secured in a stereotaxic frame and craniotomy was performed to gain access to the V subnucleus oralis (Vo) and interpolaris (Vi) and to expose the SS and the right MMA. The right temporalis muscle was partially removed to allow a more complete exposure of the MMA. The SS was isolated by slitting the dura on either side and then resting the SS in a saline-filled trough made out of polyethylene tubing. Pairs of silver ball electrodes were then placed in contact with the MMA and SS.

Tungsten microelectrodes were used to record the extracellular unit activity of Vo and rostral Vi neurons in response to bipolar electrical stimulation (0.1–0.5 ms pulses, < 16 mA, 1–3 Hz) of the MMA an/or SS. Whenever possible, cells were also examined for the existence of excitatory inputs from the facial skin and/or cornea. Mechanical (brush, pressure, noxious pinch) and radiant heat stimuli were used to characterize the cutaneous RF. Cells were then classified as nociceptive specific (NS), wide dynamic range (WDR) or low-threshold mechanoreceptive (LTM) according to standard criteria (see Davis and Dostrovsky 1986 a). Cells which responded exclusively to mechanical stimuli applied to the cornea were classified as cornea only cells. Electrolytic lesions (15 μA for 15 s) were made at selected sites and were later verified histologically (see Davis and Dostrovsky 1986 b).

Results

A total of 120 cells excited by MMA and/or SS stimulation were studied. Eighty-six cells responded to MMA stimulation and 58 to SS stimulation. Of the cells which were tested for excitation induced from both sites (**n** = 86) 28 % could be activated from both the MMA and the SS (MMA/SS cells). The average minimum latencies to activation from the MMA and SS for the entire population of cells were 12.4 ± 0.9 ms and 16.4 ± 1.1 ms respectively.

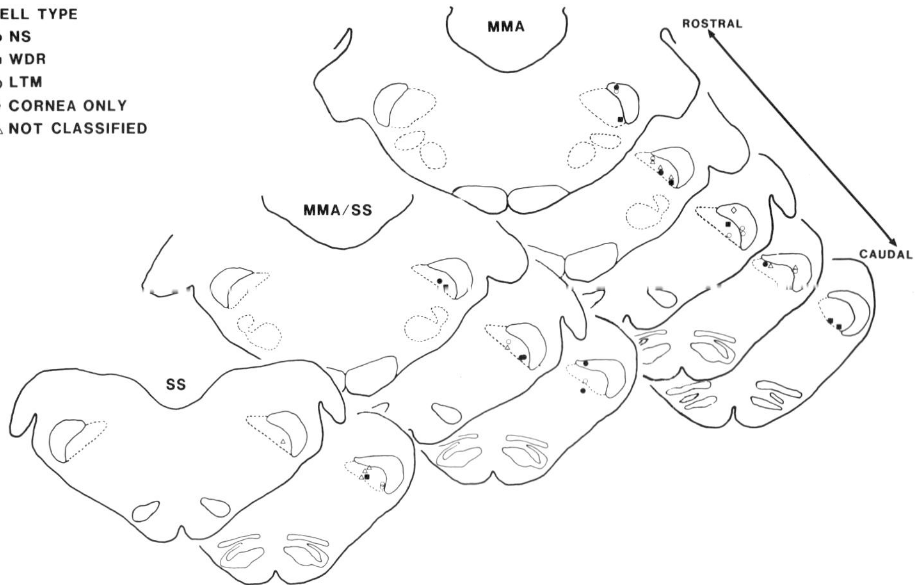

Fig. 1. Histological reconstruction of recording sites. From right to left on each set of coronal brainstem sections, the recovered recording sites of cells excited by middle meningeal artery (MMA), both MMA and superior sagittal sinus (SS), and SS stimulation are indicated

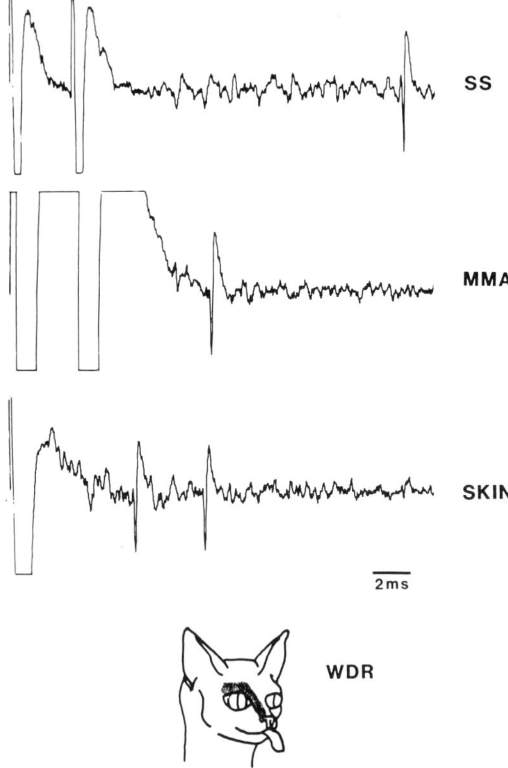

Fig. 2. Example of a MMA/SS-activated WDR neuron. Typical oscilloscope traces (from top to bottom) show excitation of the neuron following electrical stimulation of the superior sagittal sinus (SS; double pulses), middle meningeal artery (MMA; double pulses) and supraorbital skin (single pulse). The neuron's receptive field is indicated by the shaded area on the drawing of the cats face below the traces

Histological reconstruction of 36 of the recording sites indicates that most cells were located laterally and/or ventrally in either Vo or rostral Vi. Eight cells were located in the interstitial nucleus of the spinal tract of V. All of the recovered recording sites are shown in Fig. 1.

A peripheral RF was found for all cells (**n** = 64) studied in detail. Most cells (72 %) had RFs within or including the ophthalmic region. The RFs of half of these cells were confined to the ophthalmic region and for the other half the RFs involved maxillary and sometimes also mandibular regions in addition to ophthalmic regions. The remaining cells (28 %) had their RFs confined to maxillary and/or mandibular regions. Figure 2 shows an example of a WDR cell excited by both MMA and SS stimulation which had a RF that encompassed the ipsilateral nose and supraorbital skin area.

Based on the responses to mechanical cutaneous stimulation, a substantial percentage of cells excited by MMA (63 %), SS (33 %) and MMA + SS (73 %) stimulation were classified as nociceptive (i. e. WDR or NS), and the remainder were LTM neurons (see Table 1). Further-

Table 1. Classification of Vo/Vi Neurons

	No. of cells			
Cell type	MMA	SS	MMA/SS	Total
NS	10	1	7	18
WDR	12	3	4	19
LTM	13	8	4	25
Cornea only	2	0	0	2
Unclassified	25	22	9	56
Total	62	34	24	120

more, of the cells whose RFs included ophthalmic regions, 78 % of the MMA-, 80 % of the MMA/SS- and 30 % of the SS-activated cells were classified as either NS or WDR. Two cells were found which did not respond to mechanical cutaneous stimuli but responded to mechanical stimulation of the cornea.

Discussion

We have recently shown that stimulation of the MMA can excite a population of neurons in the lateral aspect of SNC (Davis and Dostrovsky 1986 a). We now report that neurons rostral to SNC can be excited by stimulation of the MMA and also the SS. The latency to activation of Vi/Vo neurons from the MMA was not significantly longer than the latency to activation of SNC cells from the MMA (see Davis and Dostrovsky 1986 a). This suggests that sensory information from the MMA most likely reaches the neurons in Vi and Vo directly, not via a relay in SNC.

A substantial number of the rostral neurons received a nociceptive input from the facial skin. This was a surprising result in light of the traditional view that the rostral V subnuclei are regions primarily involved with the processing of innocuous information and the low incidence of nociceptive neurons reported by others (see Davis and Dostrovsky 1986 b). However, there is increasing evidence that the rostral V subnuclei may be involved in pain sensibility (e. g. Vyklicky et al. 1977; Nord and Young 1979; Broton and Rosenfeld 1982, 1985; Young, 1982; Davis and Dostrovsky 1986 a; Falls 1986). The discrepancy between our results and those of others is probably due to the standard use of innocuous search stimuli by others whereas we have used MMA/SS stimulation to search for cells. Our method of locating neurons may be more selective for nociceptive neurons which could account for the relatively high proportion of nociceptive neurons found in this study.

The pattern of convergent inputs primarily from the ophthalmic skin onto the rostral V cells was similar to that found for the SNC cells, although a greater proportion of the rostral cells had maxillary and/or mandibular RFs. It has been suggested (Ruch 1961) that central neurons receiving convergent inputs from visceral and cutaneous structures could be involved in mediating the sensation of referred pain. Since many of the neurons in this study received a nociceptive input from the periorbital region, they may be involved in the referral of vascular head pain to that area of the face.

Conclusions

Neurons were found in the rostral V brain stem nuclei which were excited by stimulation of the MMA and/or SS and thus may be involved in mediating vascular head pain. Most of these cells received convergent inputs from cutaneous nociceptors in the periorbital region. Therefore, the results suggest that nociceptive neurons in the V brain stem nucleus are involved in mediating vascular head pain and provide an explanation for the referral of vascular head pain to the periorbital region.

Acknowledgements. The authors thank Mary Teofilo for her expert technical assistance. This project was supported by U.S. Public Health Service grant DEO5404.

References

Broton JG, Rosenfeld PS (1982) Rostral trigeminal projections signal perioral facial pain. Brain Res 243 : 395–400

Broton JG, Rosenfeld PJ (1985) Effects of trigeminal tractotomy on facial thermal nociception in the rat. Brain Res 333 : 63–72

Borges LF, Moskowitz MA (1983) Do intracranial and extracranial trigeminal afferents represent divergent axon collaterals? Neurosci Lett 35 : 265–270

Davis KD, Dostrovsky JO (1986 a) Activation of trigeminal brain-stem nociceptive neurons by dural artery stimulation. Pain 25 : 395–401

Davis KD, Dostrovsky JO (1986 b) Modulatory influences of red nucleus stimulation on the somatosensory responses of cat trigeminal subnucleus oralis neurons. Exp Neurol 91 : 80–101

Falls WM (1986) Morphology and synaptic connections of myelinated primary axons in the ventrolateral region of rat trigeminal nucleus oralis. J Comp Neurol 244 : 96–110

Feindel W (1954) The nervi tentorii and intracranial pain. Anat Rec 118 : 298

Feindel W, Penfield W, McNaughton F (1960) The tentorial nerves and localization of intracranial pain in man. Neurology (Minneap) 10 : 555–563

KIMMEL DL (1961) The nerves of the cranial dura mater and their significance in dural headache and referred pain. Chicago Med Sch Q 22 : 16–26

MAYBERG MC, ZERVAS NT, MOSKOWITZ MA (1984) Trigeminal projections to supratentorial pial and dural blood vessels in cats demonstrated by horseradish peroxidase histochemistry. J Comp Neurol 223 : 46–56

MCMAHON MS, NORREGAARD TV, BEYERL BD, BORGES LF, MOSKOWITZ MA (1985) Trigeminal afferents to cerebral arteries and forehead are not divergent axon collaterals in cat. Neurosci Lett 60 : 63–68

MCNAUGHTON FL (1938) The innervation of the intracranial blood vessels and dural sinuses. Assoc Res Nerv Ment Dis 18 : 178–200

NORD SG, YOUNG RF (1979) Effects of chronic descending tractotomy on the response patterns of neurons in the trigeminal nuclei principalis and oralis. Exp Neurol 65 : 355–372

NORTHFIELD DWC (1938) Some observations on headache. Brain 61 : 133–162

O'CONNOR T, VAN DER KOOY D (1986) Pattern of intracranial and extracranial projections of trigeminal ganglion cells. J Neurosci 6 : 2200–2207

PENFIELD W, MCNAUGHTON F (1940) Dural headache and innervation of the dura mater. Arch Neurol Psychiatry 44 : 43–75

RAY BS, WOLFF HG (1940) Experimental studies on headache. Arch Surg 41 : 813–856

RUCH TC (1961) Pathophysiology of pain. In: RUCH TC, PATTON HD, WOODBURY JW, TOWE AL (eds) Neurophysiology. Saunders, Philadelphia, pp 350–368

STEIGER HJ, MEAKIN CJ (1984) The meningeal representation in the trigeminal ganglion – an experimental study in the cat. Headache 24 : 305–309

VYKLICKY L, KELLER O, JASTREBOFF P, VYKLICKY L, BUTKHUZI SM (1977) Spinal trigeminal tractotomy and nociceptive reactions evoked by tooth pulp stimulation in the cat. J Physiol (Paris) 73 : 379–386

WOLFF HG (1972) Headache and other pain. Oxford University Press, New York

YOUNG RF (1982) Effects of trigeminal tractotomy on dental sensation in humans. J Neurosurg 56 : 812–818

36 Classification of Somatosensory Tract Cells by Cluster Analysis

W. D. Willis, D. J. Surmeier, J. M. Chung, D. G. Ferrington, C. N. Honda, J.W. Downie, and L. S. Sorkin

Introduction

Neurons in the spinal cord dorsal horn have been classified according to their response properties in several different ways (Willis and Coggeshall 1978). A common approach is to use the relative responsiveness to innocuous and noxious mechanical stimulation of the skin as the basis for a classification into three major types of neuron: low threshold (LT; responsive to innocuous but not additionally to noxious stimuli), wide dynamic range (WDR; responsive to innocuous but more so to noxious stimuli), and high threshold (HT; responsive only to noxious stimuli) (cf. Mendell 1966; Chung et al. 1979; Price and Dubner 1977). There are several problems with this classification scheme. First, most laboratories classify somatosensory neurons on the basis of qualitative tests of their responsiveness to batteries of stimuli that vary widely from investigator to investigator. Secondly, there is a semantic objection to the term "wide dynamic range," and this has led to the proposal that "multiconvergent" be used instead (Brown and Rethelyi 1981). Thirdly, different laboratories consider neurons with quite different response profiles to belong to this class of cell. For example, LeBars and Chitour (1983) used the term "convergent neuron" for cells that respond best to innocuous stimuli but that have an incrementing response to graded noxious stimuli. Our laboratory would consider such neurons to belong to the LT class. Finally, and most importantly, the response profiles of dorsal horn neurons vary sufficiently to make it difficult to categorize many cells on an intuitive basis (Chung et al. 1986).

It seemed to us that an objective and quantitative approach to determine natural groupings of somatosensory neurons was needed. We have begun to use a statistical approach - k means cluster analysis - for this purpose. In addition, a principal components analysis can be employed to allow us to display the groupings determined by cluster analysis in the plane that accounts for most of the variance. Cluster and principal components analysis are two of several kinds of multivariate statistical analyses that have proven useful for studies of sensory systems, especially of the chemical senses (Bieber and Smith 1986).

We applied these analytic procedures first to spinothalamic tract (STT) cells and to neurons of the ventral posterior lateral (VPL) nucleus of the thalamus in the monkey (Chung et al. 1986; Surmeier et al. 1986a,b). Next we used the analysis for dorsal horn interneurons (Sorkin et al. 1986) and STT cells in the cat cervical spinal cord (Ferrington et al. 1986), STT cells in the superficial dorsal horn of the monkey (Ferrington et al., in press), and neurons of the spinocervical tract (SCT), lateral cervical nucleus (LCN), and nucleus gracilis (NG) of the monkey (Downie et al., in preparation; Ferrington et al., in preparation). We believe that this analysis not only allows an objective classification of somatosensory neurons but also provides clues about differences in the functional properties of various ascending somatosensory pathways. Some of these differences appear to depend upon inputs from fine afferent fibers, particularly those from nociceptors.

Methods

The animals used were macaques (**Macaca fascicularis**) anesthetized with α-chloralose and sodium pentobarbital. Extracellular recordings were made with carbon filament microelectrodes (Anderson and Cushman 1981) or with electrolyte-filled (3M potassium acetate) micropipettes. All units examined were identified by antidromic activation, either from the contralateral VPL thalamic nucleus (STT, LCN and NG cells) or from the ipsilateral spinal cord dorsal lateral fasciculus at the C3 (but not Cl) segmental level (SCT cells).

After mapping the receptive field of a neuron, its responses to four mechanical stimuli were tested. These stimuli included, in sequence: BRUSH (with a camel hair brush, a tactile stimulus), PRESSURE (by application of a large arterial clip to the skin, a marginally painful stimulus in human subjects), PINCH (by application of a small arterial clip to the skin, a distinctly painful stimulus), and SQUEEZE (by compressing the skin firmly with serrated forceps, a very painful stimulus). The stimuli were each maintained for 10 s. An effort was made to apply these stimuli in a uniform fashion across trials; however, it should be recognized that there was necessarily some variation in the stimuli due in part to insufficient stimulus control and in part to differences in the region of the skin being stimulated. On the other hand, these factors were common to all of the experiments and could not account for substantial differences in responses of neurons belonging to different pathways.

Responses were recorded as pulses from a window discriminator set to detect the action potentials of only the neuron under investigation. The pulses were led to a digital computer for analysis. Background activity was subtracted from each response. The data were then treated in one of two ways. For comparisons of the responses of individual neurons to the four mechanical stimuli, the responses were normalized by assigning a value of 100 % to the largest response for each neuron and the appropriate smaller percentages to the other responses. For comparisons of the responses across the population of neurons to the four stimuli, a different procedure was used. A standard score was assigned to each response. The scores were based upon the response distribution of the pooled population to the same stimulus. The normalized or standardized response profiles were then evaluated by a k means cluster analysis, using the Systat data analysis package on a microcomputer. For the present report, the responses that were analyzed included those of STT cells in laminae I and IV-VI and neurons of the LCN and of the NG.

The normalized or standardized response profiles were also subjected to a principal components analysis. The four responses resulted in a distribution of data points in four spatial dimensions. The axis through this distribution that accounts for the largest proportion of the variance in the data is the first principal component. The second principal component is an axis orthogonal to the first and accounts for the largest proportion of the remaining variance of the data. The third and fourth principal components account for the residual variance. A two-dimensional scattergram of the data in the plane of the first two principal components (after rotation using the varimax method) yielded a satisfactory plot of the distribution of the data (accounting for about 75 %–85 % of the variance).

Results

Combined Population of Somatosensory Neurons

A k means cluster analysis of a population of 253 somatosensory neurons (150 STT cells, nine SCT and three similar spinal tract cells, 40 LCN neurons, and 51 NG cells) indicated that, based on their normalized responses to four standard mechanical stimuli, these neurons could be described as belonging to four clusters. We have elected to call these groups of neurons types 1–4. The average response profiles of these four cell types are shown in Fig. 1 A-D, and a plot of the profiles in the plane of the first two principal components is seen in Fig. 1G.

Type 1 cells were excited best by the BRUSH stimulus (Fig. 1A). Type 2 cells responded well to all of the stimuli, but relative to other classes of neuron they were particularly responsive to PRESSURE (Fig. 1B). Type 3 cells appeared to have a steep stimulus-response function, since there was a large response increment between the PRESSURE and PINCH stimuli, but the response apparently saturated and so there was no increase in the response to SQUEEZE (Fig. 1C). Type 4 neurons had small responses to the weaker stimuli, but a maximum response to SQUEEZE (Fig. 1D).

The principal component plot in Fig. 1G shows that the four clusters are relatively well separated, although there is some apparent overlap, especially between clusters 3 and 4. The apparent overlap is the result of the fact that some of the variance of the data occurs in principal components 3 and 4, which are orthogonal to the plane that was plotted. The factor loadings for the principal component plot are shown in Fig. 1E and F. The factor loadings are correlations between the factors and the stimulus-response measures. A positive loading indicates a positive correlation and a negative loading a negative correlation. Factor 1 gave positive weightings to responses to BRUSH and PRESSURE but negative weightings to responses to PINCH and SQUEEZE. Factor 2 gave large positive weightings to responses to PRESSURE and PINCH, the intermediate intensity stimuli, but small positive weightings to the responses to BRUSH and SQUEEZE.

When a k means cluster analysis was done using standardized data to allow interneuronal comparisons, again the cells could be subdivided into four clusters. Neurons in these clusters were termed types A–D. Fig. 2 A–D shows the response profiles for these classes of neurons, and the graph in Fig. 2G shows the distribution of the data in the plane of the first two principal components.

Type A cells were not very responsive to any of the stimuli (Fig. 2A). These formed the largest class. Type B cells were much more responsive than average to BRUSH and somewhat more to PRESSURE, but not to the more intense stimuli (Fig. 2B). Type C cells were more responsive than average to the three most intense stimuli (PRESSURE, PINCH, SQUEEZE), but not to BRUSH (Fig. 2C). Type D cells were very responsive to all of the stimuli, although less so for BRUSH (Fig. 2D). The factor loadings for the principal component plots had the following pattern (Fig. 2E, F): for factor 1 the weightings increased with stimulus intensity, whereas for factor 2 they decreased with stimulus intensity.

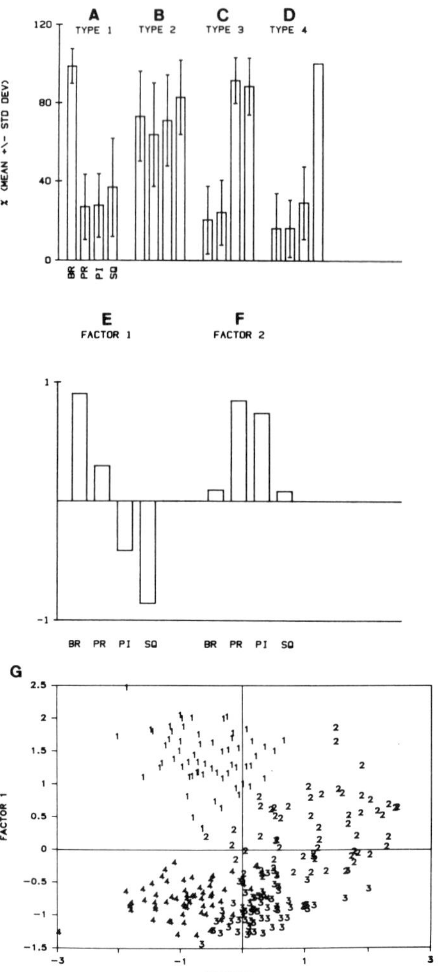

Fig. 1A–G. The histograms in **A–D** show the response profiles of the different classes of somatosensory neurons as determined from a k means cluster analysis of normalized data. The bar heights represent the mean normalized responses of each type of neuron to the different stimuli (BRUSH, BR; PRESSURE, PR; PINCH, PI; SQUEEZE, SQ), and the vertical lines show ± 1 standard deviation. The scattergram in **G** is a plot of the responses in the plane of the first two principal components. The ordinate is principal component 1 and the abscissa principal component 2 (after rotation by the varimax method). Cell types 1–4 are indicated. **E** and **F** show the factor loadings for the plot in **G**

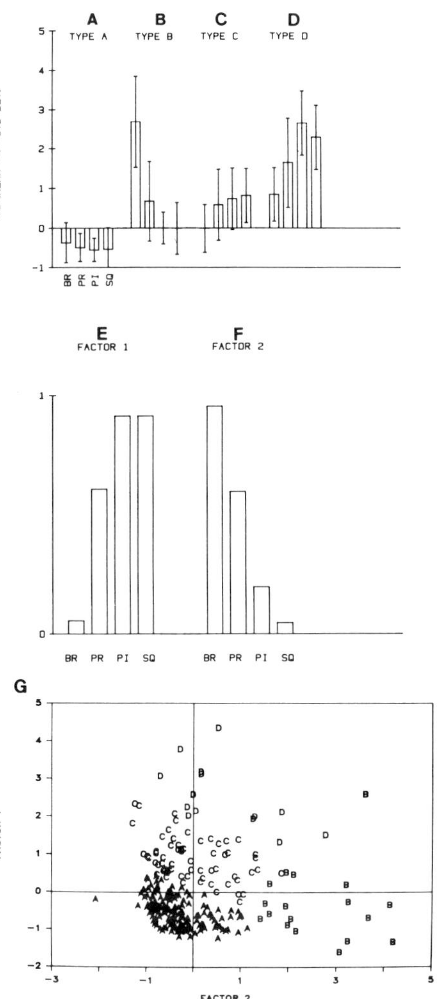

Fig. 2 A–G. The histograms in **A–D** show the means (and standard deviations) of the standard scores for responses to the four stimuli by neurons belonging to each of four response classes (types A–D). The scattergram in **G** shows the responses in the plane of the first two principal components. **E** and **F** show the factor loadings for **G**

STT Cells

The population of STT cells investigated included 37 neurons that were recorded in or near lamina I and another 113 that were in laminae IV–VI. The responses of these cells are shown on principal component plots for normalized data in Fig. 3A and B and for standardized data in Fig. 4A and B. In both analyses, there is a striking difference in the distribu-

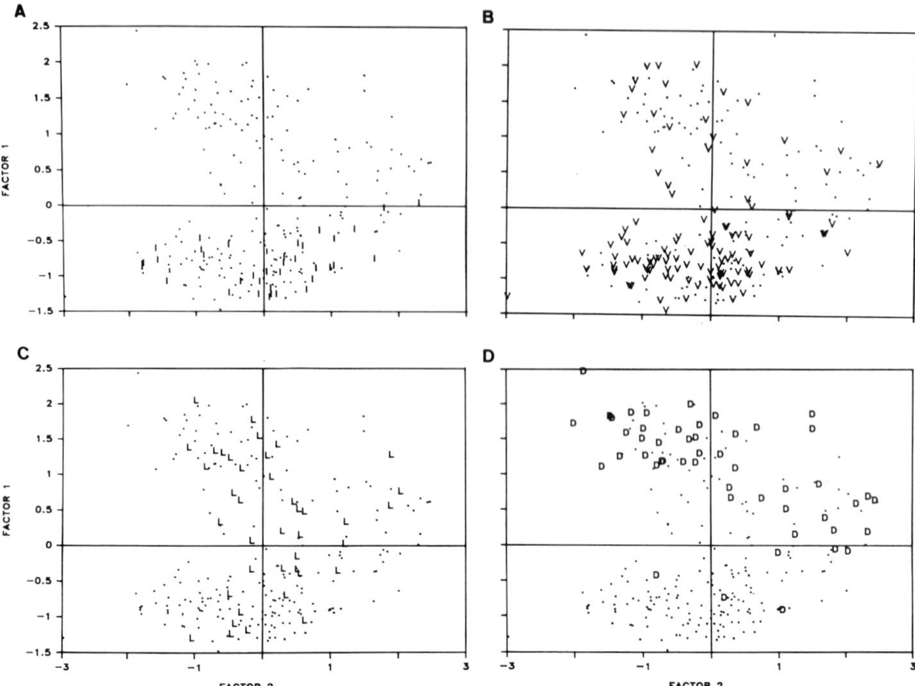

Fig. 3 A–D. Each of the scattergrams is a plot of the normalized responses of the population of somatosensory neurons in the plane of the first two principal components. In **A,** the points representing STT cells in lamina I are indicated by I, while the remainder of the cells are shown as dots. In **B,** the STT cells of laminae IV–VI are indicated by V. In **C,** LCN neurons are indicated by **L,** and in **D,** NG cells by D

tion of STT cells in or near lamina I and of those in laminae IV–VI. For the normalized data, almost all of the lamina I STT cells were plotted below the abscissa (Fig. 3A), whereas a number of STT cells in laminae IV–VI were above the abscissa (Fig. 3B). For the standardized data, most of the lamina I STT cells are to the left of the ordinate (Fig. 4A), whereas a higher proportion of STT cells in laminae IV–VI are to the right (Fig. 4B). The distribution of the STT cells by cluster is given in Table 1. STT cells in lamina I belonged to only three of four types for both normalized and standardized data, namely types 2–4 and types A, C, and D. The predominant classes were types 3, 4, A, and C. STT cells in laminae IV–VI were found to be of all types. For normalized data, types 3 and 4 were the largest groups. For standardized data, the majority of the cells were type A and the second most common group was type C.

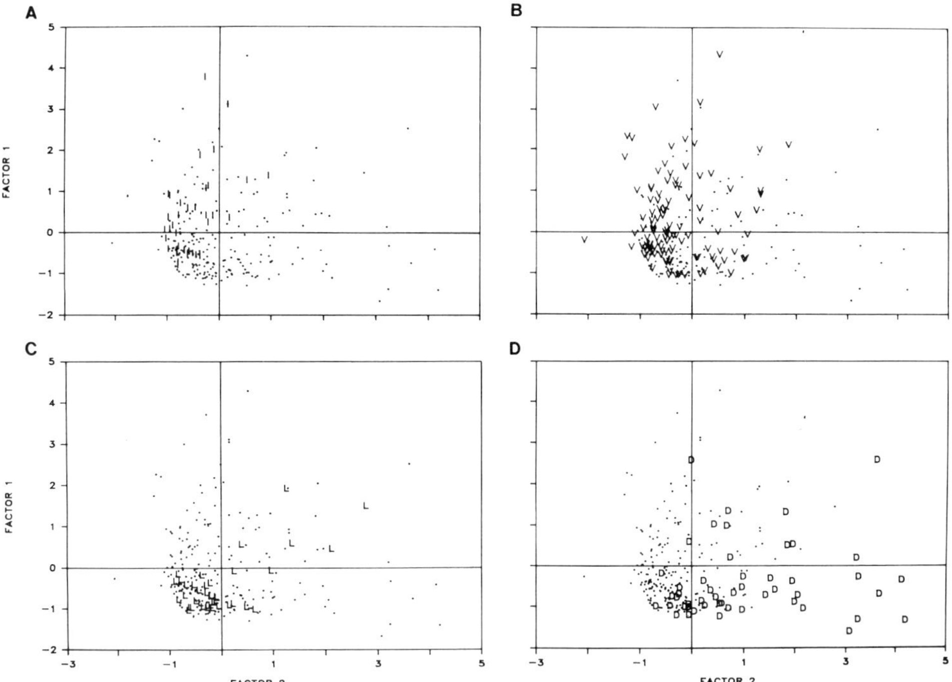

Fig. 4A–D. The scattergrams show the distribution of standardized responses in the plane of the first two principal components. The symbols are as in Fig. 3

LCN and NG Neurons

Cells of the LCN and of the NG belonged to all of the types determined from both normalized and standardized data. However, the proportions were distinctly different from those of STT cells. This is illustrated in the principal component plots in Figs. 3C, D and 4C, D and in Table 1. The most striking differences in the principal component plots for LCN and NG cells by contrast with those of the STT cells are: (1) the higher proportion of cells plotted above the abscissa in Fig. 3C and D; (2) the absence of LCN cells and the small number of NG cells in the upper left quadrant of Fig. 4C; and (3) the concentration of NG neurons in the lower right quadrant in Fig. 4D. LCN neurons were chiefly types 1, 2, and A. NG neurons were mainly types 1, 2, A, and B.

Table 1. Number (and percentage) of somatosensory neurons of the spinothalamic tract (STT), lateral cervical nucleus (LCN), and nucleus gracilis (NG) belonging to each cell type determined by k means cluster analysis

		Normalized responses				
		Type 1	Type 2	Type 3	Type 4	Total
Lamina I STT	No. (%)	0 (0)	4 (11)	22 (59)	11 (30)	37 (100)
	(%)	(0)	(8)	(31)	(19)	
Laminae IV–VI STT	No. (%)	17 (15)	15 (13)	39 (35)	42 (37)	113 (100)
	(%)	(27)	(29)	(56)	(72)	
LCN	No. (%)	15 (38)	15 (38)	7 (18)	3 (8)	40 (102)
	(%)	(24)	(29)	(10)	(5)	
NG	No. (%)	30 (59)	17 (33)	2 (4)	2 (4)	51 (100)
	(%)	(48)	(33)	(3)	(3)	
Total		62	51	70	58	241
		(99)	(99)	(100)	(99)	

		Standardized responses				
		Type A	Type B	Type C	Type D	Total
Lamina I STT	No. (%)	19 (51)	0 (0)	14 (38)	4 (11)	37 (100)
	(%)	(13)	(0)	(27)	(22)	
Laminae IV–VI STT	No. (%)	68 (60)	4 (4)	33 (29)	8 (7)	113 (100)
	(%)	(46)	(17)	(63)	(44)	
LCN	No. (%)	34 (85)	3 (8)	1 (2)	2 (5)	40 (100)
	(%)	(23)	(12)	(2)	(11)	
NG	No. (%)	26 (51)	17 (33)	4 (8)	4 (8)	51 (100)
	(%)	(18)	(71)	(8)	(22)	
Total		147	24	52	18	241
		(100)	(100)	(100)	(99)	

Discussion

The classification of cells in the complex nervous systems of vertebrates is a prerequisite for a functional analysis (Tyner 1975; Rowe and Stone 1977). The approach to classification of somatosensory neurons that we have taken is similar to that recommended for biological taxonomy (Sneath and Sokal 1973) and involves the statistical method of cluster analysis. Since we chose not to assume that our data were organized hierarchically, the k means type of cluster analysis was selected, rather than hierarchical cluster analysis, which was the technique used in studies of the chemical senses (Bieber and Smith 1986).

Cluster analyses were applied to data treated in two quite different ways. By normalizing the responses of somatosensory neurons, we were able to classify individual cells based on the profiles of activity evoked by different mechanical stimuli. The assumption underlying such an analysis is that the reactivity of individual neurons to particular types of stimuli is crucial to signalling in somatosensory pathways. However, in this analysis information is lost about the absolute responsiveness of the neurons. The other approach that we used, clustering based on standardized responses, allowed a comparison of the responses to each stimulus across the population of neurons. The analysis is based on the idea that the behavior within the population of neurons is crucial for coding.

In our initial application of a k means cluster analysis to the normalized responses of a population of primate STT cells excited by cutaneous stimuli (Chung et al. 1986), the best fit to the data was obtained when we used three clusters. However, for a subset of the data, four clusters seemed better. With a larger sample of STT cells, it now appears that four clusters offer a better description of the responses of STT cells (Surmeier et al., in preparation). For the present sample of somatosensory neurons, which includes LCN and NG cells as well as STT cells, four clusters again seem optimal. However, the addition of new variables in future work may require further subdivisions. We have already found that cells in the VPL nucleus of the monkey thalamus can be divided into at least five clusters (Chung et al. 1986).

The interpretation of the response profiles of somatosensory neurons belonging to the various categories determined by cluster analysis deserves comment. Type 1 cells respond much better to repeated BRUSH than to maintained compression of the skin (PRESSURE, PINCH, or SQUEEZE; Fig. 1A). This suggests that these neurons receive a dominant input from rapidly adapting mechanoreceptors. However, the responses of some of these neurons to intense mechanical stimuli suggest some convergent input from nociceptors. Consistent with this is the observation (not described here) that many of these cells can be activated by noxious heat stimuli. Thus, there may be a need in future to subdivide type 1 cells into purely mechanoreceptive neurons and "convergent" neurons (cf. LeBars and Chitour 1983).

Type 2 cells were very responsive to the PRESSURE stimulus (Fig. 1B). At least some of these cells in NG were found to have a dominant input from slowly adapting mechanoreceptors. However, it is possible that type 2 STT cells are activated by low threshold nociceptors, rather than by slowly adapting mechanoreceptors. Thus, there may need to be two subdivisions of type 2 after future studies.

Types 3 and 4 cells can be regarded as primarily nociceptive. Type 3 cells responded maximally to the PINCH stimulus (Fig. 1C), whereas type 4 cells required the more intense SQUEEZE stimulus for their greatest response (Fig. 1D). Both types of neuron appeared to have a convergent input from sensitive mechanoreceptors, since BRUSH usually had an excitatory action (however, it is possible that this stimulus can activate some low threshold nociceptors). We have suggested that type 3 STT cells may serve as an "early warning system" for pain, whereas type 4 cells may signal damage (Surmeier et al. 1986b).

The optimum number of clusters using standardized data was also four, both for a population of STT cells (Surmeier et al., in preparation) and for the sample of somatosensory neurons described here. Type A cells are neurons whose responses to all four stimuli that we used were below the population mean (Fig. 2A). We have suggested (Surmeier et al., in preparation) that such neurons may be better able to signal stimulation of structures other than the skin, such as muscle, viscera, or joints. Another possibility is that the circuitry in which type A cells are embedded is depressed by anesthesia or the condition of the animal. However, cells of all types could be encountered in the same animal and in any order, suggesting that some other factor determines their response categories. A third possibility depends upon the level and selectivity of descending modulatory activity, which can determine the responsiveness of somatosensory neurons.

Type B neurons showed unusually brisk responses to BRUSH but were less responsive to the more intense stimuli (Fig. 2B). Types C and D neurons responded better to the more intense stimuli than to BRUSH (Fig. 2C, D).

Table 2. Numbers (percentages) of somatosensory neurons of types 1-4 in types A-D

Type		1	2	3	4	Total
A	No. (%)	51 (33)	28 (18)	32 (21)	44 (28)	155 (100)
	(%)	(80)	(47)	(46)	(73)	
B	No. (%)	13 (52)	12 (48)	0 (0)	0 (0)	25 (100)
	(%)	(20)	(20)	(0)	(0)	
C	No. (%)	0 (0)	11 (20)	28 (51)	16 (29)	55 (100)
	(%)	(0)	(19)	(40)	(27)	
D	No. (%)	0 (0)	8 (44)	10 (56)	0 (0)	18 (100)
	(%)	(0)	(14)	(14)	(0)	
Total	No. (%)	64	59	70	60	253
	(%)	(100)	(100)	(100)	(100)	

The numbers and percentages of neurons of types 1-4 that were classified as types A-D are shown in Table 2. Type A cells are subdivided fairly evenly amongst types 1-4. Apart from type A cells, all of the remaining type 1 cells were type B. This is consistent with the previous discussion suggesting that cells of types 1 and B are likely to be tactile in function. Type 2 cells were of types A-D. If type B cells are tactile and types C and D are nociceptive, then some type 2 cells are tactile and others are nociceptive, as proposed above. Types 3 and 4 cells not classed as type A were either type C or type D. This presumably reflects their nociceptive function. It is instructive that the highly responsive type D cells comprise either type 2 or type 3 cells and not type 4 cells. This is consistent with previous work (Surmeier et al. 1986b).

We examined the possibility that neurons in different somatosensory pathways are distributed in different proportions across the various response classes (Table 1). For the normalized responses, a substantial proportion of the neurons that we sampled in the LCN and NG belonged to type 1 (38 % and 59 %, respectively), but few (15 %) of the STT cells in laminae IV-VI and none of those in lamina I were type 1. This observation is consistent with the traditional view that the dorsal column-medial lemniscus and spinocervico-thalamic pathways are the major somatosensory pathways signalling flutter-vibration but that STT cells, especially those in laminae IV–VI, can make some contribution to flutter (Willis and Coggeshall 1978; Kuru 1949; Vierck 1974).

Type 2 neurons were prominent in the samples of LCN and NG neurons, but also occurred in the populations of STT cells. Insofar as cells in these different pathways respond to slowly adapting mechanoreceptors, it can be argued that they contribute to touch-pressure (Willis and Coggeshall 1978). However, future work will be required to determine to what extent the classification of type 2 cells in different pathways depends upon an input from slowly adapting mechanoreceptors and to what extent upon low threshold nociceptors.

Neurons of types 3 and 4 were most common among the populations of STT cells (89 % of STT cells in lamina I and 72 % of STT cells in laminae IV–VI). This finding is consistent with the idea that the STT is the main pathway in primates signalling pain (Willis and Coggeshall 1978; Willis 1985). However, cells of these types were also found in the LCN (26 %) and NG (8 %). Other laboratories have reported that many SCT and postsynaptic dorsal column neurons in the cat respond to noxious stimuli (e.g., Uddenberg 1968; Brown and Franz 1969; Angaut-Petit 1975; Cervero et al. 1977; Kniffki et al. 1977; Brown et al. 1983; Lu et al. 1983; Kamogowa and Bennett 1986), as do many cat LCN cells in the absence of anaesthesia (Kajander and Giesler 1987). The possibility should be considered that such neurons form an alternative pathway for pain sensation that becomes more effective some time after interruption of the STT (White and Sweet 1969; Vierck and Luck 1979; Willis 1985). Alternatively, these neurons could be involved in activating descending control systems (Lu et al. 1983).

When we examined the classification of somatosensory neurons using standardized data, type A neurons proved to be the most common class for all of the pathways. It is not clear at present how to interpret this finding. Most type B cells were in the NG (33 % of NG cells were type B; of type B neurons, 71 % were in NG). This is consistent with a tactile function for these neurons, since type B neurons were differentially sensitive to the BRUSH and PRESSURE stimuli, and not to the most intense noxious stimuli relative to the population of somatosensory neurons. On the other hand, types C and D neurons were found most commonly in the populations of STT cells (49 % of STT cells in lamina I and 36 % of STT cells in laminae IV–VI belonged to types C and D; of types C and D neurons sampled, 90 % and 66 % respectively belonged to the STT). Since types C and D cells were differentially more sensitive to noxious stimuli and relatively less sensitive to BRUSH than was the population of somatosensory neurons, this is consistent with a nociceptive function of the STT. LCN and NG cells were less likely to be of types C and D (7 % and 16 % respectively).

This analysis of our present sample of neurons with cutaneous input suggests that cells in the ascending somatosensory pathways belong to a limited number of functional classes and that these classes of neurons are distributed in different proportions in the different ascending pathways. This viewpoint is consistent with the observation that it is difficult to disrupt particular somatic sensations by restricted lesions of the spinal cord (Willis and Coggeshall 1978).

We believe not only that these results indicate that cluster analysis can provide an objective way to recognize natural groupings of somatosensory neurons, but also that this technique can provide functional insights into the behavior of such neurons, as well as clues for further experimentation. Many of the differences between the various classes of somatosensory neurons can be attributed to differences in their responses to inputs over fine afferent fibers, especially those supplying nociceptors. Future work will be based on refinements in the types of stimuli that we have so far used and the consideration of other properties of the cells based on additional types of stimuli.

Acknowledgements. The authors thank Helen Willcockson and Griselda Gonzales for their expert technical assistance. The work was supported by NIH fellowships NS 07574 (CNH), NS 07623 (LSS), and NS 07216 (DJS) and grants NS 09743, NS 11255, and NS 18830. DGF was supported by a C. J. Martin Fellowship from the National Health and Medical Research Council of Australia.

References

Anderson CW, Cushman MR (1981) A simple and rapid method for making carbon fiber microelectrodes. J Neurosci Methods 4 : 435–436

Angaut-Petit D (1975) The dorsal column system. II. Functional properties and bulbar relay of the postsynaptic fibres of the cat's fasciculus gracilis. Exp Brain Res 22 : 471–493

Bieber SL, Smith DV (1986) Multivariate analysis of sensory data: A comparison of methods. Chem Senses 11 : 19–47

Brown AG, Franz DN (1969) Responses of spinocervical tract neurones to natural stimulation of identified cutaneous receptors. Exp Brain Res 7 : 231–249

Brown AG, Rethelyi M (1981) Reports of working parties. In: Brown AG, Rethelyi M (eds) Spinal cord sensation. Scottish Academic Press, Edinburgh, p 332

Brown AG, Brown PB, Fyffe REW, Pubols LM (1983) Receptive field organization and response properties of spinal neurones with axons ascending the dorsal columns in the cat. J Physiol (Lond) 337 : 575–588

Cervero F, Iggo A, Molony V (1977) Responses of spinocervical tract neurones to noxious stimulation of the skin. J Physiol (Lond) 267 : 537–558

Chung JM, Kenshalo DR Jr, Gerhart KD, Willis WD (1979) Excitation of primate spinothalamic neurons by cutaneous C-fiber volleys. J Neurophysiol 42 : 1354–1369

Chung JM, Surmeier DJ, Lee KH, Sorkin LS, Honda CN, Tsong Y, Willis WD (1986) Classification of primate spinothalamic and somatosensory thalamic neurons based on cluster analysis. J Neurophysiol 56 : 308–327

Ferrington DG, Sorkin LS, Willis WD (1986) Responses of spinothalamic tract cells in the cat cervical spinal cord to innocuous and graded noxious stimuli. Somatosens Res 3 : 339–358

Ferrington DG, Sorkin LS, Willis WD (in press) Responses of spinothalamic tract cells in the superficial dorsal horn of the primate lumbar spinal cord. J Physiol (Lond)

Kajander KC, Giesler GJ, Jr (1987) Responses of neurons in the lateral cervical nucleus of the cat to noxious cutaneous stimulation. J Neurophysiol

Kamogowa H, Bennett GJ (1986) Dorsal column postsynaptic neurons in the cat are excited by myelinated nociceptors. Brain Res 364 : 386–390

KNIFFKI KD, MENSE S, SCHMIDT RF (1977) The spinocervical tract as a possible pathway for muscular nociception. J Physiol (Paris) 73 : 359–366

KURU M (1949) Sensory paths in the spinal cord and brain stem of man. Sogensya, Tokyo

LEBARS D, CHITOUR D (1983) Do convergent neurones in the spinal dorsal horn discriminate nociceptive from non-nociceptive information? Pain 17 : 1–19

LU GW, BENNETT GJ, NISHIKAWA N, HOFFERT MJ, DUBNER R (1983) Extra- and intracellular recordings from dorsal column postsynaptic spinomedullary neurons in the cat. Exp Neurol 82 : 456–477

MENDELL LM (1966) Physiological properties of unmyelinated fiber projections to the spinal cord. Exp Neurol 16 : 316–332

PRICE DD, DUBNER R (1977) Neurons that subserve the sensory-discriminative aspects of pain. Pain 3 : 307–338

ROWE MH, STONE J (1977) Naming of neurones. Brain Behav Evol 14 : 185–216

SNEATH PHA, SOKAL RR (1973) Numerical taxonomy. Freeman, San Francisco

SORKIN LS, FERRINGTON DG, WILLIS WD (1986) Somatosensory organization and response characteristics of dorsal horn neurons in the cervical spinal cord of the cat. Somatosens Res 3 : 323–338

SURMEIER DJ, HONDA CN, WILLIS WD (1986a) Responses of primate spinothalamic neurons to noxious thermal stimulation of glabrous and hairy skin. J Neurophysiol 56 : 328–350

SURMEIER DJ, HONDA CN, WILLIS WD (1986b) Temporal features of the responses of primate spinothalamic neurons to noxious thermal stimulation of hairy and glabrous skin. J Neurophysiol 56 : 351–369

TYNER CF (1975) The naming of neurons: Applications of taxonomic theory to the study of cellular populations. Brain Behav Evol 12 : 75–96

UDDENBERG N (1968) Functional organization of long, second-order afferents in the dorsal funiculus. Exp Brain Res 4 : 377–382

VIERCK CJ (1974) Tactile movement detection and discrimination following dorsal column lesions in monkeys. Exp Brain Res 20 : 331–346

VIERCK CJ, LUCK MM (1979) Loss and recovery of reactivity to noxious stimuli in monkeys with primary spinothalamic cordotomies, followed by secondary and tertiary lesions of other cord sectors. Brain 102 : 233–248

WHITE JC, SWEET WH (1969) Pain and the neurosurgeon. Thomas, Springfield

WILLIS WD (1985) The pain system. Karger, Basel

WILLIS WD, COGGESHALL RE (1978) Sensory mechanisms of the spinal cord. Plenum, New York

37 Is Facilitation of a Flexor Reflex in the Decerebrated Rat Analogous to Post-Injury Pain in Humans? A Preliminary Report

E. Torebjörk and L. Lundberg

Introduction

In 1984, Wall and Woolf published a paper in the *Journal of Physiology* in which they showed that conditioning electrical stimuli at 1 Hz for 20 s at C fiber strength in muscle nerve fascicles induced prolonged facilitation of a flexor reflex in the decerebrated rat. In the introduction to their paper they implied that this flexor reflex facilitation might have a bearing on prolonged pain and tenderness resulting from deep injury in humans. Indeed, facilitation of this flexor reflex in the decerebrated rat has been interpreted as "evidence for a central component of post-injury pain hypersensitivity" (Woolf 1983).

It is conceivable that changes in excitability in the central nervous system may contribute to hyperalgesia in humans under certain clinical conditions (see Tasker 1983 for a review). However, there are obvious differences between a flexor reflex in the decerebrated rat and the perception of pain in intact humans, and it cannot be taken for granted that facilitation of a reflex in the decerebrated rat is equivalent with central enhancement of pain in human subjects.

In order to test the validity of the flexor reflex rat model for pain we have delivered similar conditioning stimuli as used by Wall and Woolf (1984) to peripheral nerves in awake human subjects and tested the effects on perceived magnitude of pain. The preliminary results indicate that the central mechanisms for pain in normal human subjects are not rendered hyperexcitable by brief conditioning stimuli which easily facilitate the flexor reflex in the decerebrated rat.

Methods

Six experiments were performed in four awake male human subjects, aged 20–33 years. The subjects sat relaxed in a reclining chair with the studied extremity comfortably supported in stable position. Intraneural electrical stimulation and recording was performed through tungsten microelectrodes (Vallbo and Hagbarth 1968) inserted percutaneously into cutaneous (n = 2) or muscle fascicles (n = 4) of the peroneal or median nerves at knee or upper arm level. Cutaneous fascicles were identified by subjective reports of cutaneously projected tactile or painful sensations during intraneural stimulation, and by observing neural responses from skin mechanoreceptors or nociceptors when the electrode was used for recording. Muscle fascicles were identified by visible muscle twitching and subjective reports of deep pain during intraneural stimulation, and by observing neural responses from muscle receptors when the electrode was used for recording. By moving the electrode in small steps it was usually possible to place the tip in such a position that pain was evoked at low stimulus amplitudes, projected to either skin or muscle.

The electrodes and the recording and display systems have been described elsewhere (Vallbo and Hagbarth 1968; Hagbarth et al. 1970). A Grass S48 constant-voltage stimulator with stimulus isolation unit delivered square wave pulses of 0.25 ms duration at amplitudes up to 5 V.

Test Stimuli

Simulus trains of 3 s duration at 10 Hz were repeatedly delivered at intervals of 2 or 5 min. The stimulation amplitude was adjusted to a level which induced moderate pain with only a minimum of concomitant tactile sensation or muscle twitching. The amplitude was then kept constant. The first train in a test series was presented as a standard and assigned a value (usually 10). Subsequent magnitude estimations were done relative to this standard on an open-ended ratio scale. The subjects were informed that they would receive electrical stimuli which might increase, decrease or remain constant during the experiment. They were instructed to pay attention to and rate the magnitude of pain perceived throughout the experimental period.

Conditioning Stimuli

After obtaining constant (or nearly constant) pain ratings to constant test stimuli over a period of 10–30 min, a few single electrical stimuli were given at increasing intensity till the subjects' tolerance level was reached. The stimulus intensity was then slightly reduced, and a conditioning stimulus train was delivered at 1 Hz for 20 s to 10 min, using pulse amplitudes up to 5 V. Then the test stimuli were resumed as before.

Results

The subjective pain ratings during the initial period of test stimuli were remarkably constant, both at 2 and 5 min intervals, and there was no indication that the test stimuli themselves caused any peripheral or central changes in the nociceptive mechanisms (Fig. 1, left). The conditioning stimuli were always perceived as very painful. If projected to skin, the pain had a dull burning quality. When projected to muscle, the pain was described as a deep severe aching, more widespread and with less distinct borders than cutaneous pain. During prolonged conditioning stimulation for several minutes, the subjective magnitude of pain progressively decreased (Fig. 1, b).

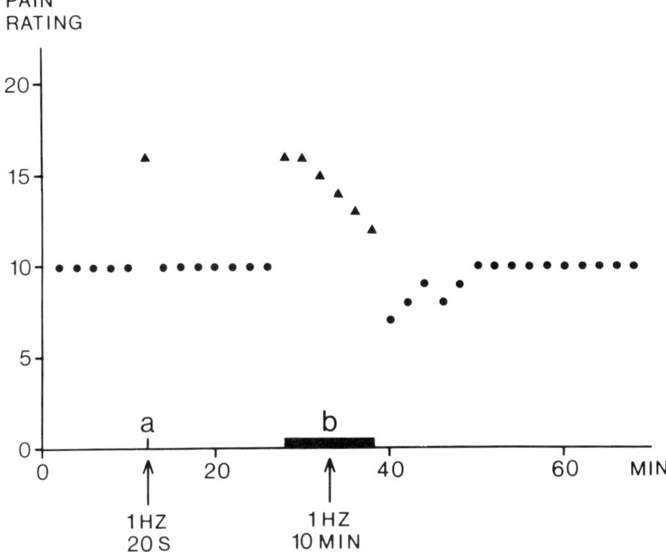

Fig. 1. Ratings of deep muscle pain projected to the lateral calf reported by a normal subject during intraneural stimulation of a muscle fascicle of the left peroneal nerve. Round symbols represent ratings elicited by test trains (10 Hz for 3 s) at constant intensity, delivered every 2 min. Triangles represent ratings elicited by intense conditioning stimuli (1 Hz) for 20 s (**a**) and 10 min (**b**). Zero on the vertical scale represents no pain. Note that the pain ratings are not exaggerated after severely painful conditioning stimuli as compared with preconditioning controls. See text for further details

Following short (20 s) trains of conditioning stimuli there was usually no change in subsequent pain ratings to the test stimuli (Fig. 1, a). After longer (up to 10 min) periods of conditioning stimulation, a reduction of pain ratings relative to control occurred during the first few minutes (Fig. 1, right) before the ratings returned to control level. No increase in pain ratings above control level was observed even after 10 min of severely painful conditioning stimulation.

No marked differences were observed from these general features in the four different subjects, and no significant differences were observed when stimulation was performed in muscle versus cutaneous nerve fascicles. No increase in pain ratings relative to control was observed following the conditioning stimuli, regardless of whether 2- or 5-min intervals were allowed between the tests.

Discussion

The present experimental set-up has a number of attractive features for the study of central modulation of pain mechanisms. First of all, the experiments are performed in awake normal human subjects who report their experience of pain. This is an obvious advantage over inferences on pain mechanisms based on studies of reflexes in decerebrated rats. Secondly, by stimulating in the nerve, rather than in the peripheral tissues, we have bypassed the peripheral nerve terminals, and hence, any change in perceived magnitude of pain cannot be explained by changes in excitability of the peripheral nerve receptors. Instead, changes in perceived magnitude of pain must reflect central mechanisms, provided that the stimulus parameters are appropriate for faithful excitation of the nociceptive fibers in the nerve. In a previous study (Torebjörk et al. 1984), various stimulus parameters were systematically tested in order to establish a reliable method to test for possible central modulation of pain. It was shown that the test trains used in the present study, 10 Hz for 3 s, was adequate for reproducible pain ratings regardless of whether the pain sensation occurred in isolation or was contaminated by mild twitching or cutaneous tactile sensations. No significant change in magnitude of pain ratings was observed during 90 min of testing when the test trains were delivered at 5- and 10-min intervals. The constancy of pain ratings observed in the present study indicates that test train intervals down to 2 min can be used without depressing the excitability of the nociceptive fibers.

Wall and Woolf (1984) observed "that a brief C-afferent fiber input into the spinal cord can produce a prolonged increase in the excitability of the flexion reflex and that muscle C-afferent fibers evoke longer-lasting changes than cutaneous C fibers." They imply that the differences in the time course of the post-conditioning effects may be related to more prolonged and widespread tenderness and pain following deep injury, while apparently equivalent cutaneous injuries result in more spatially and temporally restricted sensory disorders. In order to test this hypothesis we have reproduced their conditioning stimulus, 1 Hz for 20 s, in both cutaneous and muscle nerve fascicles in humans. In no instance did we observe any post-conditioning increase of the pain ratings. Could our negative result be explained by insufficient activation of C-afferent fibers, which, according to the results of Wall and Woolf (1984), are crucial for facilitating the flexor reflex in the decerebrated rat? Our stimuli are restricted by the subjects' tolerance, and excite fascicular contents rather than the fibers of a whole nerve. It has been shown by direct intraneural recordings (Torebjörk et al. 1984) that high intensities of intraneural stimulation, similar to those used in the present study, evoke substantial C fiber responses which are conducted centrally and elicit severe pain (Fig. 2). Furthermore, in a separate study (Torebjörk, La Motte and Lundberg, unpublished), we injected Capsaicin into the skin and evoked C nociceptor activity (documented by recording) and severe pain. Yet, as soon as the spontaneous pain from the injection had disappeared, the pain ratings of intraneural electrical test stimuli were not significantly different from controls. Thus, by activating C-afferent fibers in two different ways we have failed to document any increase in the central gain of pain in normal human subjects.

Could it be that the time course of C-afferent fiber activation was too short to elicit the proposed facilitation of central pain mechanisms in humans? Increasing the period of conditioning stimulation for up to 10 min only led to excitation failure of nociceptive fibers and concomittant reduction in pain ratings. When the fibers recovered after the conditioning stimulus the pain ratings returned to control level – but no increase in pain ratings above control was reported as testing went on for many minutes.

We admit that this is a preliminary study which should be completed using a larger sample, including testing of threshold as well as suprathreshold pain. However, even at this stage, we must conclude that central pain mechanisms in normal human subjects are not easily perturbed by a brief noxious stimulus which can induce pronounced facilitation of a flexor reflex in the decerebrated rat. This observation warrants some caution in accepting the rat model as analogous to pain in humans.

Acknowledgement: Supported by the Swedish Medical Research Council, Grants B 87-14x-05206 and B 87-14P-6153, and by ASTRA AB, Südertälje, Sweden.

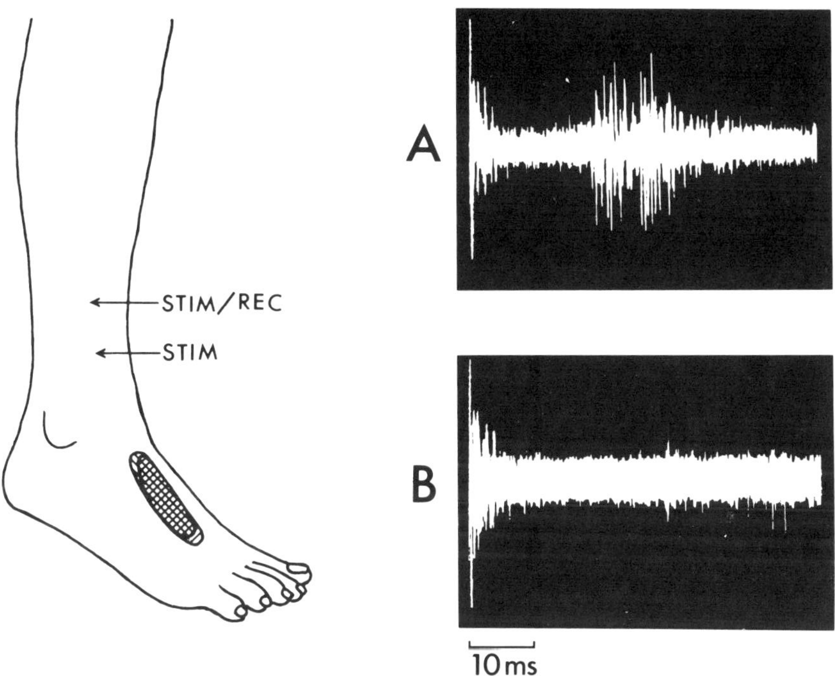

Fig. 2 A,B. Direct monitoring of C fiber response evoked by intraneural stimulation. Two microelectrodes, 4 5 cm apart, were inserted into the same fascicle of the superficial peroneal nerve, as indicated by overlap of paraesthesia induced by electrical stimulation through the proximal electrode (longitudinally hatched area) and paraesthesia induced by stimulation through the distal electrode (transversely hatched area). The proximal electrode was then used to record the response evoked by stimulation through the distal electrode. Note massive C fiber response to 5 V stimulation at 0.3 Hz in **A**, and absence of C fiber response after 30 s stimulation at 10 Hz in **B**. (From Torebjörk et al. 1984)

References

Hagbarth K-E, Hongell A, Hallin RG, Torebjörk HE (1970) Afferent impulses in median nerve fascicles evoked by tactile stimuli of the human hand. Brain Res 24 : 423-442

Tasker RR (1984) Deafferentation. In: Wall PD, Melzack R (eds) Textbook of pain. Churchill Livingstone, Edinburgh, pp 119-132

Torebjörk HE, Schady W, Ochoa JL (1984) A new method for demonstration of central effects of analgesic agents in man. J Neurol Neurosurg Psychiatry 47 : 862-869

Vallbo ÅB, Hagbarth K-E (1968) Activity from skin mechanoreceptors recorded percutaneously in awake human subjects. Exp Neurol 21 : 270-289

Wall PD, Woolf CJ (1984) Muscle but not cutaneous C-afferent input produces prolonged increases in the excitability of the flexion reflex in the rat. J Physiol (Lond) 356 : 443-458

Woolf CJ (1983) Evidence for a central component of post-injury pain hypersensitivity. Nature 306 : 686-688

38 Spinal Mechanisms in Arthritic Pain: Enhancement of Responses of Tract Neurons in the Course of Inflammation

H.-G. Schaible, R. F. Schmidt, and W. D. Willis

Arthritic diseases are a major source of pain. Consequently, various models of experimental arthritis are now used to study the neurophysiological mechanisms of nociception which lead to inflammatory pain in a joint (Coggeshall et al. 1983; Gautron and Guilbaud 1982; Grigg et al. 1986; Guilbaud and Iggo 1986; Guilbaud et al. 1982a, b, 1985; Heppelmann et al. 1985, 1986; Kayser and Guilbaud 1984; Lamour et al. 1983; Menétrey and Besson 1982; Schaible and Schmidt 1985; Schaible et al. 1987b, in press). The experiments presented here were aimed at gaining new insights into the spinal mechanisms of articular nociception. Their background is our recent study of the discharge characteristics of primary afferent fibers from normal and arthritic knees of the cat (Coggeshall et al. 1983; Grigg et al. 1986; Schaible and Schmidt 1983a, b, 1984, 1985). In chloralose-anaesthetized and paralyzed cats, ascending spinal cord tract cells were studied which could be driven by local mechanical stimulation of the knee joint. After the initial characterization of a neuron, inflammation of the knee was produced and the activity of the spinal neuron was monitored continuously for several hours to see if the neuron's discharges were changed during the early stages of the arthritis. A detailed description of the methods used (anesthesia, dissection, recording, stimulation) is given elsewhere (Schaible et al. 1987a, b, in press).

Spinal Cord Neurons with Ascending Axons and Receptive Fields in the Knee Joint

To activate neurons with ascending axons antidromically, the spinal cord was transected at the lower thoracic level and the uppermost lumbar cord was mounted on bipolar platinum electrodes for electrical stimulation. The dorsal columns were crushed caudal to the electrodes. During tracking with microelectrodes (mainly in the lumbar segments L5 and L6), electrical stimulation of the upper lumbar segment served as a search stimulus for tract cells. After identification of an ascending neuron (constant latency of the antidromic spike and collision of this spike with orthodromic spikes) the location of receptive fields was determined by manual exploration of the legs (Schaible et al. 1986).

In a sample of 160 ascending tract neurons, 25 had a receptive field in the knee joint (23 ipsilateral, two contralateral) and all 25 neurons could also be driven mechanically from skin and/or deep tissues elsewhere in the leg. They are probably a subset of the population for which articular input was identified previously by electrical stimulation of joint nerves (Schaible et al. 1986). For some of the neurons the recording site was marked with a lesion made by passing direct current through the microelectrode.

Three different patterns of convergence of afferent inputs from various tissues were found (Fig. 1). Three neurons had inputs from the skin and the knee joint (sj cells). They were located in the dorsal horn (e. g. lamina V, Fig. 1A). Another 16 neurons had convergent inputs from skin, deep tissue and the knee (sdj cells). Recording sites were in the dorsal horn (lamina V) and in the ventral horn (laminae VII and VIII, Fig. 1B). Finally, six neurons had inputs from deep tissue and the knee (dj cells). Five of these neurons were situated in the ventral horn (e. g. laminae VII and VIII, Fig. 1C).

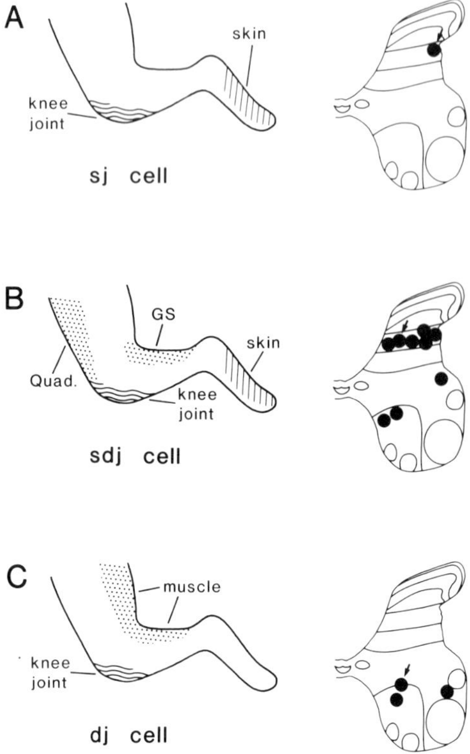

Fig. 1 A-C. Convergent inputs from articular, cutaneous and muscle receptors onto ascending tract cells. On the left, the receptive fields of three different neurons are shown. **A** Receptive fields in skin and joint (sj cell). **B** Receptive fields in skin, deep tissue [Quadriceps (Quad.) and gastrocnemius soleus (GS) muscles] and joint (sdj cell). **C** Receptive fields in deep tissue and joint (dj neuron). On the right, lesions at the recording sites of different sj, sdj, and dj neurons are illustrated. The arrows indicate the neurons whose receptive fields are shown on the left

The size of the cutaneous receptive fields of the neurons varied from small (e.g. part of thigh or lower leg) to large (e.g. from thigh to foot). They were located near and/or remote from the knee. The deep receptive fields were in the muscles of the thigh and/or the lower leg, and in some cases in the foot.

These three different types of neurons with joint input did not have clearly different thresholds to natural stimulation of their receptive fields. However, most neurons with skin input (sj and sdj cells) showed different reactions to non-noxious and noxious movements of the knee (low-frequency vs high-frequency responses). From the receptive fields in the skin, either a wide-dynamic-range response or a high-threshold response was obtained. The neurons usually displayed background activity (ongoing activity in the absence of intentional stimulation). On the other hand, three of six dj cells reacted appreciably only to noxious movements and two of these six neurons did not respond to any movement in the knee (despite their articular receptive fields to local stimulation). These cells had no background activity. Responses of a dj neuron to movements are shown in Fig. 2B. Substantial activation

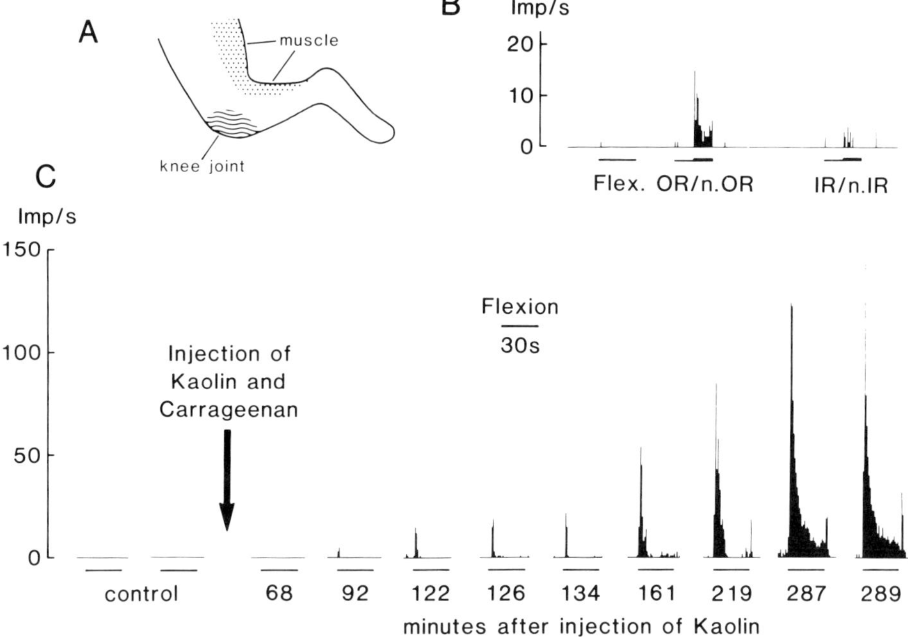

Fig. 2 A–C. Induction of responses to flexion in the knee in a dj neuron during development of arthritis. **A** Receptive fields in muscle and joint. **B** Responses to movements in the knee prior to inflammation. OR, outward rotation; IR, inward rotation; n. OR, n. IR, noxious outward and inward rotation against the resistance of the tissue (starting from mid-position of the knee joint). **C** Responses to flexion in the knee (maximal flexion starting from mid-position) in the control period and after induction of inflammation by injection of kaolin and carrageenan

was obtained only during noxious outward and noxious inward rotation of the knee. Flexion, outward rotation and inward rotation did not cause reproducible responses.

Thus, judging from the reactions to movements, noxious stimuli to the joint are signalled, first, by differential responses in highly convergent neurons, and second, by activation of neurons which have only deep inputs and elevated thresholds to mechanical stimuli.

It is appreciated that the responses of spinal tract neurons to movement may be due to convergent input from skin, muscles and joints. The specific articular contribution to such responses could not be singled out in the present experiments, where all nerves were kept intact (see, however, Schaible et al. 1986).

Effects of Experimental Arthritis on Ascending Neurons with Articular Input

In one sj, eight sdj and four dj cells it was investigated whether the responses to movements were changed during the beginning stages of an acute experimental arthritis. After characterization of a neuron's responses to non-noxious and noxious movements, we injected kaolin (0.3 - 0.4 ml of a 4 % solution) and carrageenan (0.3 ml of a 2 % solution) into the joint cavity followed by rhythmic extension and flexion to distribute the inflammatory agents in the joint. The neurons were activated by the injection for a period of time ranging from several seconds to several minutes. Thereafter, background and evoked activity returned to the control level. After induction of inflammation each neuron was kept under observation for several hours.

Neurons Without Responses to Non-noxious Movements of the Knee Prior to Inflammation

The effect of inflammation on such a neuron is shown in Fig. 2C. It was a dj cell located at the border between laminae VII and VIII which prior to inflammation reacted reproducibly only to noxious movements (Fig. 2B), non-noxious flexions evoking at the most single impulses. Significant activity during flexion commenced 92 min after the injection of kaolin. From this point on flexion evoked progressively larger responses, and there also developed a tonic component for the duration of the flexion. Similar results were obtained for two other dj cells which prior to inflammation responded only to noxious movements or not at all. In addition, one sdj cell with background activity but without responses to non-noxious movements developed responses to flexion. The results of these experiments are summarized in Fig. 3, where the average responses to flexion of the knee are shown before and during development of the inflammation.

Neurons With Responses to Non-noxious Movements of the Knee Prior to Inflammation

In seven neurons, non-noxious flexion movements evoked excitation in the control period. Five of them were sdj cells. During the development of arthritis responses to flexion were enhanced in all five of these cells. The amount and time course of the enhancement of the responses in these five neurons is illustrated in Fig. 4 (solid lines). One neuron developed strong responses to movements but the background discharges were also strongly increased, so that the difference between movement-evoked activity and background activity

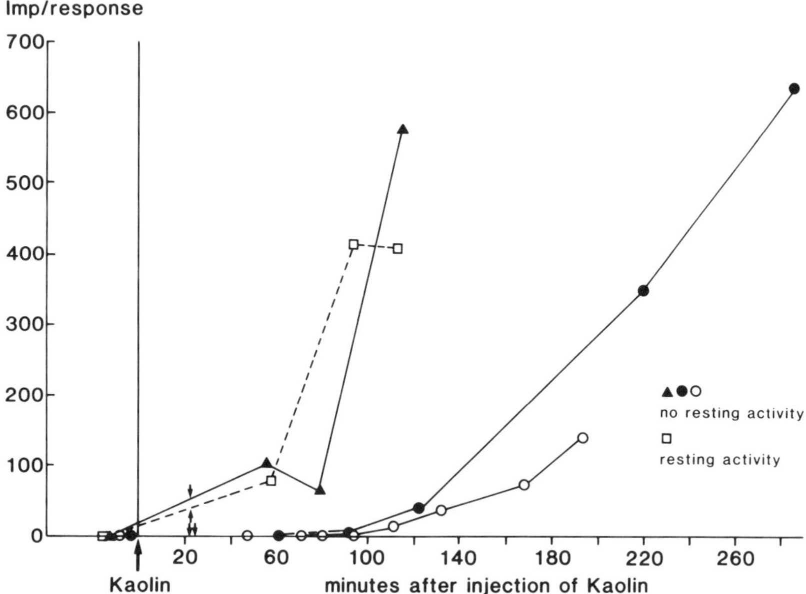

Fig. 3. Responses to flexion in the knee (maximal flexion starting from mid-position) in three dj neurons (–) and one sdj neuron (–––) during development of arthritis. The various symbols show the average responses to several trials. The small arrows indicate the time when carrageenan was injected into the knee

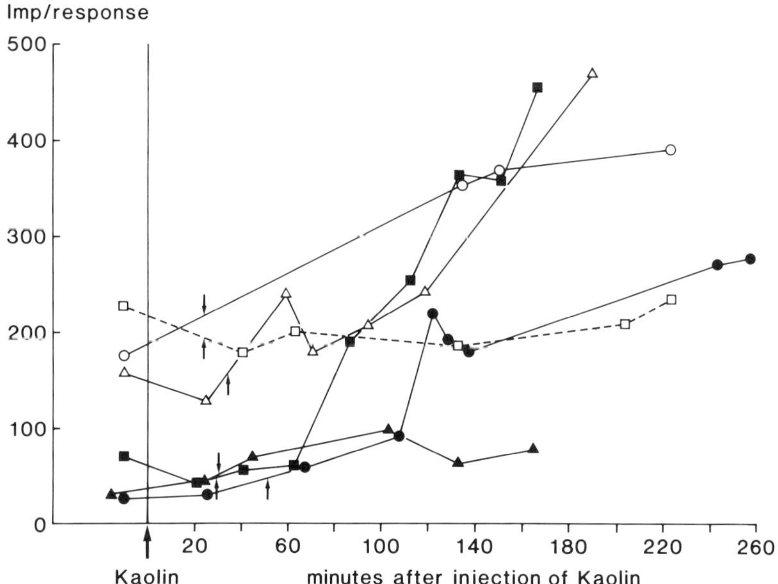

Fig. 4. Enhancement of the responses to flexion in ascending tract neurons before and after injection of the inflammatory agents kaolin and carrageenan (small arrows). The responses to several trials were averaged

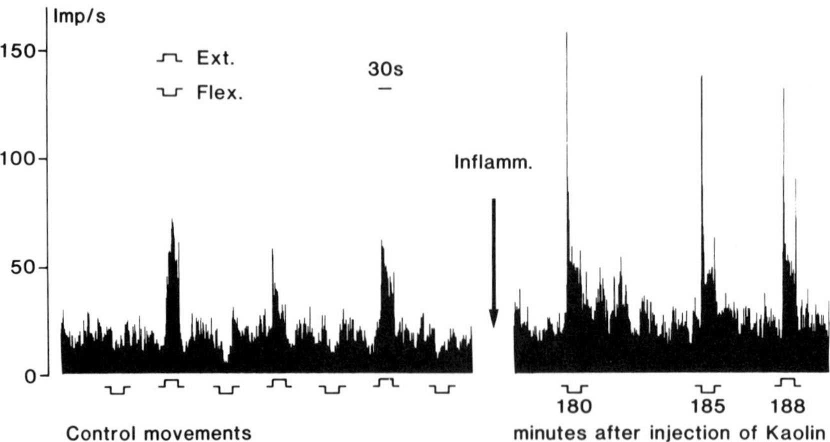

Fig. 5. Production of an excitatory response to flexion by experimental inflammation in a neuron which displayed no response or a slight inhibition on flexion in the control period

prior to the movement was not enhanced (this neuron is illustrated in Fig. 4 with a dashed line). One sdj neuron did not change its activity during the inflammation.

In two additional sdj cells, flexion movements in the control period had no effect or evoked slight inhibition, whereas extension movements led to excitation. During the development of inflammation an excitatory response to flexion was produced (see Fig. 5).

In three of these sdj neurons background and movement evoked activity was observed for about 3 h prior to the injection of the inflammatory agents. None of them showed an increase of the responses during this long control period, which excludes the possibility of spontaneous enhancement of activity of the neurons.

Comparison of the Responses to Movements of the Inflamed Leg and the Normal Contralateral Leg

In three neurons we tested whether responses to movements of the contralateral leg were altered by inflammation in the ipsilateral leg. In one of two neurons with bilateral input, responses were also increased during movements of the contralateral leg (the receptive field being located in the deep tissue of the thigh). In one neuron with unilateral input, responses increased during inflammation but no activity was evoked at any time from the contralateral leg.

Effects of Inflammation on Neurons in Which Receptive Fields in the Knee Joint Could Not Be Found

Two neurons had receptive fields in the deep tissue around the knee and, in one case, in the skin but not in the joint itself. One further neuron could be activated by pressure applied to the knee but probing of the joint structures with a glass rod did not reveal localized receptive fields there. These three neurons responded to flexion prior to inflammation. In the two neurons clearly lacking a receptive field in the knee, inflammation did not change the excitatory responses to movement, whereas in the neuron with the questionable articular receptive field, movement-evoked activity was enhanced during the development of inflammation.

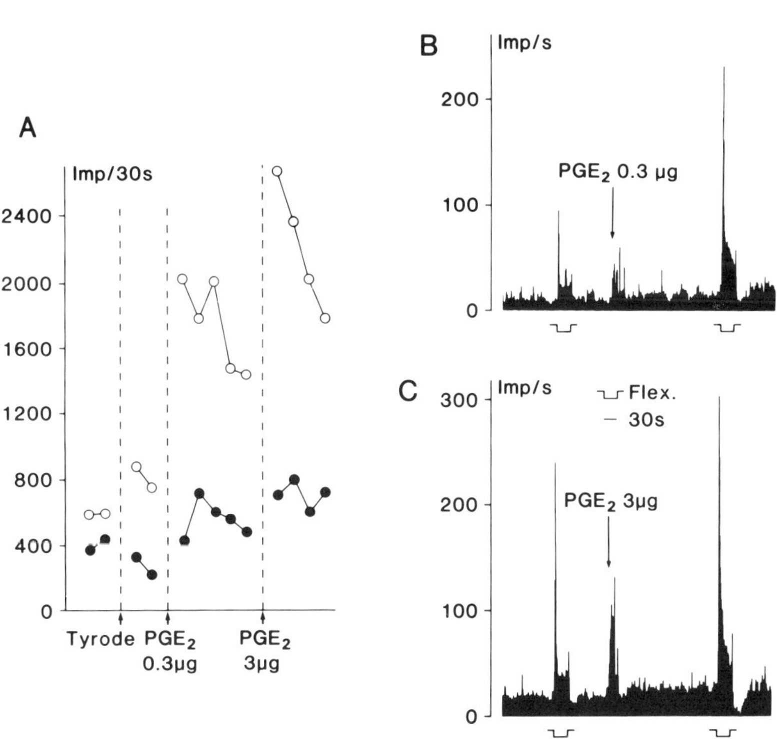

Fig. 6 A–C. Enhancement of the responses of a neuron to flexion in an inflamed knee by the intra-articular injection of prostaglandin E_2 in 0.3 ml Tyrode. **A** The closed circles show the resting activity of the neuron in the 30 s preceding flexion, the open circles show the activity during flexion. The interval between trials was 5 min. **B, C** Single trials before and after the injection of prostaglandin E_2

Effects of the Injection of Prostaglandin E_2 into the Joint Cavity on Ascending Tract Neurons

In eight experiments on eight neurons, Tyrode solution (as control) and prostaglandin E_2 were injected into the inflamed joint. The injection of Tyrode solution led to increased responses of spinal neurons to flexion in seven of the eight cats. Prostaglandin E_2 had the same effect in two neurons but elicited stronger and dose-related responses in five cases. In addition prostaglandin E_2 increased the resting activity in some of the neurons. An example is illustrated in Fig. 6.

Conclusions

These results show that experimental arthritis changes the activity in two different types of spinal cord ascending neuron with joint input: (a) in a ventrally located group of nociceptive-specific dj neurons, and (b) in various dorsally and ventrally situated wide-dynamic-range sdj neurons, both of which may contribute to the sensory consequences of an acute arthritis. Because the termination of the ascending axons was not identified, the sensory role of these neurons remains to be specified. It is, however, assumed that at least some of these cells contribute to pain sensation: the time course of the changes in the responses of these neurons fits well with behavioral experiments in which unequivocal "painful" reactions were noted mainly in the 2nd h after injection of crystals or carrageenan into a joint (Brune et al. 1974; Faires and McCarty 1962; Okuda et al. 1984; Van Arman et al. 1970).

The inflammation-induced spinal responses to movements can be related to the additional afferent input from the arthritic joint. During arthritis, many of the high-threshold or non-activated (groups III and IV) afferent units become sensitized and then respond to movements in the normal working range of the knee (Coggeshall et al. 1983; Grigg et al. 1986; Schaible and Schmidt 1985). In addition, low-threshold afferents can become more active (Schaible and Schmidt 1985). In arthritis, these increased discharges may induce responses in previously non-responsive dj neurons and enhance the background and evoked activity of responsive sdj neurons. This conclusion is supported by the findings that the intra-articular injection of prostaglandin E_2 enhanced the responses and that neurons without receptive fields in the knee were usually not affected by the arthritis. Thus the neuronal changes are confined mainly to neurons with articular input. On the other hand, a central component has to be considered for neurons which show increased responses to movements of the non-inflamed (contralateral) knee. In further experiments the balance between afferent and central sensitizing factors should be investigated.

References

BRUNE K, WALZ D, BUCHER D (1974) The avian microcrystal arthritis. I. Simultaneous recording of nociception and temperature effect in the inflamed joint. Agents Actions 4 : 21–33

COGGESHALL RE, HONG KAP, LANGFORD LA, SCHAIBLE H-G, SCHMIDT RF (1983) Discharge characteristics of fine medial articular afferents at rest and during passive movements of inflamed knee joint. Brain Res 272 : 185–188

FAIRES IS, MCCARTY DJ (1962) Acute arthritis in man and dog after intrasynovial injection of sodium urate crystals. Lancet 2 : 682–684

GAUTRON M, GUILBAUD G (1982) Somatic responses of ventrobasal thalamic neurons in polyarthritic rats. Brain Res 237 : 459–471

GRIGG P, SCHAIBLE H-G, SCHMIDT RF (1986) Mechanical sensitivity of group III and IV afferents from posterior articular nerve in normal and inflamed cat knee. J Neurophysiol 55 : 635–643

GUILBAUD G, IGGO A (1985) The effect of lysine acetylsalicylate on joint capsule mechanoreceptors in rats with polyarthritis. Exp Brain Res 61 : 164–168

GUILBAUD G, BENOIST JR, GAUTRON M, KAYSER V (1982a) Aspirin clearly depresses responses of ventrobasal thalamus neurons to joint stimuli in arthritic rats. Pain 13 : 153–163

GUILBAUD G, BENOIST JR, GAUTRON M, KAYSER V (1982b) Effects of systemic naloxone upon ventrobasal thalamus neuronal responses in arthritic rats. Brain Res 243 : 59–66

GUILBAUD G, IGGO A, TÉGNER R (1985) Sensory receptors in ankle joint capsules of normal and arthritic rats. Exp Brain Res 58 : 29–40

HEPPELMANN B, SCHAIBLE H-G, SCHMIDT RF (1985) Effects of prostaglandins E_1 and E_2 on the mechanosensitivity of group III afferents from normal and inflamed cat knee joints. In: FIELDS HL, DUBNER R, CERVERO F (eds) Advances in pain research and therapy, vol 9. Raven, New York, pp 91–101

HEPPELMANN B, PFEFFER A, SCHAIBLE H-G, SCHMIDT RF (1986) Effects of acetylsalicylic acid (ASA) and indomethacin on single group III and IV units from acutely inflamed joints. Pain 26 : 337–351

KAYSER V, GUILBAUD G (1984) Further evidence for changes in the responsiveness of somatosensory neurons in arthritic rats: a study of the posterior intralaminar region of the thalamus. Brain Res 323 : 144–147

LAMOUR Y, GUILBAUD G, WILLER JC (1983) Altered properties and laminar distribution of neuronal responses to peripheral stimulation in the SmI cortex of the arthritic rat. Brain Res 273 : 183–187

MENÉTREY D, BESSON JM (1982) Electrophysiological characteristics of dorsal horn cells in rats with cutaneous inflammation resulting from chronic arthritis. Pain 13 : 343–364

OKUDA D, NAKAHAMA H, MIYAKAWA H, SHIMA K (1984) Arthritis induced in cat by sodium urate: a possible animal model for tonic pain. Pain 18 : 287–297

SCHAIBLE H-G, SCHMIDT RF (1983a) Activation of groups III and IV sensory units in medial articular nerve by local mechanical stimulation of knee joint. J Neurophysiol 49 : 35–44

Schaible H-G, Schmidt RF (1983b) Responses of fine medial articular nerve afferents to passive movements of knee joint. J Neurophysiol 49 : 1118–1126

Schaible H-G, Schmidt RF (1984) Mechanosensibility of joint receptors with fine afferent fibres. Exp Brain Res [Suppl] 9 : 284–297

Schaible H-G, Schmidt RF (1985) Effects of an experimental arthritis on the sensory properties of fine articular afferent units. J Neurophysiol 54 : 1109–1122

Schaible H-G, Schmidt RF, Willis WD (1986) Responses of spinal cord neurones to stimulation of articular afferent fibres in the cat. J Physiol (Lond) 372 : 575–593

Schaible H-G, Schmidt RF, Willis WD (1987a) Convergent inputs from articular, cutaneous and muscle receptors onto ascending tract cells in the cat spinal cord. (in press)

Schaible H-G, Schmidt RF, Willis WD (1987b) Enhancement of the responses of ascending tract cells in the cat spinal cord by acute inflammation of the knee joint. (in press)

Van Arman C, Carlson RP, Risley EA, Thomas RH, Nuss GW (1970) Inhibitory effects of indomethacin, aspirin and certain other drugs on inflammations induced in rat and dog by carrageenan, sodium urate and ellagic acid. J Pharmacol Exp Ther 175 : 459–468

39 Responses of Ventrobasal Thalamic Neurones to Carrageenin-Induced Inflammation in the Rat

G. Guilbaud, J.M. Benoist, V. Kayser, and A. Neil

As a step towards the elucidation of clinical pain mechanisms, initiated by the use of arthritic rats (references in Guilbaud 1985), we have started electrophysiological studies in rats presenting inflammation induced by the intraplantar injection of carrageenin (Benoist et al. 1985; Guilbaud et al. 1986). Such an injection is commonly known to elicit hyperalgesia in freely moving animals (Winter and Flataker 1965: references in Kayser and Guilbaud 1987).

In a first experimental series, the responses of the same somatosensory neurones recorded in the ventrobasal thalamic complex (VB), which is known to play a role in the transmission of noxious messages (references in Guilbaud 1985), were successively studied before, and after the carrageenin injection over a period of 2 h ("acute" state). In a second series, the responsiveness of VB neurones was examined 24–96 h after a carrageenin injection. In these experiments the animals were considered hyperalgesic, as indicated by the decrease of the vocalization threshold to paw pressure, gauged just before the recording session (Guilbaud et al. 1986); this phase was named the "subacute" state.

Material and Methods

Male Sprague-Dawley rats weighing 250–300 g were used. The surgical preparation, the electrophysiological recordings, and the techniques of peripheral stimulation (mechanical, thermal) were identical to those used in the studies performed at the thalamic level (cf. Guilbaud et al. 1980, 1986).

Briefly, the recordings (via glass micropipettes filled with NaCl and pontamine sky blue) were carried out in animals immobilized by gallamine triethiodide (Flaxedil), artificially ventilated, and under moderate gaseous anaesthesia (mixture of 1/3 O_2, 2/3 N_2O 0.5 % halothane). The level of anaesthesia was stable and appeared sufficiently deep, since no signs of suffering or stress could be detected, as previously reported (Guilbaud et al. 1980). The iontophoretic application of dye at the end of each electrode track allowed the recording sites in the VB complex to be localized by examination of histological sections.

Lambda carrageenin (Satia Laboratory Paris) was used, 0.2 ml of a 1% solution being injected in the plantar paw.

In both "acute" and "subacute" phases several types of experimental electrophysiological and pharmacological series were performed. From the electrophysiological point of view we analyzed, over the first 2 h following the injection of carrageenin, the possible changes in the responsiveness of neurones located in the VB contalateral to the injected paw; these neurones were previously characterized as "non-noxious" and "noxious", using mechanical stimulation such as brushing, pressure, joint movement and pinch; the size of their peripheral receptive field, including at least the plantar region of the injected paw, was also monitored. For this first comparative study, constant pinch with a graduated forceps and hot water bath at 50° C were used as noxious stimuli of supraliminal itensity. The stimulations of 15 s duration, repeated with interval of at least 5 min, induced reproducible control responses before the carrageenin injection. Secondly, we examined the responsiveness of

VB neurones in rats presenting an hyperalgesic carregeenin inflammation over 24–96 h, at various times of inflammation.

Thirdly, using series of quantified stimuli, we studied the response threshold and the encoding capacities of the VB neurones, in both the acute and the subacute state. Indeed, we have previously shown that for such VB neurones, there was a linear relation between the thermal stimulus intensity and the number of spikes in the response (Peschanski et al. 1980).

Finally, in several neuropharmacological studies, we considered the modifying effects of aspirin, xylocaine, and naloxone on the responses induced by the carrageenin sensitization, or attempted to prevent these modifications by injection of an antihistamine. Details of these various series are given elsewhere (Guilbaud et al. 1986, 1987; Neil et al. 1986, 1987). The possible action of these various substances on the neuronal background activity has not been analyzed so far, due to the inconstancy of its changes after the carrageenin injection.

Acute Phase

Supraliminal Responses

Change in the Number of Spikes in the Response

Neither the responses nor the receptive fields (RF) of neurones classified as non-noxious (only driven by light tactile stimuli) were significantly modified during the first 2 h following the initiation of the inflammation. By contrast, for at least 90% of the "noxious" neurones, responses elicited from the contralateral injected paw were already greatly enhanced 10–15 min following the carrageenin injection (Benoist et al. 1985; Guilbaud et al. 1987). This was the case whatever the stimulus modality used, mechanical or thermal (Fig. 1). One hour after the initiation of the inflammation the mean response to mechanical stimulation was 220% ± 51% of the control value (**n** = 11, $P < 0.05$). The background activity although and temporarily increased to a greater or lesser extent for some units, was not significantly changed when the whole population was condidered (**n** = 23 in the first study).

Receptive Field Changes

An increase was also observed for responses elicited from parts of the RF remote to the injected site, such as the opposite posterior paw and/or the tail, which are often included in the RF of this type of neurones (Guilbaud et al. 1980) (Fig. 1).

In addition, in numerous cases, responses were noted from areas which were outside the RF before the carrageenin injection; for instance, in 14/23 cases it was possible to activate the neurone by stimulating the forepaws, while this stimulation did not induce a significant response during the initial tests (Fig. 1).

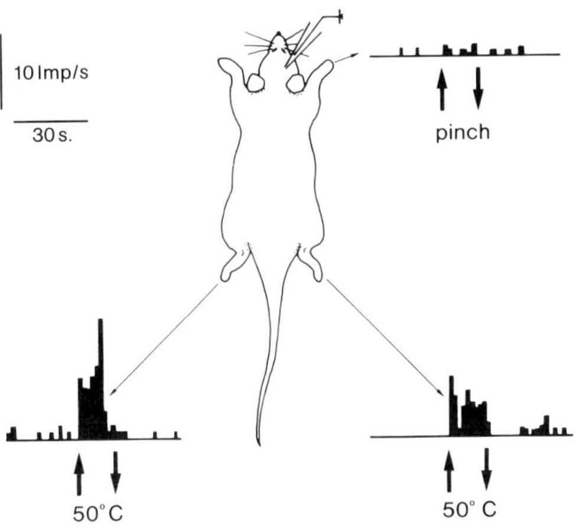

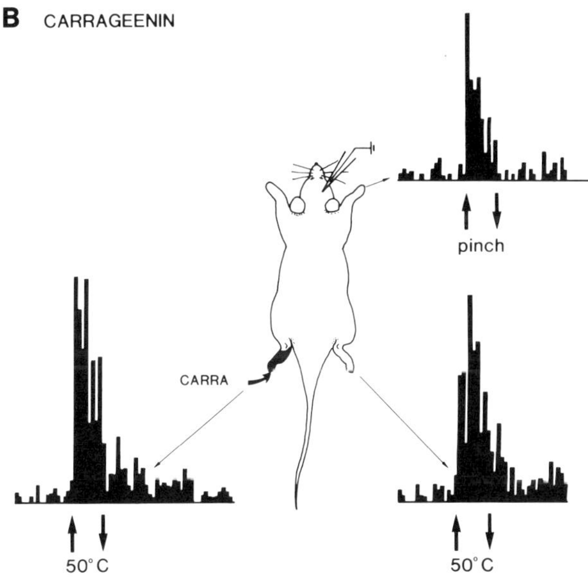

Fig. 1 A,B. Peristimulus time histograms illustrating the responses to pinch or to noxious heat of a right ventrobasal thalamus neurone of the rat before (**A**) and 25–40 min after (**B**) carrageenin injection into the left plantar paw. The stimulation duration is indicated by the thick arrows, the site of the stimulus application by the thin arrows. Ordinates: number of spikes integrated each 2 s

Effect of Lidocaine

When the local anaesthetic lidocaine was injected into the inflamed paw 30–45 min after carrageenin, neuronal response modifications were suppressed whatever part of the RF was stimulated. So, if additional phenomena of central origin are responsible for these modifications when distant areas are stimulated, they appear themselves to be triggerred by the local inflammatory process, since they are suppressed by the local anaesthesia.

These "remote" modifications, and their suppression by lidocaine, are reminiscent of the distant secondary hyperalgesia often encountered in clinical or experimental situations (Lewis 1935–1936; Hardy et al. 1967; ref. in Kayser et al. 1986). They have indeed some behavioral correlates, since in carrageenin-injected rats a clear hyperalgesia observed for paws distant from the injected site, could be relieved by an injection of a local anaesthetic in the inflamed paw (Kayser et al. 1986).

Analysis of the Response Threshold and the Encoding of the Stimulus Intensity

Response Threshold

When the response thresholds of "noxious" neurones were measured before, and 1–2 h following the carrageenin injection, we found a dramatic decrease in the response threshold with the thermal but not with the mechanical stimulation of the injected paw. The threshold temperature, (the first temperature of an ascending series, beginning at 36° C with increments of 2° C, which was able to induce a significant response), was 44.0 ± 0.6° C before vs 40.3 ± 1.4° C after carrageenin injection (n = 10). For the mechanical stimulus (indentation from 120–160 µm to 700 µm, increased by steps of 40–60 µm), the response threshold was obtained with a similar indentation of the skin before and after the carrageenin injection (300.6 ± 18.7 µm, n = 15, and 297.5 ± 8.5 µm, n = 12 respectively). Thus, the carrageenin sensitization seems to act differently on the mechanisms underlying the liminal response of a neurone to different stimulus modalities. The decrease in the threshold to thermal stimulation may account for the well-known sensitivity of an inflamed area to heat and for the decrease in the struggle threshold also observed when the carregeenin-injected paw of the rat is placed in a hot water bath (Table 1). By contrast, the decrease in the vocalization threshold to pressure on the same paw (Winter and Flakater 1965; Table 1) cannot be explained by the change of the response thresholds of the neurones that we have considered. Thus, we suggest, that at this at this early stage of the inflammation, another neuronal population poorly or not activated by somatic stimulation before carrageenin injection (therefore not selected in the study), could be activated afterwards, due to the peripheral sensitization (Guilbaud et al. 1986).

Table 1. Response thresholds of two parameters to nociceptive stimuli applied to the injected and the non-injected paw before and 1 and 24 h after carrageenin injection

Threshold	Control	Time after carrageenin 1 h	24 h
Pressure vocalization (g)[a]			
Injected paw	274.6 ± 14.2[c] n=18	185.3 ± 7.3[c] n=18	199 ± 18 n=17
Non-injected paw	261.4 ± 15.6[c] n=18	205.1 ± 7.1[c] n=18	285 ± 12 n=17
Heat struggle (° C)[b]			
Injected paw	44.3 ± 1° C n=15	40.6 ± 1.2° C n=10	39.0 ± 1.6° C n=10
Non-injected paw	44.6 ± 0.8° C n=10	43.9 ± 0.9° C n=5	40.9° C n=10

[a] Data from Kayser and Guilbaud (1987)
[b] Unpublished data from Kayser and Guilbaud (in preparation)
[c] Same series of rats

Encoding of the Stimulus Intensity

The neurones initially activated exclusively by noxious stimuli were able to encode the stimulus intensity, either before or after the carrageenin injection, whatever the stimulation modality (thermal or mechanical). An example comparing the responses to thermal stimuli of the injected and the non-injected paw is shown in Fig. 2. The stimulus-response relationship using mechanical stimuli became steeper after inflammation, while that using thermal stimuli showed no change in slope but was shifted to the left in the direction of lower thresholds (Guilbaud et al. 1986, 1987). Finally, this led to a clear increase of the responses to the supraliminal intensities as observed in the initial investigation.

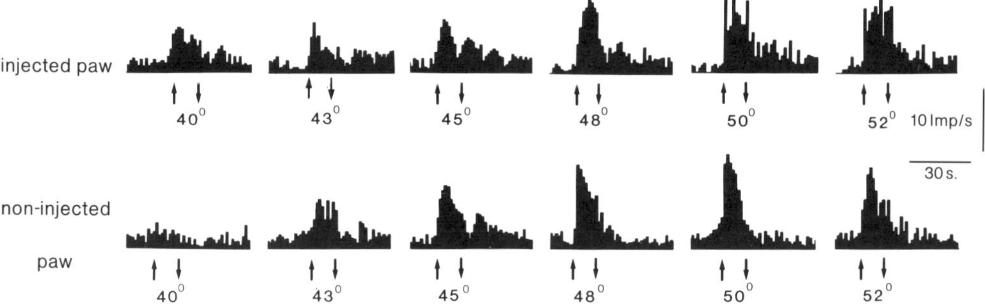

Fig. 2. Peristimulus time histograms illustrating the responses of a left ventrobasal neurone to hot water baths of progressively increased temperature applied alternately to the right injected and to the left non-injected paw. Ordinates as in Fig. 1. (To avoid additional sensitization heat stimulus was not applied before the carrageenin injection in this experimental series; see Peschanski et al. 1980)

The sensitization phenomena observed at the thalamic level resemble those seen by several authors recording peripheral fibres either in animal or humans, after noxious heat injury [see references in the more recent papers (Lynn and Carpenter 1982; Fleischer et al. 1983; Adriaensen et al. 1984; La Motte 1984; Torebjörk et al. 1984; Meyer et al. 1985)]. They also fit well with the data of Anton et al. (1985) who considered carrageenin sensitization at the peripheral level.

Pharmacological Modulation

In the acute period of the inflammation the changes in the neuronal response could be prevented by the administration of an antihistamine (Thiazinamium), but only if it was intravenously administered 10 min before carrageenin; this substance was ineffective when injected 20 min after carrageenin, and the time course of the response modifications was similar to that observed in the first part of the study: the maximal response to pinch was similarly increased by 120% when compared to the initial value 1 h after the inflammation induction (Neil et al. 1986, 1987) (Fig. 3).

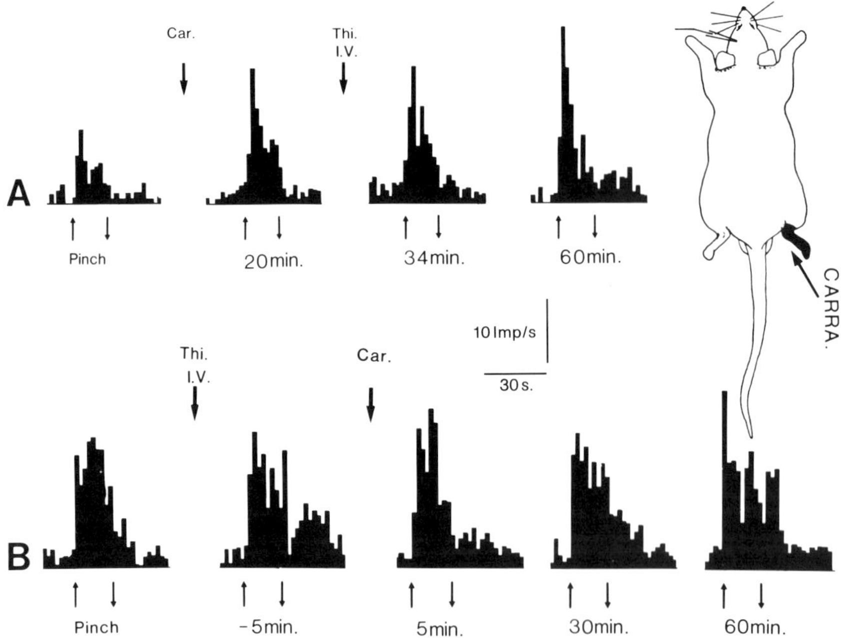

Fig. 3 A,B. Peristimulus time histograms illustrating the responses of two left ventrobasal neurones to pinches applied to the right posterior paw. **A** The sensitization due to the carrageenin injection in the right plantar paw was not reversed by Thiazinamium (Thi) (1 mg/kg i.v.), injected 20 min after; the response to a pinch applied to the injected paw continued to be enhanced compared to the control value as observed in rats non-pretreated with Thiazinamium. **B** The i.v. injection of Thiazinamium 10 min before the intraplantar injection of carrageenin prevented the increase of the response. Ordinates as in Fig. 1

In this acute state, the VB neuronal responses were modified neither by the opiate antagonist naloxone (3–10 μg/kg i.v; Kayser et al., in preparation) nor by aspirin (100 mg/kg i.v; Guilbaud et al. 1986), which blocks the cyclo-oxygenase involved in the production of prostaglandins (Vane 1971).

Therefore it appears that the modifications of VB neuronal responses observed in the acute phase of the inflammation are more likely due to the inflammatory substances released early in the exudate, such as histamine and/or serotonin, than to the prostaglandins, which are released later (3–4 h after the carrageenin injection) (Di Rosa et al. 1971; Higgs and Salmon 1979; references in Guilbaud et al. 1986). Moreover, both histamine and serotonin are known to sensitize peripheral nociceptors (Fjällbrant and Iggo 1961; Handwerker 1976; Mense 1981). Finally, during this early period, contrasting with responses to joint stimulation recorded in a situation of chronic inflammation (arthritic rats; Guilbaud et al. 1982), VB responses elicited by the stimulation of the inflamed paw do not seem to be modulated by the endogenous opioid systems, since they are not significantly modified by naloxone.

Subacute Phase

Ventrobasal Neuronal Responsiveness

In the subacute phase, lasting 24–96 h, no significant differences were found in the neuronal responsiveness according to the recording time following the carrageenin injection, but it seems worth underlining that all the tested rats were hyperalgesic just before the recording session. Among the 72 somatosensory neurones analyzed, 33 were still activated by intense mechanical stimulation, but half of these presented short duration and "fading" responses, mainly when the stimulation was repeated, as previously observed in arthritic rats at the spinal and VB level (Menetrey and Besson 1982; Gautron and Guilbaud 1982). These latter neurones were usually driven by high temperature (50° C) but their responses to this modality also "faded".

In sharp contrast, other neurones (14/72) were activated by moderate mechanical stimulation of the joints, which have been reached by the inflammation, and/or the surrounding cutaneous areas. They rarely responded to high temperature.

These two groups of neurones exhibited a background activity of 3–5 imp/s (usually the VB neurones have a resting discharge of 0-3 imp/s), and half of them presented long-lasting (15–60 s), paroxysmal discharges, occurring without intentional stimulation.

The neurones driven by light, rapid, tactile stimuli from a small contralateral receptive field were still present (25/72), without obvious change in the "classical" characteristics of their responses.

Response Threshold and Encoding of the Stimulus Intensity

Since the responses of neurones driven exclusively by intense stimuli were not reproducible, their precise threshold to a mechanical stimulus was not usually determined; when such an effort was made, the threshold was always found to be high, above 140 mN (the value of the strongest von Frey hair in the set).

By contrast, as in the early phase, the response threshold to heat applied to the inflamed hyperalgesic paw was still dramatically lowered: 38.0 ± 0.6° C (n = 12). Surprisingly, the threshold was also low following stimulation of the opposite non-injected paw: 40.2 ± 0.8° C (n = 6). Thus, these neurones can clearly account for the low threshold of a nociceptive response when the paw is plunged in a hot water bath (Table 1).

For the group of neurones driven by moderate mechanical stimulation of the inflamed paw, the liminal response was obtained with a mean indentation of 191.4 ± 17.7 μm (n = 17). Although not always activated by 50° C, these neurones could be driven by relatively low temperatures (threshold 40.4 ± 1.4° C, n = 5). When the neurones exhibited a bilateral RF, the non-injected paw was activated by heat at the limit of the noxious range (43.4 ± 1.3° C).

Therefore, this second group of neurones, not found in the VB of normal rat, could be involved in the decrease of the vocalization threshold to pressure, and possibly also in the decrease of the struggle threshold to heat (Table 1).

The low response thresholds could be due to the sensitization of peripheral receptors, reported in numerous studies, (references in the papers mentioned above; Heppelmann et al. 1985) and are probably related, 24 h after the initiation of the carrageenin inflammation, to products of the arachidonic cascade in the exudate (Di Rosa et al. 1971; Higgs and Salmon 1979).

For the two groups of neurones considered, the responses could no longer be graded when a stimulus of increased intensity was applied to the injected paw. A stimulus-response relationship was found for less than 20 % of the 19 cells tested with heat (n = 11) or with skin indentation (n = 8); however, such a relation was more frequent when the stimuli were applied to the opposite non-injected limb (present for four of the seven cells so tested). An example comparing relation between the response and the stimulus intensity, when a thermal stimulus is applied to the injected and the non-injected paw, is shown in Fig. 4.

Therefore, it appears that at this stage, VB neurones likely to be involved in the transmission of messages giving rise to the hyperalgesia or allodynia, could exhibit a relatively low threshold for responses to mechanical and/or thermal stimuli without being able to code for stimulus intensity. This fits well with some data found in clinical hyperalgesia, when peripheral fibre activities are apparently mismatched to the degree of the simultaneous pain sensation (La Motte 1984; Torebjörk et al. 1984; Meyer et al. 1985).

The fact that the capacity to code the stimulus intensity could be observed in few cases when the stimulus was applied to the non-injected paw argues for the participation of peripheral phenomena, such as tachyphylaxis, desensitization or fatigue of nociceptors, in the decline of responses to supraliminal intensity (for references see the more recent papers mentioned above); this does not necessarily mean (Fig. 4), that the neuronal response has already reached its maximum for the threshold stimulus value.

However, other observations concerning the characteristics of some neuronal responses obtained from the apparently normal paw in this subacute phase (the low threshold to a

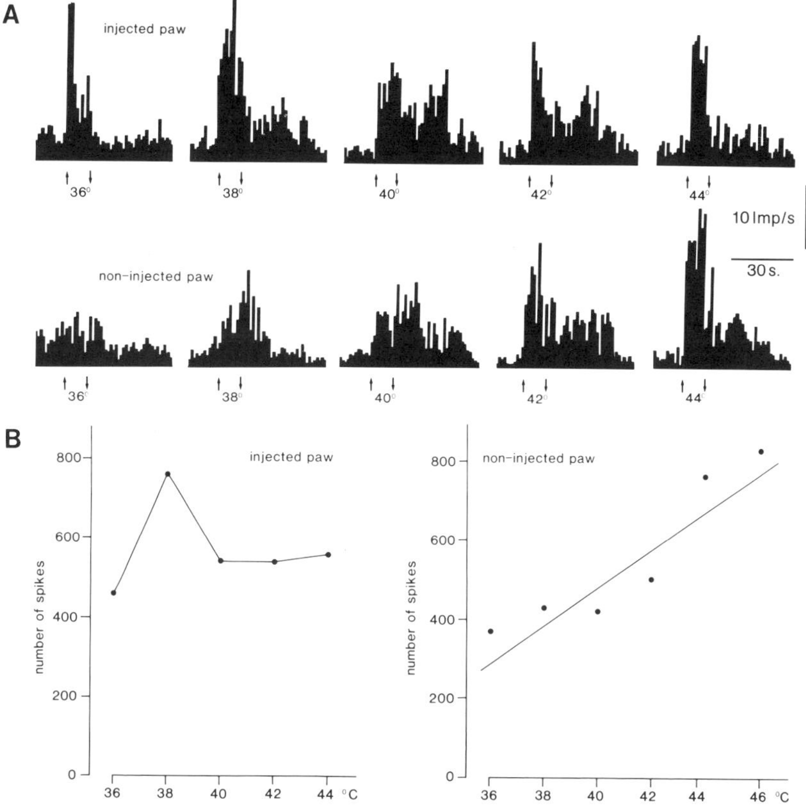

Fig. 4 A,B. Peristimulus time histograms (**A**), illustrating responses of a left ventrobasal neurone to hot water baths of progressively increased intensity, alternately applied to the right injected and the left non-injected paw, 24 h after carrageenin injection. The response threshold was below the noxious range for both hind paws (although lower for the inflamed paw). Ordinates as in Fig. 1. A significant linear relation (B) between the response and the bath temperature persisted for the non-injected paw only. (Slightly modified from Guilbaud et al. 1987)

thermal stimulus and the "fading" responses to intense stimulations) suggest the involvement of additional central phenomena. It can be speculated that both peripheral and central mechanisms might act in conjunction in a protective system able, in a first step, to warn that a stimulus of low intensity is capable of increasing the initial injury, and secondly to prevent an excessive invasion of the central nervous system by supramaximal stimuli (Guilbaud et al. 1987). Experiments, including analysis of the changes in the responsiveness of afferent fibers and central neurones during the transition period between acute and subacute stage, should be useful in determining the respective roles of the inflammatory process itself and of the various phenomena triggered by it at the central level.

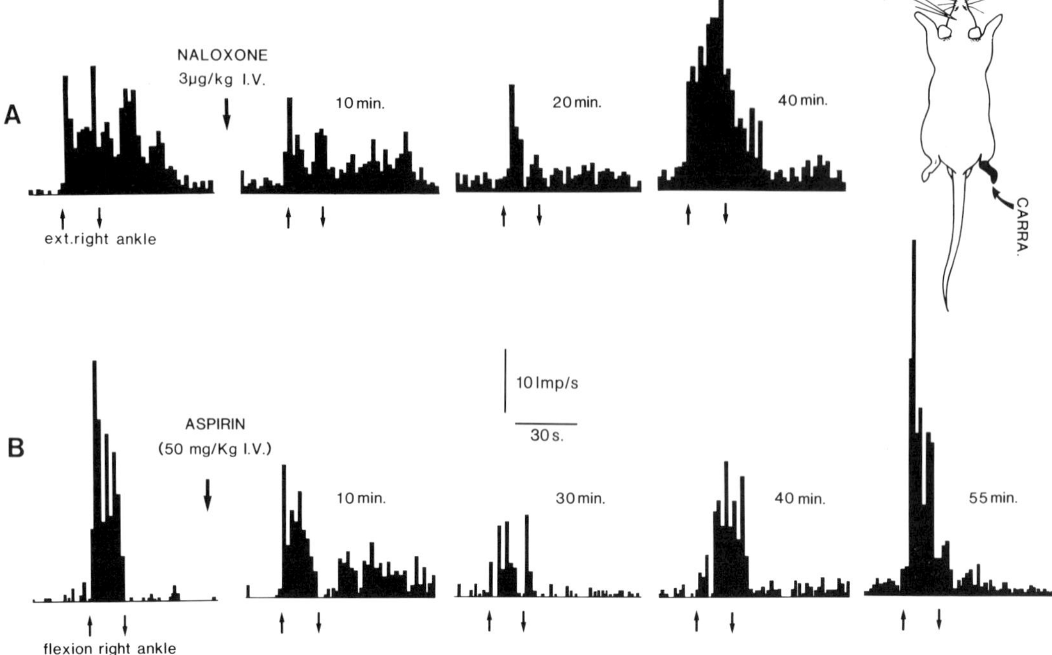

Fig 5 A,B. Peristimulus time histograms illustrating the responses of two left ventrobasal neurones recorded in two rats 24 h after carrageenin injection in the right paw, and driven by movement of the inflamed joints. Naloxone (**A**) and aspirin (**B**) strongly depressed these responses. Ordinates as in Fig. 1

Pharmacological Modulation

Aspirin, even at a dose of 100 mmg/kg i.v., was almost ineffective in modifying VB neuronal response increase in the acute phase of the carrageenin-induced inflammation. In sharp contrast, the dose of 50 mg/kg i.v. strongly depressed the responses elicited in the subacute state, by moderate stimulations (lateral pressure, flexion, or extension), applied to the inflamed paw, including joints and surrounding cutaneous areas (Fig. 5B). This agrees with data on inflammatory mechanisms showing that after carrageenin injection, aspirin is efficient against oedema development only during the late phase, when prostaglandins are released in the exudate, i.e. 3–4 h after carrageenin injection (Garattini et al. 1965; Di Rosa et al. 1971; Higgs and Salmon 1979; Holsapple et al 1980; references in Guilbaud et al. 1986). Our present data confirms that at this stage of the inflammation, the modifications of the responsiveness of some VB neurones are mainly due to the presence of prostaglandins in the tissues.

Also in this phase, naloxone was able to depress the VB neuronal responses due to moderate stimulations of the inflamed joints and surrounding cutaneous areas, when injected at the dose of 3 μg/kg i.v. (Fig. 5A). In this condition the response was 50.3 % ± 10.5 % of the initial value 15 min after the injection (n = 10). The recovery occurred at 35 min.

The depressive effect was of the same order as that observed VB neuronal responses in arthritic rats, also with low doses (Guilbaud et al. 1982). Moreover, as in arthritic rats (reference in Kayser et al. 1986), similar doses of naloxone have been shown to be analgesic in the freely moving animal, mainly when tested several hours after the hyperalgesia initiation (Kayser et al., in preparation).

Thus, in the rats rendered hyperalgesic at 24 h by the carrageenin injection, it appears that the reactivity of the endogenous opioid system might be already modified, while such effects have never been observed in normal non-hyperalgesic animals.

Conclusions

The present data indicate that carrageenin-induced inflammation could be a useful model for electrophysiological and neuropharmacological studies of the regulation and time course of inflammatory pain. They underline the differential roles in the sensitization of various substances released in the exudate.

In addition the results suggest that the final hyperalgesia might result from the interaction of peripheral and central phenomena, these latter being triggered by the initial inflammatory process, which itself adapts over the course of the inflammation. For instance, the analgesic effect of the opiate antagonist naloxone, comparable in the subacute stage to that observed in arthritic rats (references in Kayser et al. 1986), suggests a change in the reactivity of the endogenous opioid system, a change which requires several hours of hyperalgesia to be significant.

References

Adriaensen H, Gybels J, Handwerker HO, van Hees J (1984) Suppression of C-fiber discharges upon repeated heat stimulation may explain characteristics of concomitant pain sensations. Brain Res 302 : 203–211

Anton F, Kocher L, Reeh PW, Handwerker HO (1985) The effect of carrageenan induced inflammation on the excitability of unmeyelinated skin nociceptors in the rat. Neurosci Lett [Suppl] 22 : S 31

Benoist JM, Kayser V, Gautron M, Guilbaud G (1985) Changes in responses of ventrobasal thalamic neurons during carrageenin-induced inflammation in the rat. In: Fields HL, et al. (eds) Advances in pain research and therapy, vol 9. Raven, New York, pp 295–303

Di Rosa M, Giroud JP, Willoughby DA (1971) Studies of the mediators of the acute inflammation response induced in rats in different sites by carrageenan and turpentine. J Pathol 104 : 15–29

Fjällbrant N, Iggo A (1961) The effect of histamine, 5-hydroxytryptamine and acetylcholine on cutaneous afferent fibers. J Physiol (Lond) 156 : 578–590

Fleischer E, Handwerker HO, Joukhadar S (1983) Unmyelinated nociceptive units in two skin areas of the rat. Brain Res 267 : 81–92

Garattini S, Jori A, Bernardi D, Carrara C, Paglialunga S, Segre D (1965) Sensitivity of local oedemas to systemic pharmacological effects. In: Garattini S, Dukes MNG (eds) Nonsteroïdal antiinflammatory drugs. Excerpta Medica, Amsterdam, pp 151–161

Gautron M, Guilbaud G (1982) Somatic responses of ventro-basal thalamic neurones in polyarthritic rats. Brain Res 237 : 459–471

Guilbaud G (1985) Thalamic nociceptive systems. Philos Trans R Soc Lond [Biol] 308 : 339–345

Guilbaud G, Peschanski M, Gautron M, Binder D (1980) Neurones responding to noxious stimulations in V.B. complex and caudal adjacent regions in the thalamus of the rat. Pain 8 : 303–318

Guilbaud G, Benoist JM, Gautron M, Kayser V (1982) Effects of systemic Naloxone upon ventrobasal thalamus neuronal responses in arthritic rats. Brain Res 243 : 59–66

Guilbaud G, Kayser V, Benoist JM, Gautron M (1986) Modifications in the responsiveness of rat ventro-basal thalamic neurons at different stages of carrageenin-produced inflammation. Brain Res 385 : 86–98

Guilbaud G, Benoist JM, Neil A, Kayser V (1987) Neuronal response threshold to and encoding of thermal stimulus during the carrageenin-hyperalgesic inflammation, in the ventrobasal thalamus of rat. Exp Brain Res (in press)

Guilbaud G, Neil A, Benoist JM, Kayser V, Gautron M (1987) Neuronal response threshold to and encoding of the mechanical stimulus during the carrageenin-hyperalgesic inflammation, in the ventrobasal thalamus of rat. Exp Brain Res (in press)

Handwerker HO (1976) The influences of the algogenic substances serotonin and bradykinin on the discharges of unmyelinated cutaneous fibers identified as nociceptors. In: Bonica JJ, Albe-Fessard D (eds) Advances in pain research and therapy, vol 1. Raven, New York, pp 41–46

Hardy JD, Wolff HG, Goodell H (1967) Pain sensations and reactions. Hafner, New York

Heppelmann B, Schaible HG, Schmidt RF (1985) Effects of prostaglandins E1 and 2 on the mechanosensitivity of group III afferents from normal and inflamed cat knee joint. In: Fields HL, et al. (eds), Advances in pain research and therapy, vol 9. Raven, New York, pp 91-101

Higgs E, Salmon JA (1979) Cyclo-oxygenase products in carrageenin-induced inflammation. Prostaglandins 17 : 737–746

Holsapple MP, Schnur M, Yim GKW (1980) Pharmacological modulation of oedema mediated by prostaglandin, serotonin and histamine. Agents Actions 10 : 368–373

Kayser V, Guilbaud G (1987) Locate and remote modifications of the nociceptive sensitivity during carrageenin-induced inflammation. Pain 28 : 99–108

Kayser V, Besson JM, Guilbaud G (1986) Analgesia produced by low doses of the opiate antagonist Naloxone in arthritic rats is reduced in morphine-tolerant animals. Brain Res 371 : 37–41

La Motte RH (1984) Cutaneous nociceptors and pain sensation in normal and hyperalgesic skin. In: Kruger L, Liebeskind JC (eds) Advances in pain research and therapy. Raven, New York, pp 69-82

Lewis T (1935–1936) Experiments relating to cutaneous hyperalgesia and its spread through somatic nerves. Clin Sci 2 : 373–423

Lynn B, Carpenter SE (1982) Primary afferents units from the hairy skin of the rat hind limb. Brain Res 238 : 29–43

Menetrey D, Besson JM (1982) Electrophysiological characteristics of dorsal horn cells in rats with cutaneous inflammation resulting from chronic arthritis. Pain 13 : 343–364

Mense S (1981) Sensitization of group IV muscle receptors to bradykinin by 5-hydroxytryptamine and prostaglandin E2. Brain Res 225 : 95–105

Meyer RA, Campbell JN, Raja SN (1985) Peripheral neural mechanisms of cutaneous hyperalgesia. In: Fields HL, et al. (eds) Advances in pain research and therapy. Raven, New York, pp 53–71

Neil A, Benoist JM, Kayser V, Guilbaud G (1986) Quaternary antihistamine, Thiazinamium, inhibits initial nociceptor sensitization in carrageenin-induced inflammation in rat. Neuroscience [Suppl] 26 :S 526

Neil A, Benoist JM, Kayser V, Guilbaud G (1987) Initial nociceptive sensitization in carrageenin-induced rat paw inflammation is dependent on amine autacoid mechanisms: electrophysiological and behavioural evidence obtained with a quaternary antihistamine, Thiazinamium. Exp Brain Res 65 : 343–351

Peschanski M, Guilbaud G, Gautron M, Besson JM (1980) Encoding property of noxious heat messages in neurons of the ventrobasal thalamic complex of the rat. Brain Res 197 : 401–413

Torebjörk HE, La Motte RH, Robinson CJ (1984) Peripheral neural correlates of magnitude of cutaneous pain and hyperalgesia: simultaneous recordings in humans of sensory judgments of pain and evoked responses in nociceptors with C fibers. J Neurophysiol 51 : 325–339

Vane Jr (1971) Inhibition of prostaglandin synthesis as a mechanism of action for aspirin-like drugs. Nature [New Biol] 231 : 232–235

Winter CA, Flataker L (1965) Reactions thresholds to pressure in oedematous hindpaws of rats responses to analgesic drugs. J Pharmacol Exp Ther 150 : 165–171

40 Viscerosomatic Convergence onto Nociceptive Neurons in the Shell Region of Nucleus Ventralis Posterolateralis

T. Yokota, T. Masuda, H. Taguchi, and N. Koyama

Introduction

The visceral sympathetic nerve contains efferent sympathetic and afferent sensory fibers (Kuo et al. 1984; Kuo and de Groat 1985). It is suggested that at least some of these afferent fibers participate in transmission of nociceptive signals from the viscera to the central nervous system (Gernandt and Zotterman 1946; Baker et al. 1980; Cervero 1982a). Afferent impulses in the visceral sympathetic nerve can affect the activity of nociceptive neurons in the dorsal horn of the spinal cord, and these neurons may be involved in the sensation of visceral pain (Pomeranz et al. 1968; Selzer and Spencer 1969; Fields and Winter 1970; Fields et al. 1970; Hancock et al. 1973, 1975; Guilbaud and Besson 1977; Gokin et al. 1977; Foreman 1977; Foreman and Ohata 1980; Foreman and Weber 1980; Blair et al. 1981, 1982, 1984; Weber et al. 1982; Rucker and Holloway 1982; Cervero 1982b, 1983; Takahashi and Yokota 1983; Ammons et al. 1984, 1985; Foreman et al. 1984; Rucker et al. 1984; Cervero and Tattersall 1985). However, the thalamic links in the visceral pain pathway have not been vigorously studied. The present study was undertaken to examine one possible link: the nucleus ventralis posterolateralis (VPL).

Methods

Experiments were performed on 161 healthy adult cats weighing 2.5-4.0 kg. Anesthesia was induced with ketamine (20 mg/kg) and maintained with an intravenous dose of 3.5 ml/kg urethan-chloralose solution (urethan 125 mg/ml, chloralose 10 mg/ml). Animals were paralyzed with pancuronium bromide (0.4 mg/kg) and artificially ventilated. End-tidal CO_2 was maintained between 3.5 % and 4.5 %. Supplementary doses of urethan-chloralose solution were administered to maintain a deep level of anesthesia. The right femoral artery was cannulated for blood pressure measurement. Esophageal temperature was maintained at 37.5 °C with a heating pad.

In each animal, the left splanchnic and/or inferior cardiac nerve was prepared for electrical stimulation. The left greater splanchnic nerve was exposed retroperitoneally through an incision in the lumbosacral fascia at the edge of the erector spinae muscle mass. The exposed nerve was dissected free from the surrounding tissues at the level just proximal to the celiac ganglion. The left inferior cardiac nerve was exposed by a left thoracotomy in the second intercostal space. A bipolar platinum hook electrode was placed on each exposed nerve and was held in position by low-melting-point wax. The greater splanchnic and inferior cardiac nerves were tightly ligated distal to the stimulating electrodes, thus blocking efferent sympathetic impulses.

Before exploration with the microelectrode, the threshold for reflex contraction of abdominal muscles elicited by electrical stimulation of the greater splanchnic nerve was measured. The reflex is called the viscerointercostal reflex (VIR), and is due to Aδ afferent volleys (Downman 1954). Single unit activities were recorded using glass capillary microelectrodes, filled with 2% pontamine sky blue in 1 M sodium acetate. Each VPL unit was tested for both somatic and visceral inputs. Low-intensity cutaneous stimuli included displacement of single hairs and stroking as well as probing the skin. High-intensity mechanical stimuli included firm pressure, exerted by picking up a fold of skin with flattened forceps or an arterial clip, and noxious pinch with serrated forceps or an alligator clip. Visceral input was tested with electrical stimulation (0.1 ms, 2–3 V, once every 1.5 s) of the greater splanchnic or inferior cardiac nerve. The threshold of unit responses to the splanchnic nerve stimulation was compared with the threshold for the VIR. Single-unit responses to the greater splanchnic or inferior cardiac nerve stimulation were recorded by means of a transient memory and pen writer. In some units, responses were displayed by the raster-dot method.

Stereotaxic coordinates and microelectrode micrometer readings were recorded for all microelectrode penetrations. At least two spots were marked at each penetration by passing a 5-μA cathodal current through the microelectrode tip for 5 min, thus depositing a small amount of dye. Locations of all nociceptive units were marked.

At the termination of each experiment, the brain was cleared of blood and fixed in situ by perfusing 1000 ml normal saline through the beating heart, followed by 3000 ml 10% formol saline. The fixed brain was frozen and cut into 50-μm sections. Dye marks, about 50 μm in diameter, were identified in sections stained with cresyl violet.

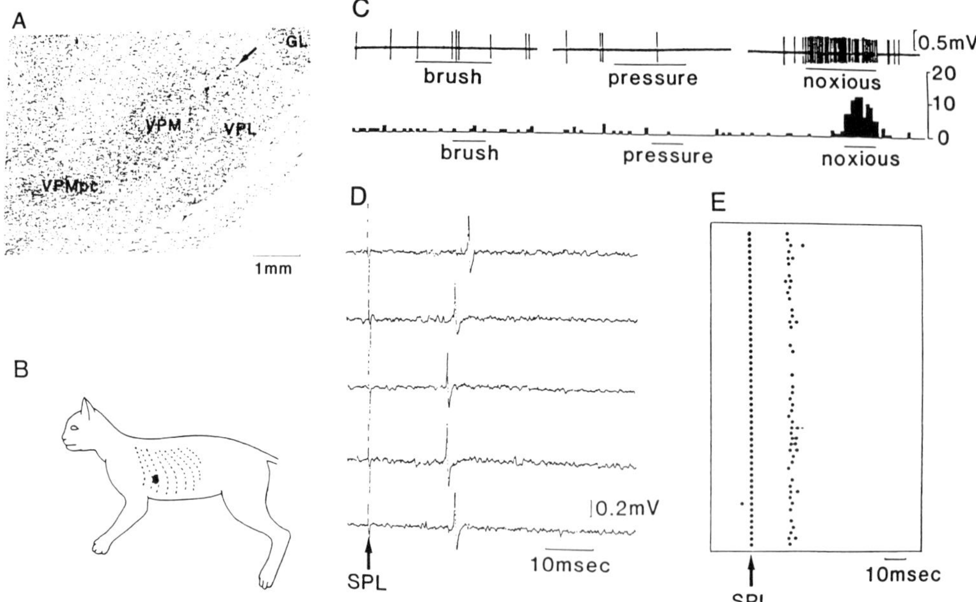

Fig. 1 A–E. A nociceptive-specific unit responsive to splanchnic afferents. **A** Location of the unit (indicated by an arrow). VPL nucleus ventralis posterolateralis, VPM nucleus ventralis posteromedialis, VPM pc parvocellular part of VPM. **B** Receptive field (marked by a black area). **C** Responses of the unit to brushing, pressure, and noxious pinch applied to the receptive field. The upper trace shows unit discharges. The lower trace shows number of spike discharges per second determined with a spike counter. **D** Responses of the unit to electrical stimulation of the greater splanchnic nerve (SPL). **E** Responses of the unit to SPL stimulation displayed by the raster-dot method

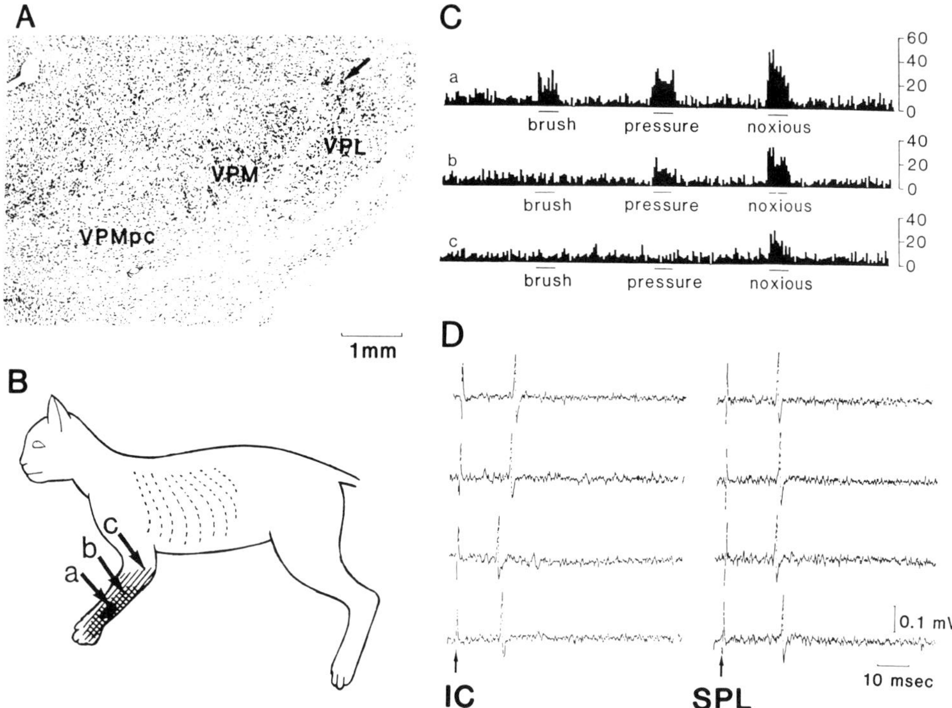

Fig. 2 A–D. A wide-dynamic-range unit responsive to visceral afferents. **A** Location of the unit (indicated by an arrow). VPL nucleus ventralis posterolateralis, VPM nucleus ventralis posteromedialis, VPM pc parvocellular part of VPM. **B** Receptive field. In black area, the unit had a graded response to brush, pressure, and noxious pinch. In the cross-hatched area, the unit did not respond to brush, but responded to both pressure and noxious pinch. In the shaded area, the unit specifically responded to noxious pinch. **C** Responses of the unit to mechanical stimulation of the receptive field. Three different small areas shown by arrows in *B* were stimulated, and traces a, b, and c represent their responses. Horizontal bars indicate periods of stimulus application. Duration of each stimulus was 10s. **D** Responses of the unit to electrical stimulation of the inferior cardiac (IC) and greater splanchnic (SPL) nerves

Results

Units recorded from the VPL responded to mechanical stimulation of the body surface. They were classified into three categories using the same criteria as employed by previous investigators (Kenshalo et al. 1980; Yokota et al. 1985). They were low-threshold mechanoreceptive (LTM) units, nociceptive-specific (NS) units and wide-dynamic-range (WDR) units. A great majority of VPL units (92%) were LTM units. They were maximally excited by gentle mechanical stimulation of a clearly defined contralateral receptive field. Units responsive to electrical stimulation of the greater splanchnic and/or inferior cardiac nerve were not found in this population. The remaining units (8 %)were identified as nociceptive responders, i.e., NS and WDR units. NS units usually responded with a maintained discharge exclusively to noxious pinch of a circumscribed contralateral cutaneous receptive field. Some responded to firm pressure, but discharged more vigorously when noxious pinch was applied. WDR units had a graded response in the center of the receptive field to brush, pressure, and noxious pinch and responded best to noxious pinch. Outside this zone was an area where they were unresponsive to low-intensity mechanical stimuli, but responded differentially to firm pressure and noxious pinch. Finally, the latter area was surrounded by a zone in which only noxious pinch resulted in unit discharges. The receptive field was confined to the contralateral half of the body surface. As reported by previous investigators (Honda et al. 1983; Kniffki and Mizumura 1983; Yokota et al. 1985), they were located in the shell region of the VPL. They showed a spatial segregation from each other, i.e., NS units were located in the dorsal as well as ventral shell regions of the caudal VPL, whereas WDR units were found in a narrow band just in front of the NS zone (Yokota et al. 1985). Units responsive to visceral afferents were included in these two classes of nociceptive units. No VPL units were encountered which were specifically driven by visceral afferents. Just outside the VPL, i.e., dorsal or lateral to the VPL, tap units with a wide subcutaneous receptive field were found. Some of them were responsive to visceral input. The threshold of their responses to the splanchnic stimulation did not exceed the threshold for the VIR, suggesting that they receive low-threshold splanchnic afferents. Since our study focused on the VPL, these tap units will not be discussed further.

Nociceptive-Specific Units Responsive to Splanchnic Afferents

In 241 NS units, responses to electrical stimulation of the greater splanchnic nerve were tested. Of these, 86 units (36 %) were driven by splanchnic afferents at 1.0-4.44 times threshold for the VIR. The shortest latencies measured at 1.5 times threshold ranged from 9.5 to 32.3 ms.

In general, NS units in the dorsal or ventral shell region had a cutaneous receptive field on the dorsal or ventral aspect of the body respectively. Receptive fields of NS units responsive to splanchnic afferents were located in the posterior forearm, posterior arm, scapular area, chest, abdomen, and anterior thigh, corresponding to tactile dermatomes C_8-L_3 (Hekmatpanah 1961). Receptive fields of NS units unresponsive to splanchnic afferents were located in the neck, shoulder, anterior arm, anterior forearm, forepaw, rump, and hind limb. There was no overlap in cutaneous receptive fields between units responsive to splanchnic afferents and those unresponsive to these afferents.

Wide-Dynamic-Range Units Responsive to Splanchnic Afferents

In 178 WDR units, responses to electrical stimulation of the splanchnic nerve were tested. Of these, 85 units (48%) were responsive to splanchnic afferents. The threshold of unit responses was 1.0–4.62 times the threshold for the VIR. The shortest latencies measured at 1.5 times threshold ranged from 9.5 to 20.5 ms.

The center of the receptive field of dorsal shell units was on the dorsal aspect of the body surface, whereas that of ventral shell units was on the ventral body surface. The receptive fields of WDR units responsive to splanchnic afferents were distributed in a wider area of the body surface than those of NS units responsive to the same afferents, and WDR units responsive to splanchnic afferents and those unresponsive to the same afferents showed a certain degree of overlap in the distribution of their receptive fields. However, all the WDR units responsive to splanchnic afferents had at least a part of their receptive fields in the area corresponding to tactile dermatomes C_8-L_3, i.e., the posterior forearm, posterior arm, scapular area, chest, abdomen, and anterior thigh, whereas those unresponsive to splanchnic afferents did not have their receptive fields in these regions.

Nociceptive-Specific Units Responsive to Cardiac Afferents

In 163 NS units, responses to electrical stimulation of the inferior cardiac nerve were tested. Of these, 75 units (46%) responded to the stimulation. The shortest latencies of the responses ranged from 10.0 to 22.5 ms. Their receptive fields were located in the forelimb, shoulder, scapular area, or chest, corresponding to tactile dermatomes C_5-T_{13}.

In 61 NS units, responses to both inferior cardiac and greater splanchnic nerve stimulations were tested. Of these, 20 units responded to both stimulations, three units responded only to cardiac nerve stimulation, and another three units responded only to splanchnic nerve stimulation. NS units responsive to both stimulations had their receptive fields in the area corresponding to tactile dermatomes C_8-T_{13}. NS units responsive only to cardiac nerve stimulation had their receptive fields in the area corresponding to tactile dermatomes C_5-C_7.

Wide-Dynamic-Range Units Responsive to Cardiac Afferents

In 120 WDR units, responses to electrical stimulation of the inferior cardiac nerve were tested. Of these, 82 units (68%) responded to the stimulation. The shortest latencies of the responses ranged from 9.0 to 19.1 ms. They had at least a part of their receptive field in the area corresponding to tactile dermatomes C_5-T_{13}.

In 60 WDR units, responses to both inferior cardiac and splanchnic nerve stimulations were tested. Of these, 29 units responded to both stimulations, four units responded only to cardiac nerve stimulation, and three units responded only to splanchnic nerve stimulation.

Discussion

The present data suggest that the shell region of the VPL constitutes a thalamic link in a visceral pain pathway. These results were predictable. First, as will be discussed in the following, nociceptive neurons in the dorsal horn of the spinal cord receive visceral input. Second, both NS and WDR units are located in the shell region of the VPL (Honda et al. 1983; Kniffki and Mizumura 1983; Yokota et al. 1985).

An important clinical aspect of visceral pain is the phenomenon of referral, in which pain originating from the viscera is referred to somatic structures. Current interpretation of the mechanism of this phenomenon is based on the "convergence-projection" theory of Ruch (1947). That is, somatic and visceral inputs converge onto neurons at some point in pain pathways. These neurons normally relay impulses from somatic structures and only rarely from the viscera. The brain learns to associate their excitation with somatic pain. When visceral impulses are transmitted via these neurons, the brain may misinterpret the true origin of the pain and refer it to somatic structures. This theory requires the existence of viscerosomatic convergence onto neurons in pain pathways. There is a good deal of experimental support for the existence of viscerosomatic convergence onto neurons in the spinal cord (Pomeranz et al. 1968; Selzer and Spencer 1969; Fields and Winter 1970; Fields et al. 1970; Hancock et al. 1973; Guilbaud and Besson 1977; Gokin et al. 1977; Foreman 1977; Foreman and Ohata 1980; Weber et al. 1982; Cervero 1982b, 1983; Takahashi and Yokota 1983; Cervero and Tattersall 1985), including neurons of the spinothalamic tract in the monkey (Foreman and Weber 1980; Blair et al. 1981, 1982, 1984; Ammons et al. 1985) and in the cat (Hancock et al. 1975; Rucker and Holloway 1982; Foreman et al. 1984; Rucker et al. 1984). Visceral noxious input converges mainly onto those neurons having a noxious cutaneous input, whereas neurons in the spinal cord driven exclusively by innocuous stimulation of the skin are rarely driven by visceral input (Guilbaud and Besson 1977; Foreman and Ohata 1980; Cervero 1983a, b; Takahashi and Yokota 1983). The results of the present study, showing convergence of visceral and cutaneous inputs onto NS and WDR units in the shell region of the VPL, lend additional support to the convergence-projection theory.

Another finding of the present study is the convergence of both cardiac and splanchnic inputs onto NS and WDR units in the shell region of the VPL. The convergence would account for some types of referred pain similar to that of cardiac origin, which may accompany certain abdominal diseases such as the splenic flexure syndrome.

Summary

Convergence of high-threshold splanchnic and cutaneous inputs onto NS and WDR units in the shell region of the caudal VPL was demonstrated in urethan-chloralose anesthetized cats. NS units responsive to splanchnic afferents had a receptive field in the area corresponding to tactile dermatomes C_8-L_3. WDR units responsive to splanchnic afferents had at least a part of their receptive fields in the same area.

Similarly, convergence of cardiac and cutaneous inputs onto NS and WDR units was demonstrated in the shell region of the VPL. NS units responsive to cardiac afferents had a receptive field in the area corresponding to tactile dermatomes C_5-T_{13}. WDR units responsive to cardiac afferents had at least a part of their receptive fields in the same area. A significant fraction of these cardiac units also received splanchnic afferents. It is suggested that the shell region of the VPL constitutes a thalamic link in a visceral pain pathway.

References

Ammons WS, Blair RW, Foreman RD (1984) Splanchnic activation of primate T_1-T_5 spinothalamic neurons. J Neurophysiol 51 : 592–603

Ammons WS, Girardot M-N, Foreman RD (1985) T_2-T_5 spinothalamic neurons projecting to medial thalamus with viscerosomatic input. J Neurophysiol 54 : 73–89

Baker DG, Coleridge HM, Coleridge JCG, Nederum T (1980) Search for a cardiac nociceptor: stimulation by bradykinin of sympathetic afferent nerve endings in the heart of the cat. J Physiol (Lond) 306 : 519–536

Blair RW, Weber RN, Foreman RD (1981) Characteristics of primate spinothalamic tract neurons receiving viscerosomatic convergent inputs in T_3-T_5 segments. J Neurophysiol 46 : 797–811

Blair RW, Weber RN, Foreman RD (1982) Responses of thoracic spinothalamic neurons to intracardiac injection of bradykinin in the monkey. Circ Res 51 : 83–94

Blair RW, Ammons WS, Foreman RD (1984) Responses of thoracic spinothalamic and spinoreticular cells to coronary artery occlusion. J Neurophysiol 51 : 636–648

Cervero F (1982a) Afferent activity evoked by natural stimulation of the biliary system in the ferret. Pain 13 : 137–151

Cervero F (1982b) Noxious intensities of visceral stimulation are required to activate viscero-somatic multireceptive neurons in the thoracic cord of the cat. Brain Res 240 : 350–352

Cervero F (1983) Somatic and visceral inputs to the thoracic spinal cord of the cat: effects of noxious stimulation of the biliary system. J Physiol (Lond) 337 : 51–67

Cervero F, Tattersall JEH (1985) Cutaneous receptive fields of somatic and viscerosomatic neurons in the thoracic spinal cord of the cat. J Comp Neurol 237 : 325–332

Downman CBB (1954) Skeletal muscle reflexes of splanchnic and intercostal nerve origin in acute spinal and decerebrate cats. J Neurophysiol 18 : 217–235

Fields HL, Winter DL (1970) Somatovisceral pathway: rapidly conducting fibers in the spinal cord. Science 167 : 1729–1730

Fields HL, Meyer GA, Partridge LD Jr (1970) Convergence of visceral and somatic inputs onto spinal neurons. Exp Neurol 26 : 36–52

Foreman RD (1977) Viscerosomatic convergence onto spinal neurons responding to afferent fibers located in the inferior cardiac nerve. Brain Res 137 : 164–168

Foreman RD, Blair RW, Weber RN (1984) Viscerosomatic convergence onto T_2-T_4 spinoreticular, spinoreticular-spinothalamic and spino-thalamic tract neurons in the cat. Exp Neurol 85 : 597–613

Foreman RD, Hancock MB, Willis WD (1981) Responses of spinothalamic tract cells in the thoracic spinal cord of the monkey to cutaneous and visceral inputs. Pain 11 : 149–162

Foreman RD, Ohata CA (1980) Effects of coronary artery occlusion on thoracic spinal neurons receiving viscerosomatic inputs. Am J Physiol 238 : H667-H674

Foreman RD, Weber RN (1980) Responses from neurons of the primate spinothalamic tract to electrical stimulation of afferents from the cardiopulmonary region and somatic structures. Brain Res 186 : 463–468

Gernandt B, Zotterman Y (1946) Intestinal pain: an electrophysiological investigation on mesenteric nerves. Acta Physiol Scand 12 : 56–72

Gokin AP, Kostyk PG, Presbrzhensky NN (1977) Neuronal mechanisms of interactions of high-threshold visceral and somatic afferent influences in spinal cord and medulla. J Physiol (Paris) 33 : 319–333

Guilbaud G, Besson JM (1977) Responses of thoracic dorsal horn interneurons to cutaneous stimulation and to the administration of algogenic substances into the mesenteric artery in the spinal cat. Brain Res 124 : 437–448

Hancock MB, Rigamonti DD, Bryan RN (1973) Convergence in the lumbar spinal cord of pathways activated by splanchnic nerve and hindlimb cutaneous nerve stimulation. Exp Neurol 38 : 337–348

Hancock MB, Foreman RD, Willis WD (1975) Convergence of visceral and cutaneous input onto spinothalamic tract cells in the thoracic spinal cord of the cat. Exp Neurol 47 : 240–248

Hekmatpanah J (1961) Organization of tactile dermatomes C1 through L4, in cat. J Neurophysiol 24 : 129–140

Honda CN, Mense S, Perl ER (1983) Neurons in ventrobasal region of cat thalamus selectively responsive to noxious mechanical stimulation. J Neurophysiol 49 : 662–673

Kenshalo DR, Giesler GJ, Leonard RB, Willis WD (1980) Response of neurons in primate ventral posterior lateral nucleus to noxious stimuli. J Neurophysiol 43 : 1594–1614

Kniffki K-D, Mizumura K (1983) Responses of neurons in VPL and VPL-VL region of the cat to algesic stimulation of muscle and tendon. J Neurophysiol 49 : 649–661

Kuo DC, de Groat WC (1985) Primary afferent projections of the major splanchnic nerve to the spinal cord and gracile nucleus of the cat. J Comp Neurol 231 : 421–434

Kuo DC, Oravitz JJ, de Groat WC (1984) Tracing of afferent and efferent pathways in the left inferior cardiac nerve of the cat using retrograde and transganglionic transport of horseradish peroxidase. J Comp Neurol 321 : 111–118

POMERANZ B, WALL PD, WEBER WV (1968) Cord cells responding to fine myelinated afferents from viscera, muscle and skin. J Physiol 199 : 511–532

RUCH TV (1947) Visceral sensation and referred pain. In: FULTON JF (ed) Howell's textbook of physiology, 15th edn. Saunders, Philadelphia, pp 385–401

RUCKER HK, HOLLOWAY JA (1982) Viscerosomatic convergence onto spinothalamic tract neurons in the cat. Brain Res 243 : 155–157

RUCKER HK, HOLLOWAY JA, KEYSER GF (1984) Response characteristics of cat spinothalamic tract neurons to splanchnic nerve stimulation. Brain Res 291 : 383–387

SELZER M, SPENCER WA (1969) Convergence of visceral and cutaneous afferent pathways in the lumber spinal cord. Brain Res 14 : 331–348

TAKAHASHI M, YOKOTA T (1983) Convergence of cardiac and cutaneous afferents onto neurons in the dorsal horn of the spinal cord in the cat. Neurosci Lett 38 : 251–256

WEBER RN, BLAIR RW, FOREMAN RD (1982) Effects of cardiac administration of bradykinin on thoracic spinal neurons in the cat. Exp Neurol 78 : 703–715

YOKOTA T, KOYAMA N, MATSUMOTO N (1985) Somatotopic distribution of trigeminal nociceptive neurons in ventrobasal complex of cat thalamus. J Neurophysiol 53 : 1387–1400

41 Nociceptive Neurons in the Ventral Periphery of the Cat Thalamic Ventroposteromedial Nucleus

C. Vahle-Hinz, I. Freund, and K.-D. Kniffki

Introduction

Recent reports have demonstrated that some neurons located in the periphery of the cat ventrobasal complex respond to noxious stimuli (Kniffki and Mizumura 1983; Honda et al. 1983; Yokota and Matsumoto 1983a, b; Kniffki and Craig 1985; Yokota et al. 1985). The present study, which is still in progress, was undertaken to confirm and to extend the previous results and to establish in more detail the functional organization of nociceptive neurons within the periphery of the cat thalamic ventroposterior nuclei, especially the ventroposteromedial nucleus (VPM).

Methods

Adult cats were anesthetized with an initial dose of 40 mg/kg i.p. sodium pentobarbital (Nembutal) and tracheal, venous (femoral), and arterial (femoral) cannulae were inserted for artificial respiration, injections, and measurement of blood pressure respectively. The animal's head was fixed in a stereotaxic holder and a small craniotomy was performed. Body temperature, mean blood pressure, and end-tidal CO_2 were monitored continuously and were kept within normal physiological limits. Before recording, the depth of the anesthesia was allowed to decrease until a moderate withdrawal reflex and just no or only slight increases in blood pressure were observed on pinching the forepaw skin. Then the animals were immobilized with pancuronium bromide (Pancuronium, Organon) and artificially respirated. During the recording session, the level of anesthesia was maintained by additional i.v. doses of Nembutal so that noxious stimuli elicited just no or only slight and short-lasting increases in blood pressure. The animals were periodically allowed to recover from the immobilization and the anesthetic level was tested. Single- and multiunit recordings were made with steel microelectrodes. Soma recordings were identified by the shape of the action potential and by the initial segment-soma inflection of the spike.

Due to the search method, only those neurons with a discharge in the absence of intentional stimulation were studied. During investigation of a unit, attempts were made to determine a receptive field on the body surface first by manual probing and with innocuous stimuli using hand-held probes (brush, forceps, tuning fork, ice cube), and then with graded noxious stimuli (pinch and radiant heat). Small electrolytic lesions were made at recording sites of identified nociceptive units.

At the termination of the recording session the animal was given additional doses of Nembutal and perfused intracardially with an aldehyde solution. The brain was then blocked with a scalpel blade inserted into the electrode holder and 50-μm serial frontal sections were taken with a vibratome and stained with Thionin. The locations of the lesion sites were determined on the sections and their histological coordinates were transferred into a standardized brain atlas according to a previously published procedure (Vahle-Hinz and Gottschaldt 1983) which is outlined in the legend of Fig. 4.

Results

The present results are based on a careful exploration of the VPM and its ventral periphery. All units recorded in VPM were only sensitive to low-threshold mechanical stimulation, except for a few neurons which were activated by innocuous cooling of the tongue. The well-known sequence of receptive fields was observed in the dorsoventral electrode tracks through VPM. When, in an electrode penetration, a sudden change in the background activity was noted, the response characteristics of the neurons also changed and in most cases the sequence of receptive fields was disrupted. Lesions made at these points revealed in the histological sections that the change in recording characteristics occurs at the ventral border of VPM. In this border region some spontaneously active neurons could not be driven by the kinds of peripheral stimulation employed, while others showed responses to noxious stimuli.

Functional Classes of Nociceptive Neurons

In 22 cats, 127 units were recorded in the periphery of VPM which showed nociceptive responses. Of these, 12 had receptive fields on the forepaw and 115 had orofacial receptive fields. The latter were classified as nociceptive-specific (40), multireceptive (34), and switching (41) neurons. Nociceptive-specific and multireceptive neurons are characterized by

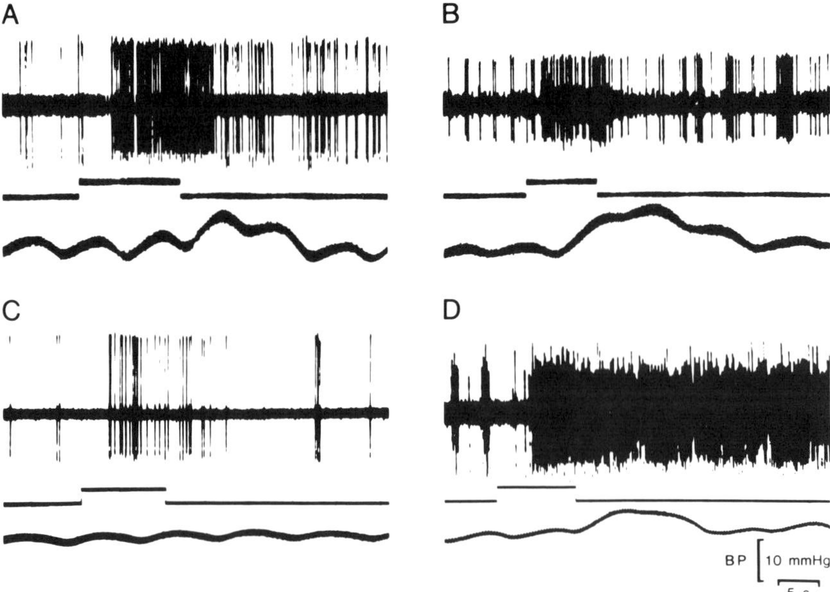

Fig. 1 A–D. Responses of four different nociceptive thalamic neurons, located in the ventral periphery of VPM, to noxious radiant heat stimuli within their receptive fields on the animal's head. Beneath each original record is shown a trace for stimulus duration and a trace for the animal's blood pressure

their ability to encode the intensity of noxious stimuli, the former responding exclusively to these stimuli, the latter also activated by low-threshold stimuli. Switching neurons, similarly, are activated either by noxious stimuli alone or by both noxious and innocuous stimuli, but in contrast to the other two classes of units their responses do not seem to represent stimulus intensity or duration. In response to a stimulus, they switch their discharge frequency to a higher level which is then maintained for up to several minutes. Because of this long-lasting excitation elicited by each stimulus, the investigation of stimulus-response characteristics and receptive fields of switching neurons is difficult. They were therefore not studied in detail.

Figure 1 shows the responses of four different neurons to noxious radiant heat stimuli within their receptive fields. The units responded to the stimuli at latencies of 2–6 s, and continued to discharge for 2–7 s (Fig. 1 A–C) after the stimuli terminated. The response latencies to the heat stimuli correlated remarkably well with the onset of pain felt by the experimenter who subjected a fingertip to the same stimuli. The large range of latencies is due to the different distances from the skin of the hand-held heat lamp for each unit tested.

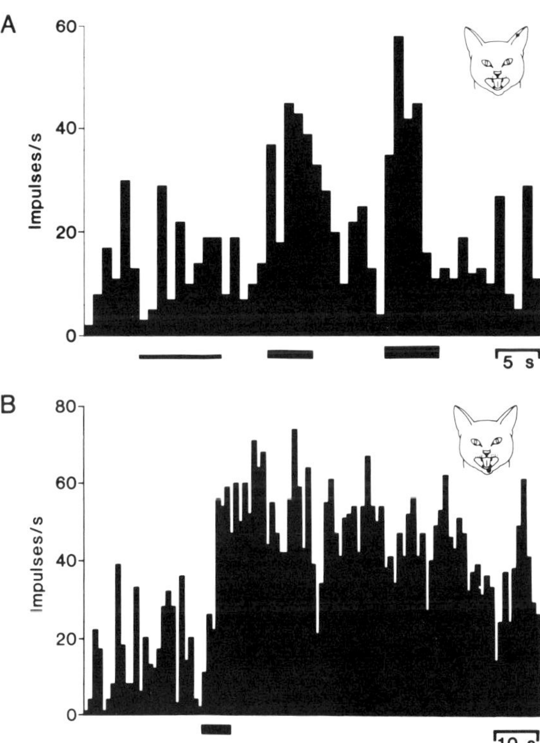

Fig. 2 A. Peristimulus-time histogram of the responses of a nociceptive-specific neuron to graded mechanical stimulation. The bars show qualitatively the increase in stimulus intensity from innocuous pressure to moderate and strong pinch applied with blunt forceps to the ear. **B** Peristimulus-time histogram of the "response" of a switching neuron to a short noxious heat stimulus (bar) on the lower lip. Note the long-lasting excitation of the switching neuron **(B)** in comparison to the stimulus-correlated responses of the nociceptive-specific neuron **(A)**

In the case of the switching units (see example in Fig. 1D), the evoked discharge continued at about the same rate for more than 30 s. This characteristic distinguishes the switching neurons from nociceptive-specific neurons, which in some cases could also exhibit an elevated level of discharge after repeated noxious stimulation. But, as can be seen in Fig. 1A, in nociceptive-specific neurons there would always be a marked drop in the discharge frequency at the transition from the end of the stimulus-response discharge to the resting discharge.

The blood pressure curves below records A, B, and D of Fig. 1 show a slight, short-lasting increase, related to the stimulus, which begins 6–14 s after stimulus onset and clearly after the beginning of the neuronal responses.

The distinct response characteristics of nociceptive-specific and switching neurons are contrasted in the peristimulus-time histograms of Fig. 2. The nociceptive-specific unit in Fig. 2A was not activated by innocuous pressure applied with blunt forceps, but showed responses to noxious pinch which increased with the intensity of the stimulus. Thus, information about parameters of noxious stimuli was encoded in the activity of this unit. The switching unit in Fig. 2B, on the other hand, merely elevated its level of discharge for over 1 min in response to a heat stimulus. This unit could be activated in the same way by noxious pinch.

Localization of Nociceptive Neurons

Lesions made at the sites of identified nociceptive units allowed us to histologically verify their locations within the area of the ventrobasal complex. Figure 3 shows an example of a frontal section through the right thalamus with two such lesion sites corresponding to a nociceptive-specific unit (lateral) and a switching unit (medial). Both were activated by pinch and noxious heat stimuli on the ipsi- and contralateral head, and the receptive field of the more medially located unit included both frontal paws, as depicted on the inset. In general, the receptive fields of switching neurons were more complex than those of the two other classes of nociceptive neurons. The lesions are located in the area between VPM proper and the external medullary lamina.

In 79% of the nociceptive units, a jump in the sequence of receptive fields was noted when the electrode entered this border region of VPM. For example, the receptive fields of units encountered in the lateral electrode track of Fig. 3 above the nociceptive unit included ipsilateral intraoral structures. The last single unit of VPM proper, whose approximate position is marked by a dot in Fig. 3, was activated by low-threshold mechanical stimulation of the upper and lower ipsilateral molars. When the electrode was advanced by 250 μm, this unit and the background activity, which could be driven by mechanical intraoral stimulation, disappeared and a single unit appeared which had nociceptive receptive fields on the ear and the nose but could not be driven by any kind of stimulus applied to the inside of the mouth. This receptive field sequence signals that the electrode has left VPM, for in VPM proper the cat's face is represented upright so that receptive fields on the upper head always lie dorsal to mouth receptive fields (Vahle-Hinz and Gottschaldt 1983). The discontinuity of the sequence of receptive fields is also true for the majority of the low-threshold receptive

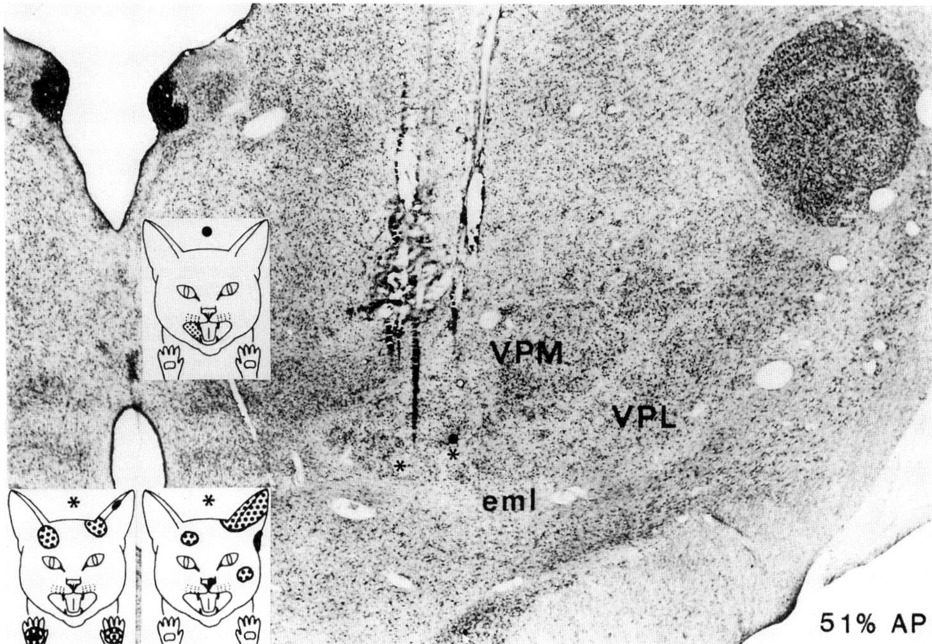

Fig. 3. Frontal section through the right thalamus showing the lesion sites (asterisks) at the recording loci of a nociceptive-specific neuron (lateral) and a switching neuron (medial). The approximate location of the last VPM neuron recorded in the lateral track before the electrode entered the nociceptive area is marked by a dot. Insets: areas from which the units could be activated by low-threshold mechanical stimulation (small stippling), by noxious radiant heat (large stippling), and by noxious pinch (black). The precise outlines of the receptive fields were not mapped. In the standardized brain atlas (see legend of Fig. 4) this section lies at anteroposterior (AP) 51%. VPM, ventroposteromedial nucleus; VPL, ventroposterolateral nucleus; eml, external medullary lamina

fields of multireceptive units. For most units these were located in the same areas as the nociceptive receptive fields or in adjacent areas, but separate areas on the face or the paws were sometimes included (Fig. 5).

Since only a few nociceptive units could be isolated and studied in each experiment, the data from all animals had to be pooled to disclose a possible somatotopic organization of the nociceptive area beneath VPM. In order to compensate for different brain sizes, a standardization method (see legend of Fig. 4) was used. Figures 4 and 5 show the lesion sites of 68 nociceptive units projected onto a horizontal plane of the standardized dimensions of the ventral periphery of VPM. Cat head outlines on which the receptive fields were marked are used instead of symbols for nociceptive-specific units in Fig. 4 and for multireceptive units in Fig. 5. The extent of the vibrissae representation in VPM is drawn in for comparison. The latter was reconstructed from the recording sites of single units with sinus hair receptive fields using the same standardization method as in the present study (Vahle-Hinz and Gottschaldt 1983). Since the vibrissae representation in a dorsoventral projection covers most of VPM, except for its medial (intraoral) part, it seems that the nociceptive neurons occupy the entire extent of the ventral periphery of VPM in the mediolateral and anteroposterior

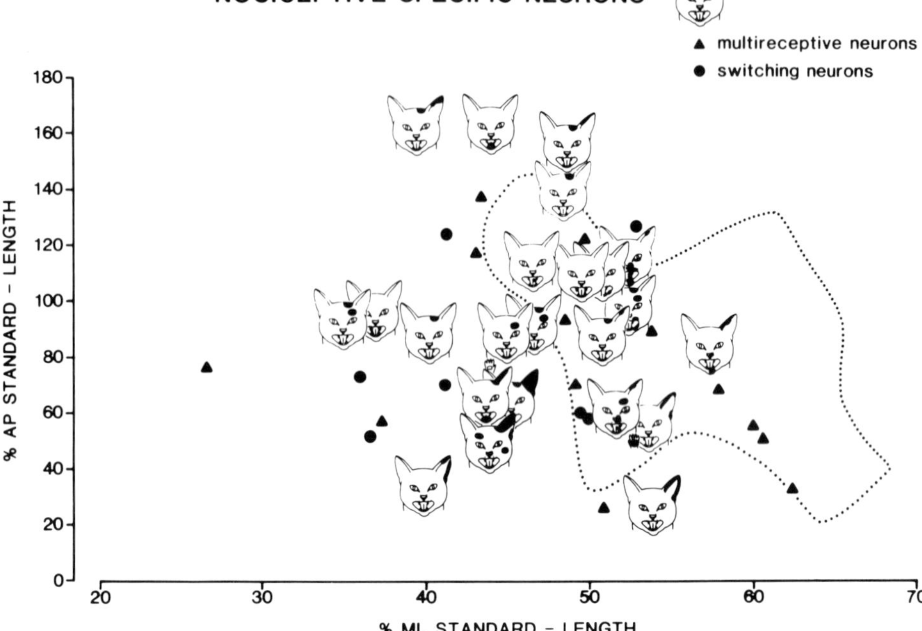

Fig. 4. Projections of the locations of the three classes of nociceptive neurons in the ventral periphery of VPM onto a horizontal plane (medial to the left, rostral up). For the nociceptive-specific neurons, cat head outlines showing their receptive fields are placed with the noses at the coordinates of the recording loci. The locations of the units were determined from the histological sections, which showed the lesions made at the recording sites, and were transferred into a standardized brain atlas using anatomical reference distances from each individual brain. The anteroposterior (AP) standard length is the distance between the rostral pole of the entrance of the optic tract into the lateral geniculate nucleus (LGN; 0%) and the rostral pole of the LGN (100%). The mediolateral (ML) standard length is the distance from the midline (0%) to the center of the LGN (100%) measured at the 50% anterior section. The scales of the axes are shown in the same proportion as the two standard lengths. The coordinates of the units are expressed in percentage of the reference distances in each individual brain. For comparison, the outline of the vibrissae representation in VPM, which was generated by the same method (Vahle-Hinz and Gottschaldt 1983) is indicated (dotted line)

dimensions. The three types of nociceptive neurons are intermingled in this area and no somatotopic organization of receptive fields can be discerned.

In Fig. 5 the low-threshold mechanical and the nociceptive receptive fields of the multireceptive units are shown. The latter include, as in Fig. 4 for the nociceptive-specific units, areas from which responses could be elicited to noxious pinch and noxious radiant heat stimuli. Although several areas on the face and paws were tested for each unit, the exact outline of the receptive fields was not mapped. Therefore, not all of the receptive fields are necessarily discontinuous as shown here, although in several cases unresponsive areas between responsive areas were clearly seen.

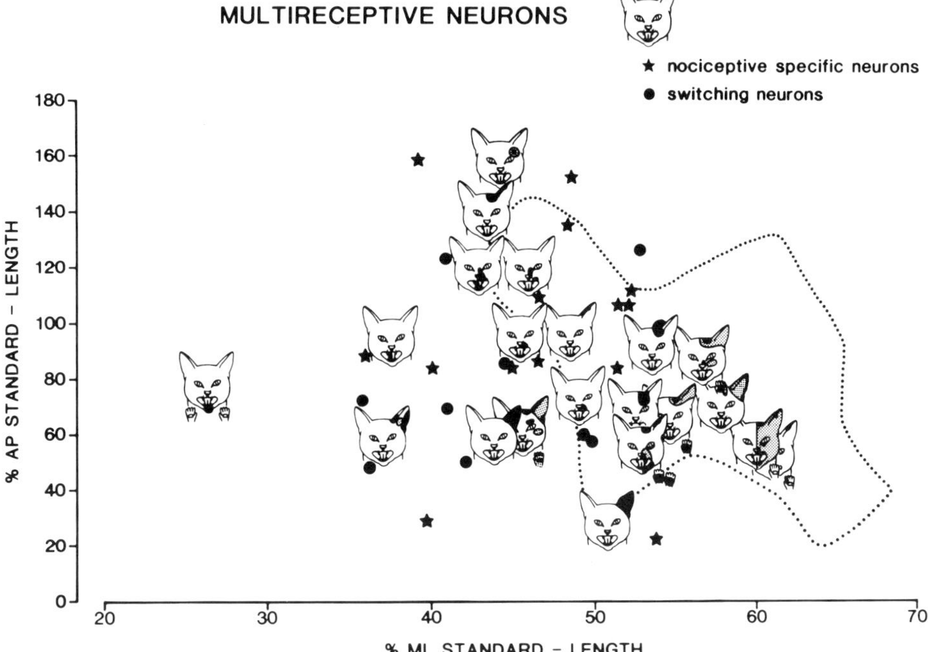

Fig. 5. Projections onto a horizontal plane (medial to the left, rostral up) of the locations of the three classes of nociceptive neurons in the ventral periphery of VPM with the receptive fields shown for the multireceptive neurons. Black areas indicate nociceptive receptive fields, stippled areas indicate low-threshold mechanical receptive fields. Same graph as in Fig. 4

Discussion

The present investigations shed additional light on the problem of how information about noxious stimuli is processed at the thalamic level. The results show that three classes of nociceptive units with receptive fields on the head can be found in the ventral periphery of VPM, located between VPM proper and the external medullary lamina. These three types of neurons, nociceptive-specific, multireceptive, and switching, occur intermingled which each other and are distributed over the entire ventral extent of VPM in the rostrocaudal and the mediolateral dimensions. A somatotopic organization of the nociceptive neurons in this area could not be discerned, and for the majority of them, the receptive fields were not in sequence with those of the overlying VPM. A specific functional role in the nociceptive system is suggested for nociceptive-specific and multireceptive neurons in the ventral periphery of VPM by their small receptive fields and their ability to encode the intensity of noxious stimuli.

The only other detailed investigation on trigeminal nociceptive neurons in the cat thalamus (Yokota and Matsumoto 1983a, b; Yokota et al. 1985) shows completely different results. Although the two classes of nociceptive-specific and multireceptive (wide-dynamic-range) units were also found, their receptive fields are shown to be very small and never comprise discontinuous components. A precise somatotopic arrangement of these units along the dorsal and ventral border of VPM is shown, which is in sequence with the somatotopy of the neighboring neurons in VPM proper. All nociceptive units are confined to the caudal part of VPM and a segregation of nociceptive-specific and wide-dynamic-range units is shown, the latter occurring only in a 300-μm-wide band on the rostral pole of the nociceptive area.

There are several possible reasons for the discrepancies between the two studies. It might be that different populations of units are described, possibly caused by a different bias of the electrodes used, metal microelectrodes vs. glass micropipettes. However, in the ventroposterolateral nucleus (VPL) different results were not obtained when using micropipettes and metal microelectrodes (Kniffki and Mizumura 1983; Kniffki and Craig 1985). A main point and a major obstacle in investigations of the nociceptive system is the anesthesia. We always took great care to maintain a constant light level of anesthesia. In some cases it was noted that after an additional dose of Nembutal was given, the nociceptive units stopped responding but the responses recovered after some time had elapsed. Certainly the anesthesia must have an influence on the receptive field configurations as well. Whether the existence of switching responses, which were not described by Yokota et al. (1985), is also dependent on the anesthesia is unclear. We failed in several cases to suppress these responses with additional doses of Nembutal; on the other hand, they were more frequently seen in some experiments than others. This might mean that the physiological conditions of the animals differed, e.g., the inhibitory control of these neurons might have been affected. The specific functional role of switching neurons is unclear. In any case, it has to be noted that these neurons do receive inputs from nociceptive afferents and have complex receptive fields, although under different conditions these inputs might be modified or even suppressed.

The lack of segregation of the two classes of units and the lack of a somatotopy in the nociceptive area found in our study cannot have been caused by the procedure used for pooling the data, because lesions at recording sites of nociceptive-specific as well as multireceptive neurons can clearly be seen to be located in histological sections through the caudal and rostral parts of VPM, and the sections from different animals aligned in the standardized brain atlas proved to be in sequence. In our view, a standardization method based on anatomical measurements is essential if data from several animals have to be pooled, because of the differences in the individual brain dimensions.

Our results on the characteristics of nociceptive neurons in the ventral periphery of VPM are in accordance with those obtained in the ventral border region of VPL by Kniffki and Mizumura (1983), Kniffki and Craig (1985), and Honda et al. (1983). In the present study we also recorded 12 nociceptive units with receptive fields on the forepaw; these were located lateral to the nociceptive representation of the head. It seems that a continuity exists between the “head” and the “fore- and hindpaw” nociceptive areas, which extend along the ventral border of VPM and VPL and curve dorsally along the lateral border of VPL. Therefore, a coarse somatotopic organization of the nociceptive neurons is present mediolaterally.

The source of the afferent input to the periphery of the ventrobasal complex (VB) is not yet clear. Sparse and scattered inputs to this area were shown to derive from those areas which have a dense projection to VB proper (dorsal column nuclei, lateral cervical nucleus, spinal cord, and spinal trigeminal nucleus) (Berkley 1980). Cervical and lumbar spinal cord injections of horseradish peroxidase caused anterograde labeling within the entire mediolateral extent of the ventral periphery of VB (Craig and Burton 1985). These anatomical projections of the spinothalamic tract seem to overlap with the area in which the nociceptive neurons were found in the present study.

The cortical projection to area 3a of the nociceptive neurons located within the ventral periphery of VPL further distinguishes this region (Craig and Kniffki 1985). Whether this is also true for the ventral periphery of VPM remains to be demonstrated.

Our results suggest that the nociceptive neurons in the ventral periphery of VPM may be part of a system which provides the basis for the sensory experience about the presence, the locus, and the intensity of noxious stimuli applied to the surface of the head.

Acknowledgements. We thank Ms. M. Meyermann for expert histological assistance and Ms. P. Haumann and Ms. C. Erhard for skillful technical assistance and preparation of the illustrations. The work was supported by the Deutsche Forschungsgemeinschaft, SPP "Nociception und Schmerz".

References

Berkley KJ (1980) Spatial relationships between the terminations of somatic sensory and motor pathways in the rostral brainstem of cats and monkeys. I. Ascending somatic sensory inputs to lateral diencephalon. J Comp Neurol 193 : 283–317

Craig AD, Burton H (1985) The distribution and topographical organization in the thalamus of anterogradely transported horseradish peroxidase after spinal injections in cat and raccoon. Exp Brain Res 58 : 227–254

Craig AD, Kniffki K-D (1985) Spino-thalamo-cortical mechanisms of nociception. In: Sharma KN, Nayar U (eds) Basic mechanisms and clinical applications. Indian Society for Pain Research and Therapy, New Delhi, pp 65–77 (Current trends in pain research and therapy, vol 1)

Honda CN, Mense S, Perl ER (1983) Neurons in ventrobasal region of cat thalamus selectively responsive to noxious mechanical stimulation. J Neurophysiol 49 : 662–673

Kniffki K-D, Craig AD (1985) The distribution of nociceptive neurons in the cat's lateral thalamus: the dorsal and ventral periphery of VPL. In: Rowe M, Willis WD (eds) Development, organization and processing in somatosensory pathways. Liss, New York, pp 375–382

Kniffki K-D, Mizumura K (1983) Responses of neurons in VPL and VPL–VL region of the cat to algesic stimulation of muscle and tendon. J Neurophysiol 49 : 649–661

Vahle-Hinz C, Gottschaldt K-M (1983) Principal differences in the organization of the thalamic face representation in rodents and felids. In: Macchi G, Rustioni A, Spreafico R (eds) Somatosensory integration in the thalamus. Elsevier, Amsterdam, pp 125–145

Yokota T, Matsumoto N (1983a) Somatotopic distribution of trigeminal nociceptive specific neurons within the caudal somatosensory thalamus of cat. Neurosci Lett 39 : 125–130

Yokota T, Matsumoto N (1983b) Location and functional organization of trigeminal wide dynamic range neurons within the nucleus ventralis posteromedialis of the cat. Neurosci Lett 39 : 231–236

Yokota T, Koyama N, Matsumoto N (1985) Somatotopic distribution of trigeminal nociceptive neurons in ventrobasal complex of cat thalamus. J Neurophysiol 53 : 1387–1400

42 A Note on the Relationship Between Site of Interruption and Somatosensory Thresholds in Lesions of Human Pain Pathway

D. Bowsher, J. Lahuerta, and L. Brock

Neurogenic pain - defined as pain due to a lesion of the peripheral or central nervous system, and not to the stimulation of nociceptors - is virtually always accompanied by a somatosensory deficit. Central neurogenic pain is frequently called "thalamic syndrome" because it was so designated by Dejerine and Roussy (1906), who described three cases with lesions in the somatosensory thalamus. Cassinari and Pagni (1969) reviewed all known cases and concluded that the condition was due to an ischaemic lesion occurring above the spinomedullary junction in the spinothalamic pathway or its terminal region, but sparing the more medially placed spino-reticulo-intralaminar-thalamic ("palaeospinothalamic") system. This would include the unique case reported by Biemond (1956), in which there was a relatively small infarct in the insular and retroinsular region of the cerebral cortex, resulting in retrograde degeneration of the ventroposterior nucleus of the thalamus. Subsequently, Agnew et al. (1983), using computed axial tomography (CAT), were able to show that a significant proportion of lesions were in the cortex.

It is not our purpose here to discuss the physiopathology of central pain, but merely to examine the relationship between site of lesion and somatosensory deficit.

Material and Methods

The material consisted of 20 patients with spontaneous pain following stroke who were subjected to CAT scanning, and 16 cases of percutaneous cervical anterolateral cordotomy in which pain due to malignant disease not involving the central nervous system was successfully alleviated by operation at the C1–2 level. The CAT scans are the only anatomical evidence of lesion sites, as all the patients are still alive (and likely to remain so for a long time). While this is not as satisfactory as postmortem pathological anatomy, it is very unlikely that any significant supratentorial lesion would have been missed by CAT scanning. Infratentorial lesions, however, often have to be inferred from the absence of any supratentorial lesion, combined with clinical evidence.

All 36 patients had a clinically evident somatosensory deficit on one side of the body, but apparently not on the other. In 15 patients of the first group, examination by CAT revealed one or more lesions in the supratentorial compartment; in three cases an infratentorial lesion was observed in the brainstem, while in two others no lesion was seen either above or below the tentorium cerebelli but the history and clinical findings pointed to the existence of an infratentorial lesion. The site of the lesions in all 20 of these patients (A to T) is shown in Table 1. Four of them, C, H, O and P, had small circumscribed lesions, were alert and cooperative, and the greatest reliance could be placed on findings obtained from them in psychophysical tests. It was fortunate that one of them was H, the only case of classical thalamic syndrome due to infarction of posterior cerebral artery territory, with homonymous hemianopia and destruction in the posterior third of the thalamus (mainly n. ventralis posterior). P had a small but radiologically visible lesion in the territory of the medullary branches of the posterior inferior cerebellar artery, affecting the anterior and lateral aspects of the medulla oblongata. The other two had small cortical lesions - C in the depths of the Sylvian fissure, O in parietotemporal cortex sparing the postcentral gyrus.

Somatosensory perception thresholds (see below) were evaluated in mirror-image points on both sides in cases of spontaneous central pain. These points were in each of the three divisions of the trigeminal nerve, the hands, and the feet. When results were assessed, however, values obtained from non-painful areas on the affected side and their mirror-image equivalents on the unaffected side were discarded. In the cordotomy patients, tests were performed in the first dorsal interosseous spaces of both hands and both feet, 2 days before and 5 days after operation. In all subjects, tests were performed after the subject had rested in a warm room for at least 30 min. Skin temperature was measured at all sites to be tested.

Perception thresholds were measured for all somatosensory submodalities, as follows: Tactile thresholds were measured by the use of von Frey "hairs". Two-point discrimination was evaluated with Weber's compasses. Vibratory sensibility was measured with a fixed-frequency (50 Hz) variable-amplitude vibrameter (Goldberg and Lindblom 1979). Amplitude was slowly increased from zero until the subject signalled that he perceived it; and then slowly decreased from a level well above threshold until the subject said that it had disappeared. Threshold was taken as the average of these two values. Warmth, coolness, hot pain and cold pain were all measured with the Marstock apparatus (Fruhstorfer et al. 1976). This is essentially a piezo-electric thermode zeroed at 30 °C; the subject has a switch which reverses current and therefore direction of temperature change. He/she is instructed first to press the button every time warmth or coolness is first felt, then when hot (pricking) pain or cold pain is felt. The results are drawn out by a calibrated X-Y plotter; the experimenter has an overriding control switch for use in case the subject makes a mistake or cannot appreciate temperature change. Tissue-damage pain was evaluated by the use of strain-gauge-coupled forceps (Lynn, personal communication) which were used to squeeze a skinfold until pain was felt.

All perception thresholds were evaluated three times at each site, and the average taken as the definitive value. In order to facilitate comparison of results, the values obtained at each control ("normal") site in each subject was expressed as 100, and data obtained from the mirror-image affected point expressed in the same terms, so that for all submodalities/tests the value can easily be seen as a number above or below (or the same as) 100. In non-painful areas, there was no significant difference between mirror-image points on the two sides; these values will therefore not be further considered.

Results

Since the subject of this symposium is the role of fine afferent nerve fibers in somatovisceral sensation, we shall mainly concern ourselves here with results obtained when testing input from fine primary peripheral afferents, i.e. the submodalities of warmth, coolness, hot pain, cold pain and tissue-damage pain. Incidental reference will of course be made from time to time to those submodalities subserved by large peripheral afferents (touch, two-point discrimination and vibration).

While perception thresholds for von Frey "hairs" (i.e. tactile sensibility) were raised, as expected, by cortical lesions, they were **not** raised in cases of cordotomy, brainstem lesion **or** in the case in which the posterior thalamus was destroyed (H), though in those cases in which thalamus was disconnected from cortex by a capsular lesion (E, G, I, S), tactile threshold was raised. Yet two-point discrimination was affected in case H, giving values of 140 for V2, 131.5 for V3, 127 for the hand and >300 for the foot. These values were about half as high as those obtained in lesions involving the postrolandic cortex; two-point discrimination was also disturbed (i.e. thresholds were raised) in cases of damage to the lateral or anterolateral medulla oblongata, and in five of the 16 cordotomy cases. Vibration thresholds were increased in the case of damage to ventroposterior thalamus, two brainstem cases (of three tested for this modality) and in the feet of 11 of 16 cordotomy cases.

Perception thresholds for warmth were raised following lesions of pericentral and/or parietal cortex; in a small capsular lesion separating lateral thalamus from cortex (S); in all cases in which the brainstem was known or suspected to be involved; and in 10 of 16 cordotomy cases (both hands and feet). But warm threshold was **not** affected in the case involving posterior thalamus (H) or in cases involving the anterior limb of the internal capsule alone (G) or in combination with other structures (B, I, R).

Hot pain threshold was raised in cases of extensive cortical lesion (L, Q, M), but not in discrete or less extensive cortical lesions (C, J, K, R) involving the pericentral area; it was, however, raised in the single case of a temporoparietal lesion sparing the rolandic cortex (O: V2 112, V3 104, hand 109, foot 91 - the foot was where the most spontaneous pain was experienced!). It was significantly raised (116) in the most painful area (V3) of the case (H) with damage to the ventroposterior thalamus, but little changed at other sites. It was raised in two cases (A, E) in which there was damage in or just lateral to the head of the caudate nucleus. One of these (E) also had presumed brainstem damage; and in the other cases of brainstem damage, hot pain threshold was also raised. It was raised in the hands of six cordotomy cases and in the feet of 10.

Threshold for coolness, on the other hand, was minimally raised by the ventroposterior thalamic lesion in some locations (V2 115 F, V3 97, hand 98, leg 110). It was raised further by the lesion (S) separating lateral thalamus from internal capsule (V3 132.2); more profound effects were seen from lesions affecting anterior thalamus (Q: V3 144.1, hand 139.8, foot 144.1; A: hand 127.6, foot 112.7; L: hand <18.5, foot <183.5; F: V2 120.4) and medulla oblongata (N: hand <164.3; P: hand <161, foot <163.6). Threshold for coolness was raised in the hands of nine cordotomy cases and in the feet of eight. Lesions affecting the caudate nucleus also results in higher coolness thresholds (E, I, K, M, R).

Higher thresholds for cold pain were found in lesions of postcentral and/or parietal cortex, including discrete lesions. Threshold was also raised in brainstem lesions, and in the hands of six and feet of 11 cordotomy cases. Values for the posterior thalamic lesion (H) were: V2 106, V3 87, hand 102.4, foot 115. Cases in which the anterior part of the internal capsule was involved (B, M, R, T) exhibited lower thresholds, as in the case of posterior thalamic V3, temporoparietal cortex (case O) hand; neither of these areas was the seat of "spontaneous" pain. Lower thresholds were also seen in the hands of three and the feet of one cordotomy case.

Tissue-damage pain (skinfold pinch) was most affected by cordotomy. Thresholds were raised in the hands of 10 and feet of 14 of these patients; the average value in the latter (against a control value of 100) was 211.8. In brainstem or presumed brainstem lesions (D, E,

Table 1. Lesions revealed by CAT scan in 20 patients with spontaneous pain following stroke

Patient	Rolandic cortex	Postrolandic parietal cortex	Insula	Caudate	Internal capsule		Thalamus			Brainstem
					Ant.	Post.	Ant.	Lat.	Post.	
A	?			+				+ (dorsal)		
B	?		+		+					
C	+									
D								?		+
E				+					?	
F	?						+			+ (atrophic)
G					+					
H									+	
I			+	+	+					
J		+	+		+					
K	+			+						
L	+	+	+				+			
M	+	+	+	+				+		
N										?
O		+								
P										+
Q	+	+	+	+	+					
R	+	+		+	+	+				
S			+			+				
T		+	+	+						+

P) thresholds were also increased; however, in case P with a demonstrable lesion, while hand threshold was raised to 424.2, the threshold in the foot, which was the site of spontaneous pain, fell to 81.4; the average raised threshold for these three cases was 212.0, not significantly different from the cordotomy result. Cases with lesions affecting the thalamus other than the ventroposterior region (e.g. F, L, M) showed slightly raised thresholds in the spontaneously painful areas (average 131.1). Most patients with cortical lesions showed raised thresholds, including those with a discrete rolandic lesion (C) and with a temporoparietal lesion sparing the postcentral gyrus (O); the average of 18 values was 170.7. However, some individual values within this group evidenced lowered threshold - the hand in cases C (83) and L (27.5); while others were unchanged - the face in cases B and Q, the hand in A and B and the foot in A and B (i.e. cases A and B showed no raised thresholds anywhere). The case (H) with a ventroposterior thalamic lesion showed no change in skinfold pinch pain thresholds.

Lowered threshold for pinch pain was seen in four other cases: I and K, in which there was a lesion of the caudate nucleus in addition to other damage; J, in which the anterior limb of the internal capsule was involved in addition to extensive cortical damage behind the postcentral gyrus; and also in the presumed brainstem case N (hand 85.7; thorax - the seat of his worst pain - 25). This is inexplicable, as it is in contrast to the other brainstem cases.

Summary

Cortical Lesions

a) Warmth thresholds are very slightly raised by small discrete postcentral or parietal lesions, but more markedly raised by more extensive lesions affecting a wider area of cortex, together with underlying white matter and sometimes the head of the caudate nucleus and/or anterior limb of the internal capsule, but not the thalamus.

b) Cool threshold was virtually unaffected by a postcentral lesion, and minimally raised by a small posterior parietal lesion. Like warmth, threshold was raised to a considerably greater extent by more extensive lesions.

c) Hot pain thresholds were not raised in cases with small discrete cortical lesions, but were in cases with the most extensive lesions.

d) Cold pain thresholds were raised in cases with small lesions, and more so in cases with extensive lesions.

e) Tissue-damage (skinfold pinch) pain thresholds were raised, more or less in proportion to the extent of the lesion.

Ventroposterior Thalamic Lesion (one case only)

a) Warm threshold was unaffected in this case and unaffected or only very slightly raised in others with other types of thalamic lesion or thalamic disconnections.

b) Cool threshold was only slightly affected by this or other thalamic lesions.

c) Hot pain threshold was only very slightly affected by this and other thalamic lesions.

d) Cold pain was only slightly affected by the ventroposterior lesion, but more so by other thalamic lesions.

e) Pinch pain thresholds were also virtually unaffected by the ventroposterior lesion but raised in other thalamic lesions.

Lateral and Anterolateral Brainstem Lesions

a) Warmth thresholds were considerably raised.

b) Cool thresholds were also considerably raised.

c) Hot pain thresholds were not greatly affected.

d) Cold pain thresholds were markedly raised.

e) Pinch pain thresholds were for the most part raised.

Anterolateral Cordotomy

a) Warmth thresholds were raised, but less than in bulbar lesions.

b) Cool thresholds were affected to a greater extent than in bulbar lesions.

c) Hot pain thresholds were virtually unaffected.

d) Cold pain thresholds were very slightly lowered on average.

e) Pinch pain thresholds were greatly elevated.

We are forced to conclude that the central pathways for sensory modalities conveyed by fine peripheral afferent fibers in man follow different routes in the central nervous system, particularly perhaps the thalamus.

References

AGNEW DC, SHETTER AG, SEGALL HD, FLOM RA (1983) Thalamic pain. Adv Pain Res Ther 5 : 941–946

BIEMOND A (1956) The conduction of pain above the level of the thalamus opticus. Arch Neurol Psychiatry 75 : 231–244

CASSINARI V, PAGNI CA (1969) Central pain: a neurosurgical survey. Harvard University Press, Cambridge, Mass

DEJERINE J, ROUSSY J (1906) Le syndrome thalamique. Rev Neurol (Paris) 14 : 521–532

FRUHSTORFER H, LINDBLOM U, SCHMIDT WG (1976) Method for quantitative estimation of thermal thresholds in patients. J Neurol Neurosurg Psychiatry 39 : 1071–1075

GOLDBERG JM, LINDBLOM U (1979) Standardised method of determining vibratory perception thresholds for diagnosis and screening in neurological investigation. J Neurol Neurosurg Psychiatry 42 : 793–803

43 Quantitative Evaluation of Itch Sensation

H. O. Handwerker, W. Magerl, F. Klemm, E. Lang, and R. A. Westerman

Introduction

The progress of sensory physiology in the last decades has led to a better understanding of the nervous apparatus subserving almost all sensory modalities of the skin. One notable exception, however, is the sensation of itch, for which a quantitative analysis is still lacking. It is even unknown whether itch is elicited by a specific subgroup of "itch" receptors or by a particular pattern of input from afferent nerve fibers subserving other sensations (e.g., pain).

A strong obstacle to a better understanding of this sensation is the lack of reliable stimuli which provoke itch sensations graded with stimulus strength. Thus a psychophysics of itch comparable to that worked out for pain sensations by Hardy et al. (1952) and by other laboratories is lacking. In pain research, psychophysical studies with rigidly controlled stimuli have been very useful in the search for and the characterization of the peripheral nervous elements mediating pain.

The aim of this study was threefold: (1) to find a quantifiable itch stimulus, (2) to establish the relationship between this stimulus and the itch sensations of healthy subjects, and (3) to find out which type of afferent nerve fibers might meet the requirements for a nervous apparatus mediating itch sensations.

Methods

Histamine was brought into the skin of healthy volunteers by iontophoresis. To this purpose 1% histamine (in the form of histamine dihydrochloride) was dissolved in a gel of 2.5% methylcellulose in aqua bidest. This jelly was placed in the cavity of an acrylic applicator having a diameter of 5 mm and a volume of 50 µl. A silver-silver chloride electrode in this applicator served for current delivery, a larger one (3 x 3 cm) in a sponge soaked with tyrode was used as reference. No air bubbles were allowed in the gel or between gel and skin, since they were found to interfere with the reliability of the stimulation.

Constant current pulses (10 s) from an isolated stimulator (WPI/305 B) were used. Current strength was varied from 0.01 to 3 mA for the application of different quantities of histamine. Stimulus strength is proportional to the product of current and time, i.e. to the charge.

These stimuli usually induced a wheal and a flare reaction developing slowly after termination of the stimulus. Both wheal and flare were marked with pens 10 min after each stimulus and redrawn on translucent paper for planimetric evaluation. To assess time courses and the relative increases in blood flow in the course of the flare reaction, a laser Doppler flowmeter (Periflux/PF1) was used.

Itch sensations evoked by these stimuli usually started within 20 s after termination of the stimulus and lasted for several minutes. They were assessed by the subjects on a horizontally placed visual analogue scale. The left and right ends of the scale were defined as "threshold" and as "maximal imaginable itch" respectively. In some preliminary experiments a further mark at one third of the scale was defined as "itch strong enough to induce scratching." Ratings of the actual strength of itching were made by the subjects on acoustic signals at 10-s intervals for 10 min.

Differential blocks of superficial radial nerves were performed at the right forearm by two dangling weights of 5 kg via a sleeve pressing the nerve to the radius bone (Torebjörk and Hallin 1973). Two states of block were distinguished: one in which only the sensitivity to low von Frey hair (0.1 N force) stimulation was abolished in the skin field innervated by the nerve (block of Aβ fibers), and another one in which also the cold sensitivity failed (block of Aβ and Aδ fibers). In both states C fibers were still conducting, shown by the persisting sensitivity to pin pricks.

Six skin fields (20–50 cm^2) at the inner sides of the forearms of four subjects were desensitized with capsaicin. To this purpose the respective skin areas were painted first with dimethylsulfoxide (DMSO) followed by a solution of 1% capsaicin in 85% ethanol at intervals of 2–3 h. This treatment had to be repeated at least 10 times until capsaicin no longer provoked a burning sensation. (Method communicated by J. Szolcsanyi, who also served as a subject. The other subjects participating in the capsaicin experiments were coauthors of this study.)

Microneurography was performed following standard routines described elsewhere (Gybels et al. 1979).

Data evaluation was accomplished at the Computer Center of the University of Heidelberg using the Statistical Analysis Systems (SAS) package.

Following the declaration of Helsinki all subjects were informed about the risks of the respective experiment in which they participated and gave their consent.

Results

Correlations of Itch Sensations with Physiological Reactions to Histamine

In a pilot study on 48 subjects (27 male, 21 female) in which the stimuli were applied to the inner side of the forearm, the correlations between the stimulus size (charges), the radius of the wheal (RWH), the radius of the flare (RFL), and different parameters of the subjective itch responses were evaluated. The correlation coefficients between the two physiological parameters (RWH and RFL) vs the logarithm of charges were 0.88 each ($p < 0.0001$). The thresholds for both reactions were 0.04 mC (flare) and 0.05 mC (wheal). Figure 1 shows specimen records from one experiment. The figure indicates a strong correlation of the wheal size, the flare size, and the increase in blood flow (flux) to the subjective itch responses.

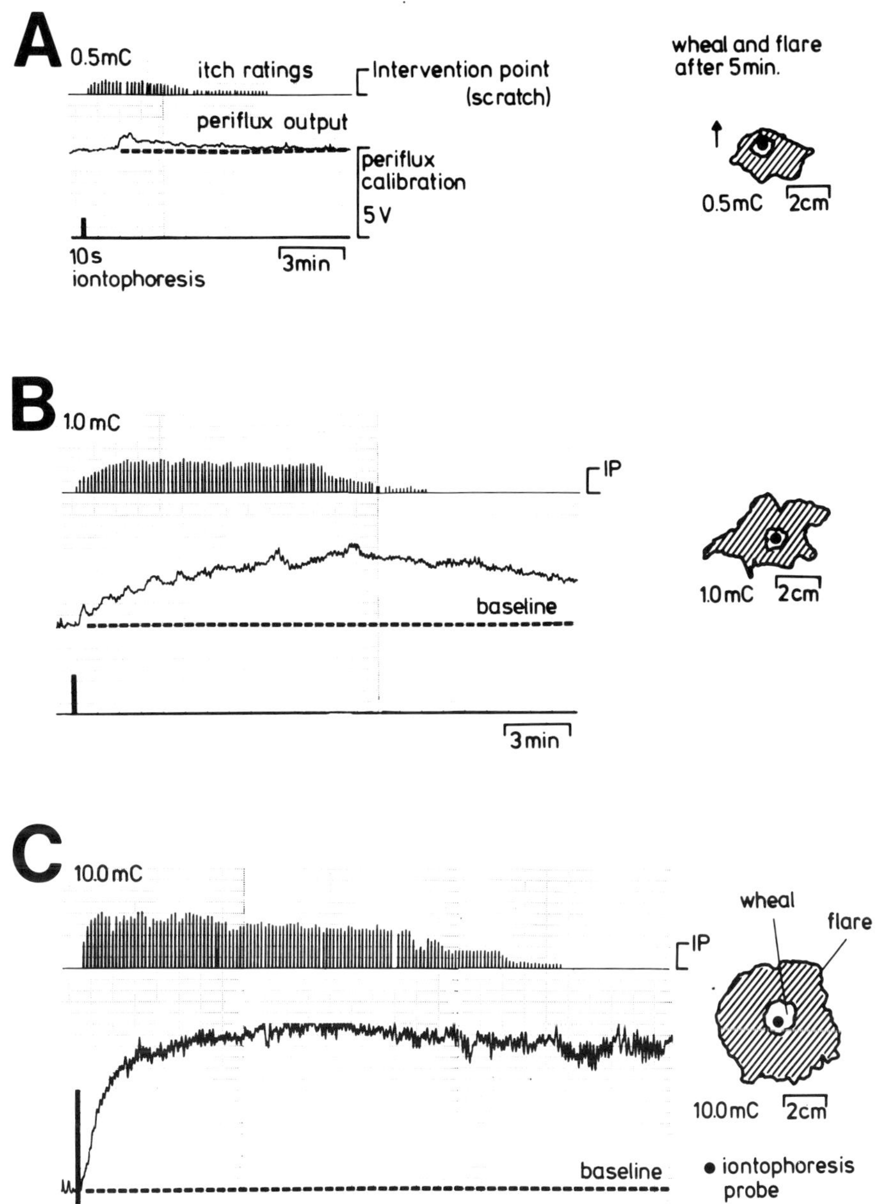

Fig. 1 A–C. Specimen recordings from an experiment with histamine iontophoresis applied to the inner side of the forearm. Three different charges were applied to different skin sites. Upper traces: ratings of the intensity of itching given by the subject on a visual analogue scale at 10-s intervals. Middle traces: relative increases in blood flow in the flare region measured with a PERIFLUX laser Doppler flowmeter. Lower traces: duration and magnitude of current application. The sizes of the wheal and flare reactions are shown at the right side of the figure

In a more carefully designed study in 22 subjects (12 female, 10 male) these results were corroborated. Five stimulus levels (0, 0.156, 0.625, 2.5, and 10 mC) were applied in randomized order to the inner side of the forearm. As in the pilot study, the subjects were blind with respect to the stimulus magnitude. In this second study, again the correlation coefficients of the logarithms of the charges with RWH were 0.88. The respective correlations between the logarithms of the charges and mean fluxes were 0.72. The RWH parameter, for example, seems to be a better predictor of itching than the stimulus level. When itch responses were standardized on the basis of a first training stimulus of medium size, the correlation coefficient of RWH and itch was as high as 0.66 ($p < 0.0001$).

Time courses of the mean itch responses to a given charge are characterized by maxima occurring approximately 1 min after the end of the current application. The responses declined exponentially with time constants of 155–205 s.

Eight percent of the stimuli elicited no itch (9 of 110). These misses occurred at different stimulus levels.

The Influence of Nerve Blocks and of Capsaicin Pretreatment

Differential blocking of nerve fibers is one approach to identify those fibers which transfer the itch signals.

A pressure block of the superficial radial nerve was performed in 16 subjects (9 male, 7 female). The average values of the blood fluxes in the flare region and of the itch responses obtained in the course of this procedure are shown in Fig. 2.

None of the small changes in average responsiveness observed in the course of the blocking experiment were statistically significant. A first control stimulus delivered to the back of the right hand induced a somewhat smaller flux and an itch response which declined more slowly. Itch responses obtained during the blocking procedure were rather similar in the skin field at the right hand undergoing the blocking and in the contralateral field. We have also tested whether the itch sensations did change qualitatively in the course of the blocking. Some subjects (5 of 16) reported an increase of burning sensations under blocking conditions. It was, however, hard to discriminate whether this burning was induced by the pressure block itself or by the histamine stimuli, in particular since more prominent burning sensations in the course of the experiment were reported by those subjects who also exhibited block-induced aftersensations for some days. The majority of the subjects (11 of 16) had no block-induced aftersensations. When their data were analyzed separately, a small decrease of the itch response was found ($p < 0.05$) under total A-fiber blockade.

It is well established that a subgroup of afferent C fibers containing neuropeptides is characterized by a selective sensitivity to capsaicin (methyl-vanillyl-nonenamide) (for a review see Szolcsanyi 1985). We tried to block the receptive endings of capsaicin-sensitive C fibers by repetitively painting skin fields with this agent. It has been shown previously that C fibers sensitive to chemical stimuli can be temporarily blocked by this treatment. Painting was repeated until the substance no longer induced burning in the treated skin area, a stage reached after 2–3 days. Allowing some time for the subsidence of the signs of inflammation, this skin field showed a strongly increased threshold to heat stimuli, whereas the sensitivity

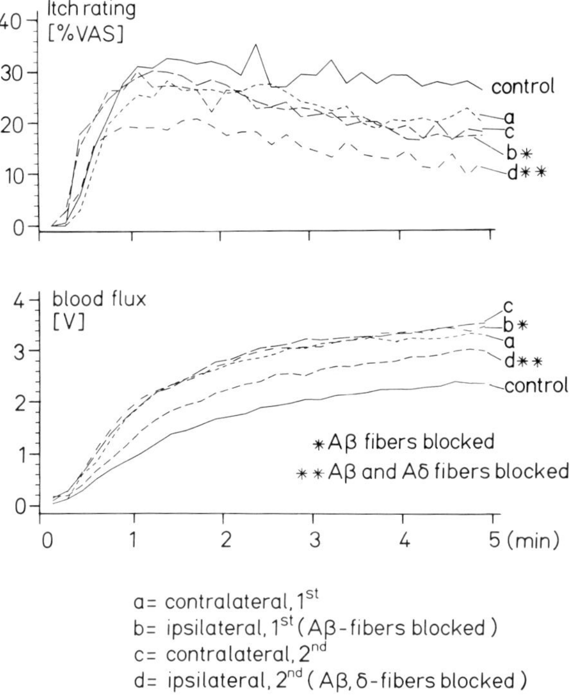

Fig. 2. Mean itch ratings (upper diagram) and mean blood flux measurements in the erythematous zone after histamine iontophoresis obtained in experiments with pressure blocks of the superficial radial nerve. VAS, visual analogue scale; V, Periflux reading in voltage

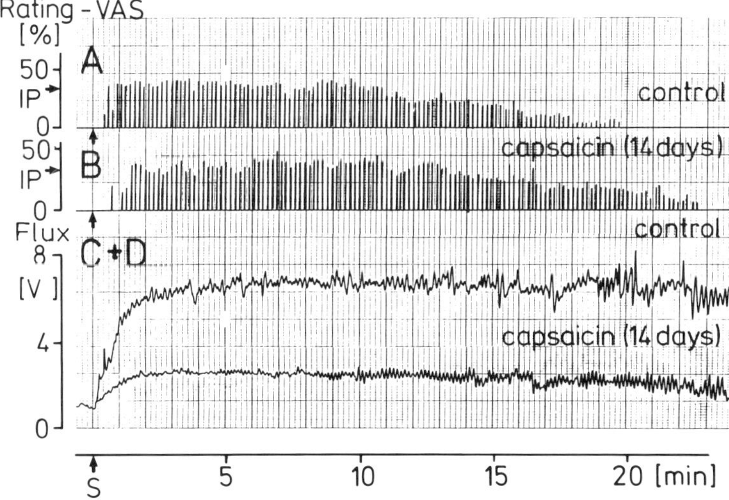

Fig. 3 A–D. Itch reaction and the respective flare reaction (blood flux measured with the Periflux) obtained from a skin site at the inner side of one forearm 2 weeks after capsaicin treatment **(B, D)** and from the contralateral untreated forearm **(A, C)**.VAS, visual analogue scale; IP, intervention point (scratch); V, Periflux reading in voltages; S, stimulus (histamine)

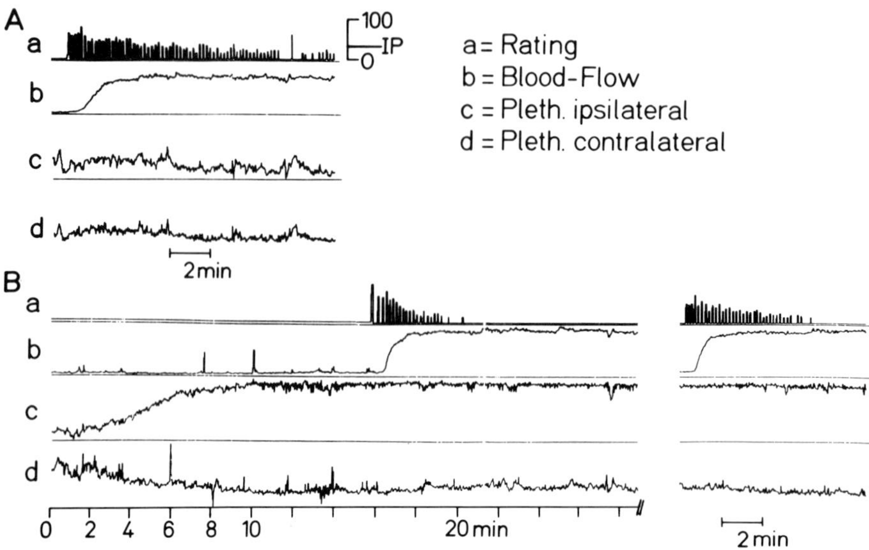

Fig. 4 A, B. Specimen recordings from an experiment in a patient undergoing a stellatum blockade. **A** Control recordings of itch and flux reactions. **B** Recordings obtained after development of the block which is documented by the increase in blood flow documented by finger photoplethysmography in trace C. **a** Ratings of itch intensity. IP, intervention point (scratch). **b** Blood fluxes through the skin affected by histamine iontophoresis measured with a laser Doppler flowmeter. **c, d** Finger plethysmograms from the middle fingers of both hands

to cold and to Frey hair stimulation was not altered. Vasodilatation following transcutaneous electrical stimulation strong enough to excite C fibers was reduced to 5 % of control values (Westerman et al. 1986). Histamine iontophoresis in a capsaicin-treated skin field no longer provoked itch sensations. The flare was also abolished, whereas the wheal reaction was unchanged. If the iontophoresis electrode was placed close to the border of the pretreated skin field (e.g., in a distance of 2–3 mm), a flare sometimes developed outside of the capsaicin-treated area. In these cases itch was felt by the subject, and it was localized in the flare region. Within 2 weeks after termination of the capsaicin treatment the itch response to histamine iontophoresis recovered completely. However, the flare response remained diminished for a longer period. Figure 3 shows an experiment conducted 2 weeks after capsaicin in a treated skin field and at the contralateral forearm.

According to occasional clinical observations, pathological itch states may be relieved by a block of the sympathetic chain. We were able to test three patients who had to undergo a blockade of the ganglion stellatum, which temporarily interrupted the sympathetic outflow to one arm. In none of these patients were we able to demonstrate a diminished itch response to histamine after blockade of the sympathetic innervation, which was proven by finger plethysmography revealing an increase in blood flow. Figure 4 shows an experiment with sympathetic blockade.

Microneurographic Recordings During Histamine Iontophoresis

A direct approach to the presumed "itch fibers" is by use of the microneurographic technique. We have tried to record impulse activity in different types of nerve fibers from the superficial radial nerves of volunteers and to apply histamine iontophoresis to the receptive fields. Ideally, one should be able to compare directly impulse patterns of afferent C fibers with subjective itch sensations, and thus to find the best candidates for the coding of itch.

We found, however, that under the conditions of microneurography itch is more rarely induced by histamine iontophoresis than under the conditions of a purely psychophysical experiment. We assume that this is due to the prolonged immobilization of the arm, which may induce an altered responsiveness of central sensory neurones. Furthermore, the manipulation of the nerve itself may induce a suppression of itch.

When recording from polymodal C fibers we were surprised that most of them did not respond to histamine. In some others we found a bursting discharge of low frequency which was hard to discriminate from background sympathetic discharges. Our sample of afferent C fibers (identified by the conduction delays to electrical stimulation in their receptive fields) is still too small to estimate the exact percentage of polymodal C fibers which show prolonged afterdischarges - albeit of low frequency - after histamine iontophoresis. The proportion of responding C fibers is, however, apparently less than 20 %. In a parallel study on anesthetized rats with a similar iontophoresis technique we found an even lower responsiveness of polymodal C fibers in this species. Ten "polymodal" C units and four C mechanoreceptors were tested. None of them responded to histamine with prolonged afterdischarges. Figure 5 shows the discharge pattern of a polymodal C fiber (recorded in man) to histamine iontophoresis in the receptive field. In the course of the recording additional sympathetic activity was recruited.

Another fiber group was much easier driven by histamine iontophoresis than the C fibers: the slowly adapting mechanoreceptors (SA) with fast-conducting myelinated fibers. Of 10 fibers tested, five showed regular (SA II units) or irregular (SA I units) discharges lasting for several minutes after termination of the iontophoresis. Figure 6 shows such a recording from an SA II fiber.

Discussion

Histamine iontophoresis as used in this study induced predominantly the sensation of itching. However, other sensory attributes, such as "burning" and "stinging," were also used by the subjects to characterize the stimuli. It is noteworthy that the incidence of sensory reports out of the semantic spectrum of pain (Mumford and Bowsher 1976) did not increase with higher current densities within the chosen range of stimuli. Thus, itching apparently does not turn to burning with stronger stimulation, in agreement with a report on electrically induced itching (Tuckett 1982).

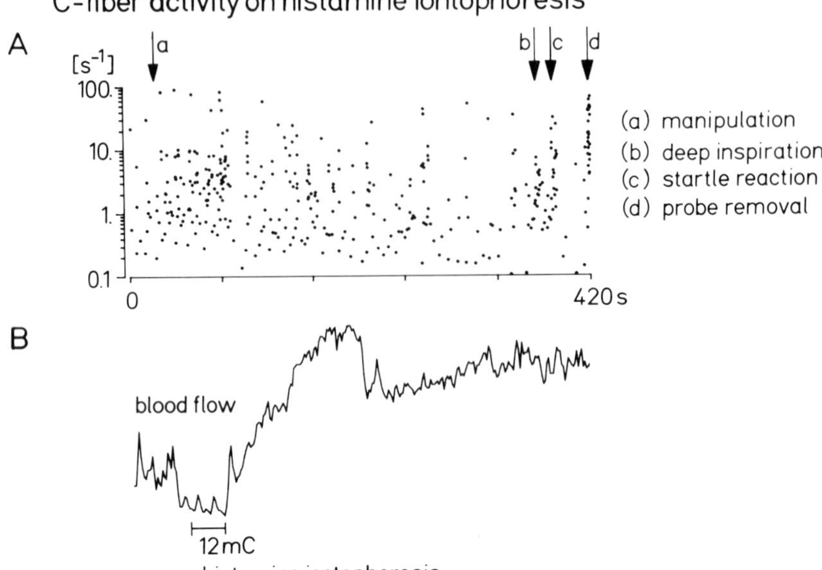

Fig. 5. Discharge patterns of a polymodal C-fiber unit after histamine iontophoresis, obtained in microneurography and the respective blood flux increases measured with the Periflux laser Doppler flowmeter. The recordings of an identified afferent polymodal C fiber were contaminated at the end of the recording by sympathetic activity (note tests b and c)

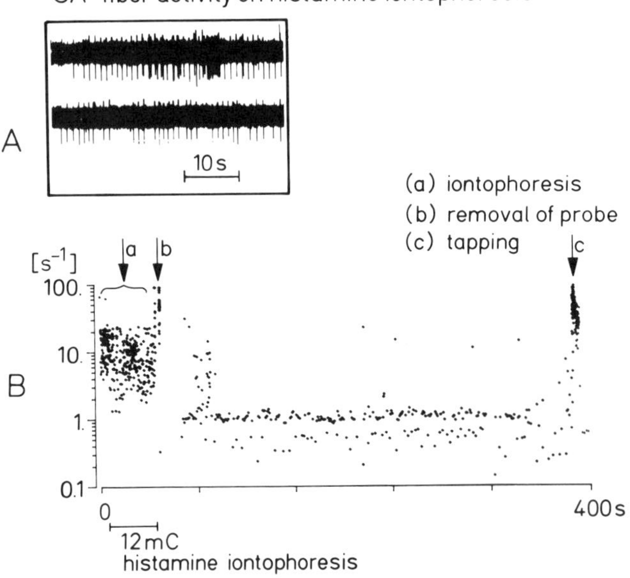

Fig. 6 A–C. Specimen recordings **A** of an SA II unit after histamine iontophoresis and **B** of the discharge pattern of an SA II unit during and after histamine iontophoresis obtained in a microneurographic experiment

The primary objective of this work was a quantitative analysis of itching with an appropriate stimulus method. We found that the subjects were well able to distinguish between different levels of itch in relation to the stimulus strength. The physiological reactions to the histamine iontophoresis, wheal and flare, turned out to be good predictors of the intensity of itching.

Another objective was to find the nervous elements mediating the sensations induced by the histamine iontophoresis. The results of our blocking experiments indicate that C fibers are the most relevant - if not the only - fiber group mediating the sense of itch. This is also indicated by the experiments of Bickford (1938) using ischemic and cold blocks of skin nerves. Furthermore the experiments with capsaicin painting of skin fields have shown that these C fibers are sensitive to this agent, a characteristic of peptidergic C fibers (Jancso et al. 1967, 1985; Lembeck and Gamse 1982). Among the different functional subgroups of C-fibers, in particular the "polymodal" C fibers are sensitive to capsaicin (Szolcsanyi 1985), i.e., those which are sensitive to strong mechanical stimulation, to heat, and to chemical stimulation (Bessou and Perl 1969). It has been shown in animal experiments that some of these fibers are sensitive to close arterial bolus injection of histamine (Fjällbrandt and Iggo 1961; Juan and Lembeck 1974). However, histamine is far from being the most effective substance for driving this fiber group. No group of exclusively chemosensitive fibers has yet been described in animal or in human experiments. One has to keep in mind, however, that search stimuli in single-fiber experiments are more often mechanical than chemical stimuli.

Though the indirect evidence of our blocking experiments indicates that polymodal C fibers are most probably the sensors for itch, little evidence was found in our microneurography experiments for an excitation of C fibers by histamine iontophoresis. Similar weak effects of histamine on polymodal C fibers have been observed previously in the cat (Fjällbrandt and Iggo 1961). We ourselves have seen no clear C fiber afterdischarges in the rat when a similar technique of histamine iontophoresis was used as in human psychophysics and microneurography.

Since most of the polymodal C fibers do not respond at all, it is rather unlikely that itch is mediated just by a weak excitation of the whole population of C fibers. It is much more likely that a small subgroup of the C fibers mediates itch. Most probably these "itch fibers" have their receptive endings in the most superficial layers of the epidermis (Shelley and Arthur 1957; Keele and Armstrong 1964), since a sufficiently high concentration of histamine is induced by the iontophoresis primarily in these superficial layers. It is well known that injection of histamine into deeper skin layers with a vaccinating pistol induces not itch, but pain (Lindahl 1961).

One side aspect of our microneurography experiments was the finding of the high sensitivity of myelinated SA fibers to histamine iontophoresis. It is unclear whether these SA fibers respond directly to the chemical stimulation or indirectly to the changed turgor of the skin. Since the impulses of these SA fibers were most probably blocked in our pressure block experiments, this part of the iontophoresis-induced input is lacking under blocking conditions. This apparently does not change the itch sensation to a greater extent. It is astonishing that this barrage of nervous impulses in a group of myelinated fibers seems to have so little impact on the itch sensation.

Acknowledgements. This work was supported by the Deutsche Forschungsgemeinschaft and by the Wilhelm-Sander-Stiftung. We wish to thank these institutions.

We wish to thank C. Forster, who participated in the microneurography experiments and was helpful in the statistical analysis, and Prof. Szolcsanyi for his help in the capsaicin experiments. Prof. Frosch kindly provided us with a laser Doppler flowmeter. We are grateful to D. Bechtle and M. Weinrich for typing the manuscript and to all subjects who volunteered for our experiments.

Note added in proof:

The results on the lack of flare and itching after histamine application in capsaicin pretreated skin has been confirmed recently by Toth-Kasa et al. (1986).

Toth-Kasa I, Jancso G, Bognar A, Husz S, Obal F (1986) Capsaicin prevents histamine-induced itching. Int J Clin Pharmacol Res 6 : 163–169

References

Bessou P, Perl ER (1969) Response of cutaneous sensory units with unmyelinated fibers to noxious stimuli. J Neurophysiol 32 : 1025–1043.

Bickford RG (1938) Experiments relating to the itch sensation, its peripheral mechanism, and central pathways. Clin Sci 3 : 377–386

Fjällbrant N, Iggo A (1961) The effect of histamine, 5-hydroxytryptamine and acetylcholine on cutaneous afferent fibers. J Physiol (Lond) 156 : 578–590

Gybels J, Handwerker HO, van Hees J (1979) A comparison between the discharges of human nociceptive nerve fibers and the subject's ratings of his sensations. J Physiol 292 : 193–206.

Hardy JD, Wolff HG, Goodell H (1952) Pain sensations and reactions. Williams & Wilkins, Baltimore

Juan H, Lembeck F (1974) Action of peptides and other algesic agents on paravascular pain receptors of the isolated perfused rabbit ear. Naunyn Schmiedebergs Arch Pharmacol 283 : 151–164

Keele CA, Armstrong D (1964) Substances producing pain and itch. Arnold, London

Jancso G, Obal F, Toth-Kasa M, Katona M, Husz S (1985) The modulation of cutaneous inflammatory reactions by peptide containing sensory nerves. Int J Tissue React 7 : 449–457

Jancso N, Jancso-Gabor A, Szolcsanyi J (1967) Direct evidence for neurogenic inflammation and its prevention by denervation and by pretreatment with capsaicin. Br J Pharmacol Chemother 31 : 138–151

Lembeck F, Gamse R (1982) Substance P in peripheral sensory processes. In: Substance P in the nervous system. Ciba Found Symp 91 : 35–49

Lindahl O (1961) Experimental skin pain. Acta Physiol Scand 51 (Suppl 179)

Mumford JM, Bowsher D (1976) Pain and protopathic sensibility. A review with particular reference to the teeth. Pain 2:223–243

Shelley WB, Arthur RD (1957) The neurohistology and neurophysiology of the itch sensation in man. AMA Arch Dermatol 76:296–323

Szolcsanyi J (1985) Sensory receptors and the antinociceptive effects of capsaicin. In: Hakanson R, Sundler F (eds) Tachykinin antagonists. Elsevier, Amsterdam, pp 45–56

Torebjörk HE, Hallin RG (1973) Perceptual changes accompanying controlled preferential blocking of A and C fiber responses in intact human skin nerves. Exp Brain Res 16:321–332

Tuckett RP (1982) Itch evoked by electrical stimulation of the skin. J Invest Dermatol 79:368–373

Westerman RA, Low A, Pratt A, Hutchinson JS, Szolcsanyi J, Magerl W, Handwerker HO, Kozak WM (1986) Electrically evoked skin vasodilatation: a quantitative test of nociceptor function in man. Clin Exp Neurol 23:81–89

44 Intrafascicular Nerve Stimulation Elicits Regional Skin Warming That Matches the Projected Field of Evoked Pain

J. L. Ochoa, W. J. Comstock, P. Marchettini, and G. Nizamuddin

Background

It was recently reported that prolonged repetitive electrical stimulation at high, painful intensities, using Vallbo-Hagbarth tungsten microelectrodes impaling individual median or ulnar skin nerve fascicles, normally and consistently results in warming of discrete coherent regions of the human hand, as conveniently detected by liquid crystal contact thermography (Comstock et al. 1986).

The warming effect was interpreted as due to substance P-dependent vasodilatation induced by antidromic excitation of unmyelinated C sensory fibers. The argument rested neither on actual demonstration of antidromic impulse conduction nor on chemical or cytological evidence of neurotransmitter release. The proposition was based on powerful analogy with known evidence of involvement of C nociceptor fibers in antidromically triggered neurosecretion of vasoactive substances (Bayliss 1901; Hinsey and Gasser 1930; Lewis 1937a,b; Chapman et al. 1961; Jancso et al. 1967; Lembeck 1981; Chahl et al. 1985). One alternative explanation for the observed warming was considered and tested by human experiment. This was the possibility that the repetitive stimulation might have induced frequency-dependent excitation failure in C fibers and block of sympathetic efferent activity. Suppression of vasoconstrictor neural outflow would then result in paralytic vasodilatation. The observation that the regional warming effect was not abolished weeks after postganglionic sympathetic denervation of the tested skin ruled out this alternative explanation (Comstock et al. 1986).

Purpose of this Report

In the present report, we aim at providing an actual thermographic record of the phenomenon of antidromically induced neurogenic warming. In doing so, we will propose that the phenomenon carries both anatomical and physiological significance. In addition, we will discuss clinical implications of the phenomenon itself and of its thermographic illustration.

Figure 1 shows a photograph and a liquid crystal contact thermogram of the palmar aspect of the hand of a normal volunteer, both exhibiting the effects of painful repetitive intraneural stimulation sustained for 20 min within an ulnar nerve fascicle through Vallbo-Hagbarth tungsten microelectrodes. The area where the evoked sensation was perceived, the **projected field**, is delineated in red ink on the photograph. It strikingly matches the region of evoked skin warming, colored blue in the thermogram. This is a consistent result in normal human volunteers.

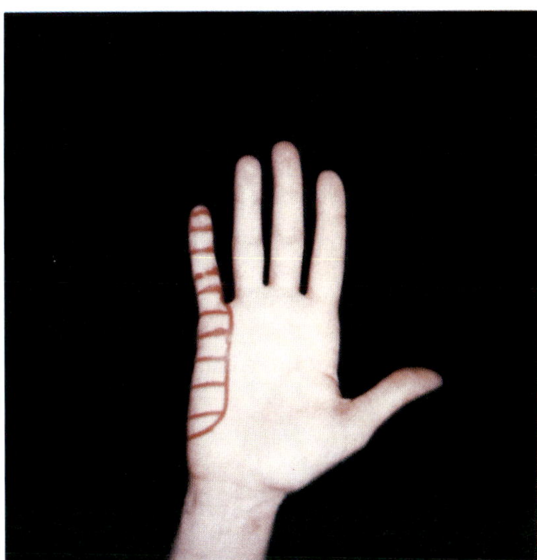

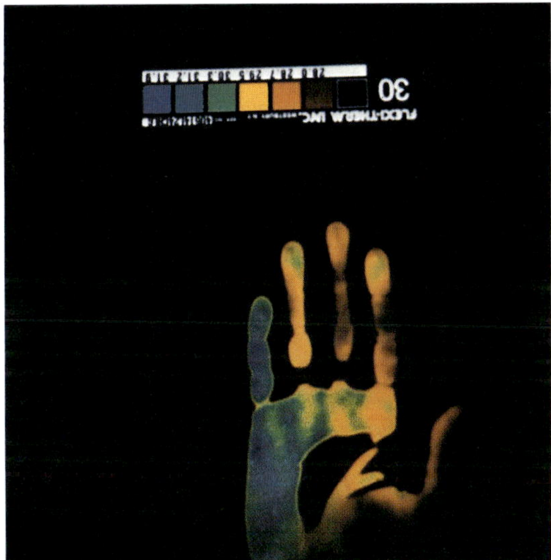

Fig. 1. Left panel shows liquid crystal thermogram of the palm of the hand portrayed on the right. The baseline thermogram before stimulation displayed a uniformly yellow color. Following prolonged painful intrafascicular stimulation, regional warming developed (blue). The projected field of sensations evoked during painful intraneural stimulation are marked in the skin of the hand. See text. (From Ochoa 1987)

Anatomical Relevance

If it is accepted that the regional warming induced by painful intraneural stimulation reflects neurosecretory consequences of antidromic excitation of the unmyelinated fibers of nociceptor sensory units, then the warmed region constitutes a representation of the cutaneous innervation territory of those fibers. Thus the present observation has the value of a neuroanatomical tracing equivalent, providing prime documentation of how C nociceptor units contained in individual nerve fascicles are distributed into partial domains within the total nerve territory. This is a novel contribution to minor neuroanatomy.

Implications for Sensory Physiology

The observed phenomenon also carries implications for sensory physiology. These surfaced when Wall and McMahon (1985) questioned the claim by Schady et al. (1983) that the projected field of sensation evoked by intraneural stimulation of human skin nerve fascicles was a representation of the anatomical receptive field of those fascicles. Wall and McMahon dismissed the areas of projected sensation as condensed abstractions of the brain rather than real fragments of the total nerve territory. The objective evidence provided here settles that controversy.

Clinical Implications

In the realm of neuropathic pain the implications of this natural phenomenon, which involves C nociceptor fibers, are potentially vast. Indeed, excitation of those fibers may cause pain associated with objective physical vasomotor signs. Such sensory and cutaneous vascular events are reminiscent of causalgia – reflex sympathetic dystrophy (RSD; see review by Bonica 1979) – and are traditionally explained through incrimination of the autonomic system as a pathogenetic agent. However, decisive evidence has recently been contributed in support of vintage proposals (Lewis 1937a, b; Jung 1941) that at least a subgroup of patients with RSD suffer from irritative phenomena in primary C nociceptor units, leading to afferent sensory plus antidromic neurosecretory clinical manifestations (Ochoa 1986).

On the other hand, the implications of this natural phenomenon in the realm of diagnostic technology are unexpectedly transcendental. Indeed, early 1987 witnesses fierce controversy about the usefulness of thermography as a diagnostic tool. Even if it had been unscientifically misused, there should remain no doubt that in itself the technique is impeccable and that it is sensitive enough to detect changes in skin temperature of neurogenic origin, and anatomically precise in mapping them. This statement is unambiguously illustrated, in color, in Fig. 1.

Acknowledgement. Supported by NINCDS grant NS 24740-01.

References

Bayliss WM (1901) On the origin from the spinal cord of the vasodilator fibers of the hand limb, and on the nature of these fibers. J Physiol (Lond) 26 : 173–209

Bonica J (1979) Causalgia and other reflex sympathetic dystrophies. In: Bonica JJ, Liebeskind JC, Albe-Fessard DG (eds) Advances in pain research and therapy, vol 3. Raven, New York, pp 141–166

Chahl L, Szolcsanyi J, Lembeck F (eds) (1985) Antidromic vasodilation and neurogenic inflammation. Akademiai Kiado, Budapest

Chapman L, Ramos A, Goodell B, Wolff H (1961) Neurohumoral features of afferent fibers in man. Arch Neurol 4 : 617–650

Comstock W, Ochoa J, Marchettini P (1986) Neurogenic warming of human hand provinces by activation of the unmyelinated population of single skin nerve fascicles. (Abstr Soc Neurosci 12 (1) : 331

Hinsey J, Gasser H (1930) The component of the dorsal root mediating vasodilation and the Sherrington contracture. Am J Physiol 92 : 679–689

Jancso N, Jancso-Gabor A, Szolcsanyi (1967) Direct evidence for neurogenic inflammation and its prevention by pretreatment with capsaicin. Br J Pharmacol 31 : 138-151

Jung R (1941) Die allgemeine Symptomatologie der Nervenverletzungen und ihre physiologischen Grundlagen. Nervenarzt 14 : 493–516

Lembeck F (1981) Substance P and the primary afferent neuron. Adv Pharmacol Therap 2 (1) : 115–126

Lewis T (1937a) The nocifensor system of nerves and its reactions. Lecture I. Br Med J 194 : 431–435

Lewis T (1937b) The nocifensor system of nerves and its reactions. Lecture II. Br Med J 194 : 491–494

Ochoa J (1987) The newly recognized painful ABC syndrome. Thermology 2 (2)

Schady W, Ochoa J, Torebjork H, Chen S (1983) Peripheral projections of fascicles in the human median nerve. Brain 106 : 745–760

Wall P, McMahon S (1985) Microneurography and its relation to perceived sensation. Pain 21 : 209–229

Index